The Women of Anna Freud's War Nurseries

In this volume, Christiane Ludwig-Körner describes the lives and work of the staff members of the War Nurseries set up and run by Anna Freud and Dorothy Burlingham during the Second World War.

The Women of Anna Freud's War Nurseries looks in turn at each of the women who helped run the homes in Hampstead: Alice Goldberger, Sophie and Gertrud Dann, Manna Friedmann, Anneliese Schnurmann, Ilse Hellman and Hansi Kennedy. As young women, they narrowly escaped the Holocaust and dedicated themselves to children who had suffered the same fate. Few arrived with any knowledge of psychoanalytic theories or methods; this volume charts their education from Freud and Burlingham, which eventually lead to both Freud's independent psychoanalytic child therapy training and the young women's embarkment on careers as professional analysts. Using case studies throughout, Ludwig-Körner illustrates the intense relationships often experienced between children in care and their analysts/carers, and uses the children of the War Nurseries as examples for how contemporary psychoanalysts can work with children today.

This book is essential reading for psychoanalysts, especially those working with children, as well as scholars and professionals interested in the history of child analysts and childhood trauma.

Christiane Ludwig-Körner is a psychologist, psychoanalyst, training analyst and supervisor for the IPA. She has taught developmental and clinical psychology at the University of Applied Sciences in Potsdam, and at the International Psychoanalytic University Berlin (IPU), Germany, where she now holds a senior professorship.

The Women of Anna Freud's War Nurseries

Their Lives and Work

Christiane Ludwig-Körner

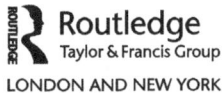 Routledge
Taylor & Francis Group

LONDON AND NEW YORK

Designed cover image: © Freud Museum London

First published in English 2024
by Routledge
4 Park Square, Milton Park, Abingdon, Oxon OX14 4RN

and by Routledge
605 Third Avenue, New York, NY 10158

Routledge is an imprint of the Taylor & Francis Group, an informa business

© frommann-holzboog Verlag e.K. · Eckhart Holzboog, Stuttgart-
Bad Cannstatt 2022

Translated by Tara Loeber. Unless otherwise indicated, all quotations from
German sources and original interviews were translated for this edition.

The right of Christiane Ludwig-Körner to be identified as author of this work has
been asserted in accordance with sections 77 and 78 of the Copyright, Designs
and Patents Act 1988.

Published in German as *Und sie fanden eine Heimat. Leben und Wirken der
Mitarbeiterinnen von Anna Freud in den Kriegskinderheimen* by frommann-holzboog
Verlag e.K. · Eckhart Holzboog, Stuttgart-Bad Cannstatt 2022.

British Library Cataloguing-in-Publication Data
A catalogue record for this book is available from the British Library

Library of Congress Cataloging-in-Publication Data
Names: Ludwig-Körner, Christiane, author.
Title: The women of Anna Freud's war nurseries : their lives and work /
Christiane Ludwig-Körner.
Other titles: Und sie fanden eine Heimat. English.
Description: Abingdon, Oxon ; New York, NY : Routledge, 2024. |
"First published in English 2024." | Includes bibliographical references and index.
Identifiers: LCCN 2023041245 (print) | LCCN 2023041246 (ebook) |
Subjects: LCSH: Freud, Anna, 1895–1982. | Hampstead Nurseries—Biography. |
Child psychoanalysts—20th century—Biography. | Women psychoanalysts—
Great Britain—20th century—Biography. | World War, 1939–1945—Children—
Great Britain. | Jewish refugees—Great
Britain—Biography. | Holocaust survivors—Great Britain—Biography.
Classification: LCC RC339.52.F73 L83 2024 (print) | LCC RC339.52.F73 (ebook) |
DDC 618.92/89170922—dc23/eng/20231211
LC record available at https://lccn.loc.gov/2023041245
LC ebook record available at https://lccn.loc.gov/2023041246

ISBN: 978-1-032-51779-7 (hbk)
ISBN: 978-1-032-51754-4 (pbk)
ISBN: 978-1-003-40390-6 (ebk)

DOI: 10.4324/9781003403906

Typeset in Times New Roman
by codeMantra

Contents

List of Photos   vii
Preface   ix

Introduction: From the Edith Jackson Nursery
to the War Nurseries   1

1   Alice Goldberger (15.8.1897–22.2.1986) – Mother of the
    Lingfield House Children   21

2   Sophie (3.3.1900–18.12.1993) and Gertrud Dann
    (27.5.1908–2.4.1998) – Home for the Children from
    Theresienstadt   37

3   Manna (Marta) Friedmann (8.1.1915–16.11.2013) –
    Surviving to Ensuring the Survival of Others   63

4   Anneliese Schnurmann (31.1.1908–21.9.2006) – Wanderer
    Between Worlds   114

5   Dr Ilse Rosa Hellman-Noach (08.09.1908–03.12.1998) –
    'From War Babies to Grandmothers'   141

6   Hansi (Hanna) Kennedy (6.1.1923–30.10.2003) – A Life
    for the Hampstead Child Therapy Clinic   162

7   Anna Freud – Interweaving Life, Work and Research   189

References and Bibliography   203
Index of Persons   215
Index of Terms   219

Photos

1   The six children from Theresienstadt (credit: Gertrud Dann
    and USHMM)   8
2   Alice Goldberger 1951 (credit: Gertrud Dann and USHMM)   24
3   Alice Goldberger on a walk with children (credit: USHMM)   30
4   Manna Friedmann and Alice Goldberger in Weir Courtney
    (credit: Manna Friedmann and USHMM)   31
5   The siblings Elisabeth, Lotte, Sophe and Gertrud Dann 1919
    (credit: Gertrud Dann)   40
6   Sophie and Gertrud Dann at the opening of the Freud Museum
    (credit: Gertrud Dann and AFC, reproduced with permission)   42
7   Sophie Dann in her early days (credit: Gertrud Dann)   43
8   Poster of Gertrud Dann's kindergarten in Augsburg (credit:
    Gertrud Dann)   44
9   Gertud Dann in Augsburg (credit: Gertrud Dann)   46
10 Hansi Kennedy (left) and Sophie Dann (credit: Gertrud Dann and
    AFC, reproduced with permission)   50
11 Sophie Dann with the children from Theresienstadt, summer
    1946 (credit: Gertrud Dann and AFC, reproduced with permission)   54
12 Father Dann typing (credit: Gertrud Dann)   57
13 Gertrud Dann and her parents with their car (credit: Gertrud Dann) 58
14 Manna Friedmann, 6 years old, and her brothers Albert and Salo
    (credit: Manna Friedmann)   64
15 Manna Friedmann with children (credit: Manna Friedmann
    and AFC, reproduced with permission)   80
16 Manna Friedmann dancing with children (credit: Manna
    Friedmann and AFC, reproduced with permission)   81
17 The married Friedmann couple (credit: Manna Friedmann)   86
18 Oscar Friedmann in Bad Gastein with his sister Male (left) and
    Alice Goldberger (credit: Manna Friedmann)   87
19 Manna Friedmann while working (credit: Manna Friedmann and
    AFC, reproduced with permission)   90
20 Anna Freud at the loom (credit: Manna Friedmann)   104

21   Manna Friedmann, 1996 showing her photo album
      (credit: Christiane Ludwig-Körner)   107
22   Manna Friedmann in a wheelchair together with Andra Bucci
      (credit: Getty Images)   111
23   Anneliese Schnurmann with her nanny 'Loline' (Louise Blei) in
      Karlsruhe, 1908 (credit: Anneliese Schnurmann)   114
24   Anneliese Schnurmann with her sister Leonore, 1911/1912
      (credit: Anneliese Schnurmann)   116
25   Anneliese Schnurmann, 6 years old, with her dog (credit:
      Anneliese Schnurmann)   117
26   Anneliese Schnurmann with Walther Dress and Susanne Dress,
      born Bonhoeffer, 1950 in Berlin (credit: Andreas Dress)   124
27   Anneliese Schnurmann, black dress (credit: Anneliese Schnurmann)   126
28   Anneliese Schnurmann at her desk (credit: Anneliese Schnurmann)   135
29   Anneliese Schnurmann, London, 15 September, 1996 (credit:
      Christiane Ludwig-Körner)   138
30   From left to right: Ernst, Bernhard and Ilse Hellmann in
      traditional clothing, 1912 (credit: Paul Hellmann)   143
31   Ilse Hellman in Vienna, 1930 (credit: Paul Hellmann)   145
32   Ilse Hellman with her brothers Ernst and Bernhard in London
      (credit: Paul Hellmann)   147
33   Sophie Dann, Ilse Hellman, Josefine Stross, Hansi Kennedy, in
      the background Clifford Yorke, with Princess Alexandra of Kent
      at the opening ceremony of the Freud Museum 1986 (credit:
      Gertrud Dann)   154
34   Ilse Hellmann as an old woman (credit: Paul Hellmann)   157
35   Susie and Hanna Engl, 1924 (credit: Hansi Kennedy)   163
36   Hansi Engl, about 15 years old, in Vienna (credit: Hansi Kennedy)   164
37   The Kennedy couple, 1988 (credit: Hansi Kennedy)   171
38   Hansi Kennedy next to Ted Cohen, 1992 (credit: Hansi Kennedy)   179
39   Hansi Kennedy on 28 April, 1997 (credit: Christiane Ludwig-Körner)   184
40   Anna Freud (left) and Sophie Dann feeding babies (credit:
      Gertrud Dann and AFC)   193

Preface

One feels impulses to write a book like this. Having been inwardly preoccupied for some time with the theme of 'lesser-known women within psychoanalysis', when I was in Augsburg in 1995 with Anne-Marie Sandler for a technical–casuistic conference of the German Psychoanalytic Society (DPG), I visited the synagogue there and discovered an exhibition on Augsburg Jewry.

My gaze was caught by the name Anna Freud on the display panels, and with astonishment I read the short text about the sisters Gertrud and Sophie Dann, who were forced to flee Augsburg and whose later lives were connected to Anna Freud. Fragments of memories of the war children's homes that Anna Freud and Dorothy Burlingham had set up in London emerged. But I knew nothing of the staff who did the day-to-day work on the spot and soon found that most of my colleagues felt the same way.

I was met by the desire to learn more about these women and their lives, accompanied by a sense of shame at having repressed the fact that there were, of course, people on Anna Freud's staff who were also displaced during the Nazi era and had to find a new home. Unfortunately, it took a long time before I was able to finish writing this book, which occupied me inwardly for more than twenty-five years, after I had conducted conversations with the still living female employees from 1996 onwards. I felt the passing time like a burden because I wanted the still living staff to see their 'silent work' appreciated, at least at the end of their lives. I used every free minute, and even on some holidays the staff of the War Nurseries accompanied me without them knowing it. Sophie Dann and Alice Goldberger had already died, and I could only get information about them through Gertrud Dann, Anneliese Schnurmann, Manna Friedmann and Hansi Kennedy. Ilse Hellman died shortly after I began my research, and, in the meantime, unfortunately, none of the interviewees is alive anymore. It was possible to commemorate her accomplishments with an article (Ludwig-Körner, 2000), which everyone was pleased about, but this book is now being published after her death.

These women gave me an insight into their personal lives, but they also helped me to close my own wounds. Born during the war, I belong to the generation of those whose parents' shared responsibility for the Holocaust. As a non-Jewish

German, I now met Jewish women who had all been expelled from Germany or Austria and had lost their family or relatives in concentration camps.

In this book, only a few selected life stories of the many female co-workers of Anna Freud and Dorothy Burlingham can be recorded. They are Gertrud and Sophie Dann from Augsburg, Manna Friedmann from Cologne, Alice Goldberger from Berlin, Anneliese Schnurmann from Karlsruhe and Berlin respectively, and Ilse Hellman and Hansi Kennedy from Vienna. By presenting their work in the children's homes during the war and in the institutions that followed, the book also records the beginning of child analysis as developed by Anna Freud. From this point of view, it is also a history of Anna Freud's analytical child and adolescent psychotherapy.

This book could not have been written without the support of many. Thanks are due to Anne-Marie Sandler, who helped me pave the way to the interviewees, Prof. Dr. Dr. Inge Pretorius, former Anna Freud Centre staff, Dr Regine Lockot for her many suggestions and support, Katrin Bärhold, assisted by Heiko Liegmann, who transcribed more than just interviews for her diploma thesis and sorted data, my husband, Jürgen Körner, who often had to share his holidays with 'old ladies' mostly unknown to him, and Paul Hellman, Sophie Williams, Steven Kennedy, Jan Wiener, Prof. Dr Claudia Schnurmann, Eran Wolkowski, and Helen Cohen for their additionally provided photographs and hints, as well as Roger Richter for support with the photos.

Thanks also go to the Moritz Straus Foundation for their funding for translating the book into English and preparing the photos and image rights, and to Tara Loeber for the translation of my text as well as quoted materials, Zoë Meyer, Editor – Psychoanalysis – Mental Health at Routledge and Jana Craddock, Alanna Donaldson and Yvonne Doney for their great help at the publishing house.

Christiane Ludwig-Körner
Berlin, June 2023

Introduction

From the Edith Jackson Nursery to the War Nurseries

When Anna Freud had to leave Vienna after the annexation of Austria in 1938, she had to abandon many things dear to her heart. This included the Jackson crèche, which was built in February 1937 thanks to a generous gift by the American doctor Edith Banfield Jackson, a teaching analysand of Sigmund Freud, who had her cases supervised by Anna Freud. In this, Anna Freud had just begun to realize her lifelong dream of a psychoanalytic nursery (crèche) for socially disadvantaged children up to the age of two (Kennedy, 1988; Krivanek, 2014). In the growing atmosphere of antisemitism the crèche was not officially allowed to be run under Anna Freud's name, so the project was specifically linked with the prestigious Montessori Society – Anna Freud held the work of Maria Montessori in high esteem – whose premises they also used. The staff members were the principal of the Montessori kindergarten, Hilde Fischer, her assistant Mizzi Milberger, and the director of the crèche, Hertha Fuchs-Wertheim (Zwiauer, 2001; Johler et al., 2016). The person responsible for the children's meals was Julia Deming, an American psychiatrist who had been in training analysis with Anna Freud, while health care was provided by the pediatrician and psychoanalyst Josephine Stross[1] (Mühlleitner & Reichmayr, 1992).

'Anna Freud visited frequently as an observer and she and Dorothy Burlingham attended the once-weekly staff meetings where the individual children's progress and problems were discussed' (Kennedy, 1988, p. 272). Looking ahead, it can be said that Anna Freud chose the same approach in the War Nurseries.

It had been Edith Jackson's, Dorothy Burlingham's and Anna Freud's desire to gather more experience of early life – particularly the second year of life – which they regarded as particularly important for the step from primary to secondary process function, as well as for superego development, drive control, and the formation of object relations:

> ... gather direct information about ... earlier ages, particularly the second year of life, which we deemed all-important for the child's essential advance from primary to secondary functioning; for the establishment of feeding and sleeping habits; for acquiring the rudiments of superego development and impulse control [and] for the establishment of object ties to peers.
>
> (A. Freud, as cited in Young-Bruehl, 1988, p. 218)

DOI: 10.4324/9781003403906-1

For the young psychoanalytic colleagues who emigrated to England, like Kate Friedlander (originally Käthe Friedländer), the arrival of the Freud family in London was a consolation during such hard times. A statement made by Kate Friedlander to Barbara Lantos during the war years shows how much it meant to her to be able to work with Anna Freud.

> It is terrible what we had to go through and still have to go through, but isn't it a godsend that, in the midst of all this misfortune we have the opportunity to work in the same place as Anna Freud.
>
> (Haager, 1986, p. 28)

The Hampstead Nurseries

When the bombing of London forced many families to take refuge in the underground railway station tunnels, homes for children were urgently needed. 'So in Great Britain alone 734,883 children were evacuated' (Wolf, 1945, p. 389). In October 1940, Anna Freud and Dorothy Burlingham began preparations to build a children's home. They rented a furnished house at 13 Wedderburn Road, London, NW3, which had previously housed Swedish students, so that, in January 1941, the first of three 'wartime children's homes', was opened. It was a 'day nursery run for the children from the residential nursery and some outsiders' (Freud & Burlingham, 1943, p. 13).

'The basement of the house was converted into a reinforced shelter to sleep some twenty-five people in the relative safety of Hampstead' (Kennedy, 2009, p. 307). Supported by donations, finance from The American Foster Parents Plan for War Children (AFPPWC), and equipped with furniture from the former Jackson crèche in Vienna, which Anna Freud brought with her to London, in February 1941, twenty-five children were already being cared for in this house, and, by April 1941, they housed thirty children (Kennedy, 2009, p. 309). In the summer of 1941, two further houses were opened, all of which were financially supported by AFPPWC under the name Hampstead War Nurseries. The house in 5 Netherland Gardens, London, NW 3, which opened in June 1941 and was called the Babies Rest Centre, was a large residential nursery for babies and young children and cared for up to 50 children (Midley, 2017). Two months later '"New Barn", Lindsell, near Chelmsford, Essex, a country house for evacuated children from 3–6 years' was rented' (Freud & Burlingham, 1943, p. 13).

> On the average the Hampstead Nurseries catered to eighty to ninety children at any one time, more or less equally divided between Netherhall Gardens and the Country House. Wedderburn Road became a staff hostel and a nursery school for the older London children.
>
> (Kennedy, 2009, p. 309)

> It can be safely said that all the children who were over two years at the time of the London 'Blitz' have acquired knowledge of the significance of air raids. They all recognize the noise of flying aeroplanes; they distinguish vaguely between the sounds of falling bombs and anti-aircraft guns. (…) They fully

understand the significance of taking shelter. Some children who have lived in deep shelters will even judge the safety of a shelter according to its depth under the earth. The necessity to make them familiar with their gas masks may give them some ideas about a gas attack, though we have never met a child for whom this particular danger had any real meaning.

(Freud & Burlingham, 1943, pp. 15–16)

Anna Freud (1973) writes:

Thirty-five children were regular shelter sleepers before they came to us. The shelters used were the Tilbury shelter [Commercial Road E1, where as many as 8,000 people slept during the Blitz], and some of the tube stations, for instance, Oxford Circus, Piccadilly Circus, and Paddington Station. Some of the pregnant mothers slept in these shelters up to the last night before the birth and returned to the same place ten days later with their new-born babies. All other children slept in their own homes, either in Anderson shelters, on ground floors, in basements, or under the stairs.

Anna Freud needed numerous female staff because she had to work from a ratio of one adult to three or four children. Thus, she employed mainly young German-speaking women to whom she could offer only a small salary. Many of the women employed by Anna Freud and Dorothy Burlingham had been displaced from their countries and had often lost close relatives in concentration camps. For them, the work with Anna Freud and her circle offered support, and, for some, it was at times a kind of family substitute (Interviews with Hansi Kennedy, 23 April, 1997; Manna Friedmann, 21 November, 1996; Kennedy, 1996, 2009).

In the archives of the Anna Freud Centre, in addition to the women reported on here, there are personnel sheets of an additional thirty women from Austria and Germany and one young man who were employed as trainees in the War Nurseries in 1941, as well as many others from other countries. Most of them had already worked as nurses, kindergarten teachers, after-school carers, and teachers, or were in training when they had to flee Nazi persecution. Almost all of them were Jewish women whose families were still in Austria or Germany and who often knew nothing about the fate of their families left behind.

Our staff at the moment consists of: a pediatrician, Josephine Stross, M.D., who is in attendance two or three hours every day; a head nursery school teacher, Miss Hedy Schwarz, with two assistants and two trainees; a baby nurse; a cook, Miss Sofie Wutsch; a social worker, Mr. James Robertson, a bookkeeper, Miss Julia Weiss; various help for laundry, clearing etc. This seems a large number, but they are all kept busy owing to the helplessness of the infants we are dealing with. Four members of the staff are British; the rest are refugees from Austria, Germany, Czechoslovakia and Holland. Four important members of the staff are volunteer workers.

(Freud, A., 1973)

Hedy Schwarz, who had already run a Montessori kindergarten in Vienna, told Hansi Engl, then 17 years old (later married to Gerald Kennedy; see Chapter 6), that another house – the 'Babies Rest Centre', located at 5 Netherhall Gardens – was to be opened near the first house. Hansi Kennedy worked in the War Nurseries from 1941 to 1945, eagerly absorbing all the knowledge offered to her in the regular staff meetings and training. It was a large facility where fifty infants and toddlers received care.

Joyce Robertson (1919–2013)[2] and James (Jimmy) Robertson (1911–1988),[3] a Quaker and conscientious objector, also learned through Hedy Schwarz that Anna Freud was looking for associates. As a young married English couple, they were an exception among the many mostly single Jewish women who had been forced into exile. Their opinions were important to Anna Freud because, both coming from working-class families, they could 'help translate' not only language differences but also cultural differences. James Robertson was a man of all trades in the War Nurseries, helping to remove incendiary bombs, extinguishing fire outbreaks, taking on handyman tasks and, as one of the few men, he was an important figure of identification for the children. In 1948, he took up a post at the Tavistock Clinic in John Bowlby's research project on the separation reactions of young children, where he remained until 1975. His psychoanalytic training, which began at the same time, was sponsored by Anna Freud. After his retirement, he and his wife set up the Robertson Centre with the aim of making their more than 50 years of professional experience surrounding attachment and separation known to a wider public beyond professional circles. In addition to Dorothy Burlingham and Anna Freud, psychoanalysts Ruth Thomas and Claire Winnicott were among the founding members of this institution (Ludwig-Körner, 2000).

Sisters Sophie and Gertrud Dann belonged to the staff of the wartime children's homes (Chapter 2). Sophie Dann, a trained educator, children's nurse and midwife, and her sister, Gertrud Dann, a trained nursery and infant nurse, were forced to flee from Augsburg to London in 1939 and had to earn their living as housekeepers until they both found lifelong work with Anna Freud. Sophie Dann was responsible for the care of the babies, the mothers, the milk kitchen and later also for the infirmary; Gertrud Dann looked after the infants.

> Practical problems of daily organization and the wish of the Center staff to exchange experiences and observations had prompted to us to start the habit of a short, nearly daily, staff meeting in the middle of the day.
>
> (Freud, A., 1973, pp. 22–23)

Anna Freud attached great importance to close observation of the children; for example, how they reacted to separation from their mothers and fathers, how they interacted with each other, their stage of development, etc. All staff members, whether educators, nurses, or students, were involved in these meetings and were encouraged to write down their observations of the children on small cards; she had already started doing this at the Jackson Nursery in Vienna (Pretorius, 2012; Midgley & Pretorius, 2014). In this way, Anna Freud both followed her research

interest and was able to deliver obligatory monthly reports to the sponsor organization, the AFPPWC. She later processed these records with Dorothy Burlingham
(Burlingham & Freud, 1942) in *Young Children in War-Time: A Year's Work in a
Residential Nursery*. In her search for suitable additional staff, Anna Freud also
asked the psychologist and social worker Dr Ilse Hellman (Chapter 5), a former assistant of Charlotte Bühler from Vienna, if she would take over the management of
the Babies Rest Centre in 5 Netherland Gardens and the care of infants, which she
ran from March 1941 until the closure of the home in September 1945.

Anna Freud was already of the opinion at that time that an early separation of
mother and child could have pathogenic effects and was therefore endeavouring to
involve the parents as much as possible in the work. Mothers of newborns were encouraged to live and work in the house. Likewise, siblings were admitted together
to foster their relationship with each other.

Contrary to the prevailing opinion that children should be left and not visited for
one or two weeks 'to ease the pain of separation' and cause less disruption, Anna
Freud encouraged mothers to stay, feed and put their children to bed on the first day
and, if possible, for the next week or two. The beneficial effect was evident and led
her to address it in her twelfth monthly report to America (Freud, A., 1973).

> The quickness of the child's break with mother contains all the dangers of ab-
> normal consequences. Gradual separation may bring more visible pain, but it
> is less harmful because it gives the child time to accompany the event with
> reactions – to work through his own feelings over and over again and find out-
> ward expression for his state of mind.
>
> (Kennedy, 1988, p. 274)

The home was open day and night for visits by family members. Anna Freud had
serious objections to evacuating young children without a mother. Gudrun Fuchs
(1992, p. 61) writes:

> She refers to all children evacuated without a mother as 'war orphans' or 'arti-
> ficial orphans', because young children do not react to temporary absence any
> differently than to the death of their parents. For the infant, then, the only thing
> that matters is the physical presence or absence of the mother, while the ques-
> tion of life or death in the real world lies beyond its affective understanding.

After only one year, the War Nurseries were restructured in such a way that each
group of four or five children was assigned a carer according to their individual
wishes and attachments, that is, 'family groups' were introduced. Already at that
time, Anna Freud recognized and incorporated into practice the fundamental importance of the mother–child relationship and bonding. If one reads Anna Freud's
accounts of her work in the wartime children's homes (A. Freud, 1987), one would
like to proclaim her as the founder of attachment theory. She describes in detail the
different separation reactions of children and pleads strongly against separating

mother and child in the early years. We know, however, that René Spitz also held this view and conducted his research on deprivation against this background, as did Charlotte Bühler. Edith Jackson, after her return to the USA, focused her research on the impact of the separation of infants and young children from their mothers in hospitals and was a proponent of rooming-in (Jackson, 1946, 1948a, b; Jackson & Thoms, 1947). James and Joyce Robertson were later able to use their experience in the War Nurseries when they worked with John Bowlby in attachment research from 1948 in the Tavistock Clinic. Certainly, Anna Freud also received inputs from her co-workers, who, for example, made it unmistakably clear through practical action that mother and child belong together – an attitude vehemently advocated by all the female workers listed here.

After the bombings increased, it was necessary to weigh up which could be the greater danger for the children: possible physical damage from the bombs or psychological damage if they were evacuated to the countryside and thus separated from their attachment figure. When a house in the country, named the 'Country House', at New Barn, Lindsell, near Chelmsford, Essex, became available in August 1941, it was mainly the older children who were taken there as they were thought to be able to cope more easily with the separation. There were thirty children between the ages of three and six who were able to stay in their familiar groups, accompanied by staff they knew, so that the evacuation was easier for them to cope with. A short distance from this home (a four-minute walk across the fields), another small house was rented – the 'Farmhouse'. Both houses were considered to belong together. Hansi Kennedy (2009) describes very vividly in her posthumously published speech on the occasion of Anna Freud's 100th birthday how, for the first time, the children were no longer forced to sleep in a crowded shelter and how they playfully processed this time by building shelters for their dolls and animals, asking the staff for crocheted nets so that no one would fall out.

New Barn was run by Alice Goldberger (Chapter 1), a welfare worker and after-school care worker from Berlin. Anna Freud and Dorothy Burlingham could only visit the homes in the countryside once a month on Sundays, whereas in the war children's homes in London, they were present every day (Dann, interview, 14 July, 1996).

Sophie Wutsch was one of the few staff members without a Jewish background. Gertrud Dann reported (interview, 20 November, 1996) that she came from a 'very simple background' in Austria. She had worked in Vienna with the Herzberg family as a domestic helper and – like Paula Fichtl in the Freud family – was taken with them to London when they emigrated. Martha Herzberg had taken over the management of the Hampstead Nurseries and was aware of the many and varied skills of her employees. Gertrud Dann describes Martha Herzberg as a very charming lady.

But she did not take care of the children, more so the maids. And also made sure that if she saw a young girl looking bad, she took care of the girls. Sophie very soon started making dolls' dresses for the Herzberg children. And in general – she must have been very good.

(Dann, interview, 20 November, 1996)

Starting in 1942, Anneliese Schnurmann (Chapter 4), a sociologist, also volunteered at the War Nurseries in London.

With the end of the war, the purpose of the Hampstead War Nurseries was fulfilled, and the children's homes were dissolved by September 1945 (Pretorius, 2020). The number of children residing in the Hampstead War Nurseries varied, as there were always children being discharged or new ones being admitted. In May 1945, at the end of the war, Anna Freud's 52nd Monthly Report lists 100 children who were being cared for, including 62 children under care: 28 in London and 34 in New Barn (Freud, A., 1973).

Of the total of 191 children cared for in Anna Freud's children's homes during the war, 101 were able to return to their parents. From Anna Freud's final report, we can see that among them were 24 children who were 1–4 weeks old when they were admitted, 74 children aged 1–12 months, 33 children were 1–2 years old, 22 children were 2–3 years old, 26 were 3–5 years old and only 12 children were over five years old. Ten of the children had lived in the children's home for more than five years (Freud, A., 1973).

Responsibility for repatriating the 62 children fell to James Robertson, who divided them into six groups. The first group consisted of thirteen children who were able to return home immediately, as their parents were able to care for them again at home after the end of the war. The second group consisted of three children who could not immediately return to their mothers and had to stay at the War Nursery and then continue to be cared for in daycare at Wedderburn Road. Group three comprised ten children whose mothers worked in the War Nurseries, so it was necessary to wait until their employment there ended. For seventeen children from the fourth group, the move out was delayed because their parents or relatives were either living abroad or the parents were living in small, crowded apartments. In the case of three children (group 5), Anna Freud and the staff tried to delay repatriation as long as possible, knowing that they would be returning to very poor slum conditions, where there were an additional six other siblings. Group six included sixteen children with unexplained fates. They were war orphans, one intellectually disabled child, or children whose parents refused to take them home again. In their case, much time was spent in dealing with the welfare institutions to find creative solutions for the children.

Child transports

Between December 1938 and September 1939, the Refugee Children's Movement (RCM) brought roughly 1,000 mostly unaccompanied Jewish children from Germany, Austria, Poland, and Czechoslovakia to England through various aid organizations. They were to be temporarily accommodated in English families. This had been preceded by negotiations, among others, by the British Prime Minister Neville Chamberlain in November 1938 with delegations of influential British Jews and Quakers and the commitment of the Jewish community to bear the costs of travel and resettlement for each child. The children were to receive good educations in towns all over England and, later, were to be reunited with their families and given a new home in British-administered Palestine. Shortly after this, the British government relaxed the entry regulations, and an appeal was made for English families who were willing to take in a foster child. The organization took over the Inter-Aid Committee for Children. The British government hoped that, although it had already met its immigration quota for refugees, it would become a role model for the USA to relax its strict entry regulations – which unfortunately did not happen (Thüne, 2019).

Very quickly, the number of places offered for care was no longer sufficient and many young people were exploited as free service personnel. It can unfortunately be assumed that this is still practised worldwide today. Many children and adolescents were interned in temporary refugee camps, accompanied by far too few carers who could hardly absorb the children's suffering. Either they were too young to understand the context of their separation, or they were alone with their worries about their relatives back home (Meyer, 1989).

In laborious negotiations with Adolf Eichmann, the Dutch banker's wife Geertruida Wismuller-Meyer, for example, succeeded in gaining permission for children to leave under strict conditions up until the outbreak of the war. The children, who were each given a number, were only allowed to bring one suitcase, a bag and 10 Reichsmarks with them – no books or toys and only a photograph.

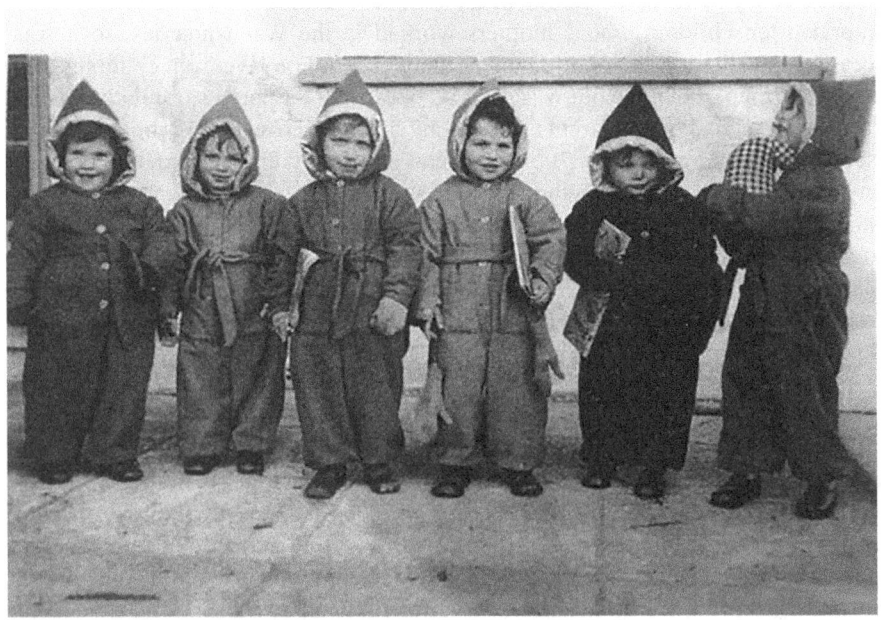

'Bulldogs Bank children' from Theresienstadt (credit: Gertrud Dann and US Holocaust Memorial Museum, Alice Goldberger Collection)

Not all the children whose parents wanted to take them to safety in this way were allowed to leave, however. The children were selected in an inhumane manner not only based on their own state of health, but also on the basis of the families' medical histories. Rejections on the English side were based on chronic illnesses (e.g., diabetes, mild asthma) or disabilities of any kind (including strabismus, bed-wetting or scars). People were probably afraid of not finding a suitable family in England or that the English state would incur additional costs for medical treatment (Penz, 2013, p. 68f). Göpfert (1999) and Curio (2006) describe the background of the child transports; for example, that Jewish communities also allowed some 'unsuitable' children to leave in order to save them, about which the responsible authorities in London complained. The Viennese authorities in turn referred to the difficult Jewish living conditions, which hardly made perfect health possible (Penz, 2013).

> Although the children's stay was only planned as a temporary measure, they were to be anglicised as soon as possible. Placement in foster families was seen as the most suitable option, as this would allow the children to be socialised into British families. Behind the plan of anglicisation was the desire for the children to be as inconspicuous as possible. The children were not to attract attention and were to be virtually invisible in British society. It was feared undue attention would provoke anti-Semitic and generally hostile feelings against refugees. The desire for this 'invisibility' was the basis for all decisions (RCM) and influenced everything from the selection to the accommodation of the children.
>
> (Penz, 2013, p. 71)

Initially, those interested in providing foster care were instructed to present themselves at a central reception point at a specific port of arrival and to choose a child on the spot; however, this system was soon abandoned.

> … as it was perceived by many children as similar to a cattle market. Instead, information about the foster families began to be matched with that of the children and assign the children to a family in advance, who could then collect the child as soon as they arrived in England.
>
> (Penz, 2013, p. 72)

But even in Weir Courtney, where rescued children from concentration camps were cared for (see below), people who wanted to adopt came to visit again and again to choose 'their' child. Here, children hoped to finally be chosen or were afraid of being torn away from their now familiar, trusted group of children.

Although, of course, no comparison can be made between the current refugee policy and that of the past, there are similarities. Fortunately, refugee children are no longer selected for their health status, but we allow children in need to grow up under difficult conditions in camps or on the streets, knowing what it means for their development.

An impression of the child transports by Wolf Blomfield is given here as representative of many others, especially since he appears again later in Chapter 1 (Alice Goldberger).

I came to Britain when I had just turned ten. I was a *Kindertransport* boy and came over on a train full of German Jewish children, on 15 March, 1939. All we were allowed to bring was a small suitcase that we could carry, so for a ten-year-old it wasn't very much. My father put me on the train in Berlin and had tried to explain what was happening. I think I was too bewildered to completely grasp it. Just before the war my family and I were going to go to America via England but when war broke out the U-boats were sinking the boats coming from Europe to the States, so I stayed in England. My mother had already left Germany and gone to Shanghai. She had remarried and her husband was in a concentration camp and the only way she could get him out was by emigrating and Shanghai was an open city. They took people when they weren't accepted anywhere else.

We arrived in England with little placards round our necks saying who we were. None of us spoke English, and when we arrived, there were kind ladies behind trestle tables offering us a drink, which I'd never seen before. I was very suspicious of it, but it was only tea with milk. We were all sent to children's homes, and I was allocated to one in Croydon. It was staffed by German Jews so the food I got was familiar, which was helpful. It really would have added to the trauma if we were given food that we didn't recognise.

My father worked for a Jewish refugee organisation and he was able to put my name down on the *Kindertransport* list, which was very hard for him. We were very close and we loved each other very much. He thought I would be safer in England. He stayed in Berlin for a while, but then he was sent to a concentration camp in Poland where he died. We were able to correspond with each other for a short while, via the Red Cross, but then the letters ceased. Then at the end of the war I checked with the Red Cross lists of names of who had died where it was confirmed that he died in 1942. My mother stayed in Shanghai and then got a work permit to come to England and worked as a domestic, to her horror, and then got a better job and worked in an old people's home. She stayed in this country for about 20 years but eventually she went back to Germany, where she died aged 93 years old (Holocaust Memorial Day Trust, n.d.).

Care for the children rescued from concentration camps

When Jewish children who had survived the concentration camps were to find a new home in England in 1945, suitable carers were sought under whose care these children could come to terms with their traumatic experiences. Lola Hahn-Warburg and Leonhard Montefiore, two prominent Britons, approached the British Home Office, the representative of the Jewish community, in the spring of 1945 to make good on a promise to help Jewish children who had survived in the concentration camps.

Proved through their work with the wartime children's homes, Anna Freud's staff offered themselves for this task. Oscar Friedmann (Chapter 3) and Alice Goldberger (Chapter 1) were entrusted with the task of putting together a suitable team, since more than 1,000 children were expected. They had a group of 35 staff members and prepared to receive the children, who were to arrive first in May, then in July and finally in August 1945. Many of the children and young people were so malnourished and ill that they could not make the journey from the death camps to England immediately. Those who arrived in England no longer had adult relatives on the continent who could care for them. For the group of thirteen four- to nine-year-olds, Sir Benjamin Drage provided his beautiful Weir Courtney home in Lingfield, Surrey.

Alice Goldberger took over this group, supported by Sophie Wutsch. Eight months later, another eleven children were integrated into this group who, hidden in Germany, had survived the Nazi regime, so that there were twenty-four children between the ages of three and fifteen to look after. In 1946, Manna Friedmann (Chapter 3) joined the group as another staff member. Together with Alice Goldberger, she looked after this group of children for three years. The last of the six little ones from Theresienstadt, who could not be adopted from the Bulldogs Bank home, were also integrated after one year. This Weir Courtney children's home was not led directly by Anna Freud; however, due to the close relationship between Alice Goldberger and Anna Freud's other employees, there was a close exchange. The employer was the West London Synagogue, where Alice Goldberger was the director of a home for children from the concentration camps as matron and superintendent from 1945 to 1952.

Start of psychoanalytic training: Hampstead Child Therapy Training Course and Clinic

As early as November 1941, Anna Freud and Dorothy Burlingham decided to offer an informal training programme for the twenty or so young women working in the Hampstead Nurseries. The training involved female staff with a variety of professional skills: Josephine Stross, a paediatrician, gave introductory courses in anatomy, first aid, nutrition, childhood diseases and hygiene. The latter was soon taken over by Sophie Dann, and Sophie Wutsch, the main cook in the children's homes, taught nutrition. Claire Nettl,[4] a nurse, gave courses in gymnastics with babies and toddlers. Hedy Schwarz, the head of the kindergarten, taught the Montessori method, the psychologist Ilse Hellmann taught developmental psychology and test methods (Bühler-Hetzer Developmental Test). Hedwig Hoffer, together with Dorothy Burlingham, taught a course on the writings of Freud, and Kate Friedlander taught 'Basic concepts of psychoanalysis' (Ludwig-Körner, 2000).

Anna Freud picked up the threads from her Vienna days in the 1920s with the beginning of a training course for female staff in the War Nurseries, through which she held her famous seminar 'On the Technique of Child Analysis'. Together with Siegfried Bernfeld and Willi Hoffer, she had created a psychoanalytic working group at that time in Vienna called the 'Children's Seminar', which met regularly in Berggasse. It was a group of people interested in working with children, including August Aichhorn, Dorothy Burlingham, Berta Bornstein, Hedwig Hoffer, Muriel Gardiner and Edith Jackson. Back then, there had been no established training in child analysis in Vienna, but she followed up on the courses for the youth welfare office of the City of Vienna. In a two-year course for training candidates and welfare workers, she had at that time – under the direction of Willi Hoffer – imparted psychoanalytic pedagogical knowledge alongside August Aichhorn, Siegfried Bernfeld and Editha Sterba (Laible, 1978, p. 43f).

With the training programme, Anna Freud succeeded in recruiting many women who worked in the Hampstead War Nurseries as trainees for a small wage, while board and lodging and training were free. The demand for this training was so great that waiting lists of female applicants were created and many had to be turned down.

> Apart from the Heads of Department, who acted as the teaching staff, and three or four paid assistants who functioned during 1941–1942, the children's work in the Nurseries was done entirely by students who worked full time for the training they received, in addition to board, lodging, and pocket money. Three student hostels in London and a cottage and farmhouse in Lindsell provides accommodations.
>
> (Freud, A., 1973)

The theoretical teaching was directly linked to the practical work in the children's homes, similar to how Anna Freud and Dorothy Burlingham had run the Jackson Nursery. The practical training included various workstations: infants from ten days to three months, infants from three to twelve months, milk kitchen, toddlers from one to two years, kindergarten (two to five years), and school children (five to nine years). In addition, there were periods of helping in the infirmary and air raid shelters. In the beginning, there was no official training in the Nurseries, but Anna Freud imparted her knowledge in the course of her daily work through what she observed theoretically.

By the time the Hampstead Nurseries closed, 66 candidates had already been trained, 28 of whom had received training ranging from two to over four years (Freud, A., 1973). Many of the staff who had acquired basic psychoanalytic knowledge in Anna Freud's training courses wanted to acquire further skills, as they often reached the limits of their abilities with the traumatized children. It was Kate Friedlander who convinced Anna Freud to offer her own independent training after the British Psychoanalytic Association decided in 1946 that only those trained in its own courses could be officially recognized as analysts. In a letter by Anna Freud to Jutta Haager on 14 November, 1980, she wrote: 'Kate Friedlander was very interested in training young female psychologists to work in the child guidance clinics, and for this reason she persuaded me to set up the Hampstead Child Therapy Course. I gave in to her urging' (Haager, 1986, p. 79).

The Hampstead Child Therapy Training Courses were first offered in 1947 to candidates with a university degree in psychology or related fields. They were trained as 'Child Experts'. Six of the staff from the War Nurseries took part in the first course: Hanna Engl (later: Hansi Kennedy), Johanna (Hanni) Köhler (later Benkendorf), Lizzy Wallentin (later Rolnick), Sara Kut (later Rosenfeld), Alice Goldberger and Anneliese Schnurmann. They were joined by Lili Neurath, who had worked at the Psychoanalytic Publishing House in Vienna before the war. The first seminars took place either in Anna Freud's house or in Kate Friedlander's flat in Upper Harley Street; on Wednesday evenings, according to tradition, they met in Freud's house. There was also a bookcase there, from which the training candidates could borrow books (Kennedy, 1995, p. 351). In London, therefore, the Viennese tradition of Wednesday evening seminars was taken up, in which colleagues who had already trained in Vienna or Berlin met regularly, and from this circle Anna Freud recruited teachers for her child psychoanalyst training. For example, there were her old friends Eva Rosenfeld, Dorothy Burlingham and the Hoffer couple from Vienna, Kate Friedlander from Berlin, and Barbara Lantos and Julia Mannheim from Budapest. Teaching and control analyses as well as theoretical and clinical seminars were conducted by members of the British Psychoanalytic Society (Schnurmann, interview, 24 November, 1996). In the years that followed, the initial three-year training was formalized and was soon transformed into a four-year course and today a four- to five-year full-time programme. Even in the early days, the entire course was accompanied by a five-hour teaching analysis.

With the financial support of the Field Foundation in New York, the house at 21 Maresfield Gardens was acquired in 1951, a stone's throw from the site of the former Hampstead Children's Home and, after the renovation work was completed, the Hampstead Child Therapy Clinic was opened in February 1952 under the direction of Anna Freud. The house already contained six treatment rooms, a playroom for children, offices, a small library, and a classroom for training candidates. Four years later, a second house – 14 Maresfield Gardens – was purchased through the support of the New Land Foundation and opened in May 1956 to commemorate Freud's 100th birthday. Donations from the California-based Foundation for Research in Psychoanalysis enabled a third building to be commissioned in 1967 (Kennedy, 1982, p. 131). In 12 Maresfield Gardens there was space for a kindergarten on the lower floor, in which the furniture from the Jackson crèche was used. It was mainly the extensive work of the Anna Freud Centre, which took place within these houses, such as the Hampstead Child Therapy Training Course and Clinic – renamed in 1984 in memory of Anna Freud, two years after her death – which encompassed the three interlocking areas: training, therapy, and research.

In 1954 Dorothy Burlingham was able to realize her long-cherished wish to open a kindergarten for blind children. A small extension to 21 Maresfield Gardens was erected, designed and built for the blind by Ernst Freud. A counselling service for parents of blind babies was added, and the staff carried out home visits to observe the children in their home environments. In addition, a maternity counselling service (Well Baby Clinic) was set up with the aim of counselling young mothers on how to deal with their babies, whether in medical, psychological or educational subjects such as sleeping and eating habits, weaning, teaching cleanliness, etc. The responsibility for this lay with Josephine Stross, the head paediatrician at the clinic. In the mornings, a playgroup for toddlers and their mothers was offered. This meant that mothers who had previously attended the Well Baby Clinic could continue to receive care there with their children. When Anna Freud succeeded in raising money for a nursery as part of the Educational Unit of the clinic in 1956, she offered Manna Friedmann the directorship, which she held until her retirement in 1978.

The child guidance centres

Kate Friedlander had a great interest in 'making analytic knowledge accessible to the widest possible public'. Through lectures for social workers, seminars for teachers and judges and publications in accessible journals, she tried to communicate psychoanalytic insights to lay people. One of her concerns was to bring psychoanalysis into public institutions, for which child guidance centres were very suitable (Haager, 1986, p. 65).

> This idea of psychoanalytically oriented child guidance services was then pursued by Kate Friedlander with her characteristic obsession. She informed herself about comparable institutions in the United States, spoke again and again with those responsible for community health services and submitted her plans to them. In January 1942, Edward Glover, Ernest Jones, and D. W. Winnicott wrote letters of recommendation for her application for the post of consultant psychiatrist to the Education Committee on the Middlesex County Council. All these letters were a mark of respect for her high professional qualifications and inexhaustible commitment. For such a position in an administration, however, formal criteria had to be met. The Diploma of Psychological Medicine was a prerequisite for appointment. In October 1943, Kate Friedlander passed the examination for the Diploma of Psychological Medicine.
>
> (Haager, 1986, p. 65 f.)

Kate Friedlander was commissioned by the West Sussex County Council in October 1944 to set up a child guidance centre in an area where nothing comparable existed at the time (Haager, 1986, p. 67). As a psychoanalyst, she experienced it as a challenge to apply psychoanalytic knowledge in a different way than in individual treatment, that is, to develop modified treatment methods (Friedlander, 1946; Haager, 1986). She wrote in an article:

> Child guidance services have a different task than the individual treatment of children in private practice or outpatient clinics: such a counselling centre must deal with the problem of the mentally disturbed child in a community as a whole. In addition to the psychiatric and psychological aspects of its work, it must also include social and preventive aspects. It should therefore have opportunities

for public relations work on the one hand and for researching and testing new methods of treatment on the other, for the aim of a child guidance centre must ultimately be the prevention of psychological disorders in childhood.

(Haager, 1986, p. 67)

The treatment method in the child guidance centre was by no means merely an abbreviated process of individual therapy (Friedlander, 1947, p. 454). The open-mindedness towards new therapeutic concepts and the insight into the limited possibilities of psychoanalysis as a method of treatment earned Kate Friedlander the reputation of not being so 'Anna Freud orthodox'. Anna Freud herself expressed great respect for her colleague in her letters, but she explicitly noted that her own efforts were always more engaged with child analysis in the narrower sense than family counselling, as understood by Kate Friedlander (Haager, 1986, p. 76).

Lydia Jacobs, a psychiatric social worker who had been trained in psychoanalysis and knew Kate Friedlander from working groups around Anna Freud, was one of the first staff members of the child guidance centres. All staff were to have psychoanalytic knowledge, therefore the designated staff trained and developed concepts in weekly discussion groups over the course of a year before the first two child guidance centres opened in Horsham and Chichester in January 1946 – the third was added in Worthing in February 1947. The child guidance centres were all located about 50km apart in the county and easily accessible for everyone (Haager, 1986, p. 71). Each child guidance centre consisted of a team: a psychiatrist, child psychologist or child therapist, a psychiatric social worker and a secretary. Anne-liese Schnurmann and Hansi Kennedy were among the first staff members of the child guidance centres in Chichester. Hansi Kennedy worked there for four years as a child therapist.

Employment in the child guidance centres enabled good clinical experience, as not all candidates who attended the seminars at the Hampstead Training Courses could work there. In addition, the training candidates needed patients, some of whom were provided by the child guidance centres, but also by Dr Augusta Bonnard and Dr Liselotte Frankl. Both also taught in Anna Freud's training programme and were able to offer three further placements at the East London Child Guidance Clinic (Kennedy, 1995, p. 350). Liselotte Frankl, a medical doctor and psychologist, had joined after the untimely death of Kate Friedlander in 1949. She became the responsible psychiatrist in charge of further education and was later also employed at the Hampstead Child Therapy Clinic.[5]

The struggle for official recognition of the training

There was an agreement with the British Psychoanalytic Society (BPaS) that those trained by Anna Freud could not call themselves analysts. In 1960, Anna Freud expressed her regret to the International Psychoanalytic Association that her training in child analysis, unlike that of the BPaS, was not recognized. Again and again, she and numerous colleagues presented their work at various psychoanalytic congresses – for example, international congresses in Rome, Vienna, Paris, and Geneva – and sought recognition by the International Psychoanalytic Association (IPA; Geissmann & Geissmann, 1998, p. 200 f.). When the Hampstead Child Therapy Training Course and Clinic applied to the IPA to become an IPA Study Group, the BPaS felt threatened that a second English psychoanalytic society might be recognized, and so a compromise was reached. Thereafter, from 1972 on, training candidates and qualified members of the British Psychoanalytic Society could also acquire their child analytic training at the Hampstead Clinic (Kennedy, 1982a, p. 130). In addition, some of those who had acquired their training at the Anna Freud Centre went on to complete additional training in adult analysis at one of the International Psychoanalytic Association's centres (Ludwig-Körner, 2000).

Hampstead Child Therapy Clinic – Anna Freud Centre – Anna Freud National Centre for Children and Families (AFNCCF)

The work that Anna Freud, Dorothy Burlingham, and their many collaborators had begun in the Hampstead War nurseries left a worldwide mark, but also changed over time.

> The opening of the Hampstead Clinic in 1952 was made possible by former colleagues, analysands, and supervisees from Vienna, now working in the United States, who helped to obtain the necessary financial support. For the next thirty years, Anna Freud's tireless leadership and infectious enthusiasm ensured that the organization became a renowned psychoanalytic center offering comprehensive child training, services, and research facilities.
>
> (Kennedy, 1983a, p. 504f)

Hansi Kennedy (1978b, p. 7) describes the work during the time when Anna Freud was still living:

> The clinical services include psychoanalytic treatment on a five times weekly basis for some 50 children and adolescents at a time. In a few cases both mother and child are in analysis; with other children in intensive treatment, the therapist's contact with the mother varies from weekly interviews with the younger age groups to less regular and sometimes only telephone contact with parents of older children. A much smaller number of children are in once weekly therapy. The developmental difficulties of very young children are occasionally dealt with by working only with the mothers in so-called 'mother guidance' treatment.

Another focus was on diagnostic work and preventive and educational services.

> The Clinic's preventive and educational services play an equally important part in the three aspects of our work – training, service and research. The Well-Baby

Clinic offers a medical and psychological service to mothers and young children with the aim of helping mothers cope better with problems arising in connection with sleeping and feeding habits, the processes of weaning and toilet training and the repercussions of these and other experiences on the child's development. The Baby Clinic has a case-load of approximately 40 families. Very young babies are seen weekly, others less frequently by the paediatrician and other staff members, all of them psychoanalytically trained. Often home observations are also made by students. Apart from the service aspect, the Well-Baby Clinic's work affords opportunities of making long-term observations from birth onwards.

The weekly Mother/Toddler Group, originally an offshoot of the Baby Clinic, offers toddlers opportunity to explore new territory and make their first tentative contacts with other children while their mothers exchange experiences with each other and the staff. Here students can observe the one to two-year-old age group.

(Kennedy, 1978b, pp. 7–8)

Officially registered as a charitable institution, the name 'Hampstead Child-Therapy Course and Clinic' was changed in 1971 to the more suitable name: Hampstead Centre for the Psychoanalytic Study and Treatment of Children (Kennedy, 1978b, p. 10). After the death of Anna Freud, it was renamed the Anna Freud Centre (AFC) in 1984 and the Anna Freud National Centre for Children and Families (AFNCCF) in 2016. Up until the turn of the millennium, the work at the Anna Freud Centre was divided into the following areas: training of psychoanalytic child therapists in theoretical and technical seminars, clinical work with children and adolescents under supervision, psychoanalytic diagnostic work, research, and prevention. As of 1999, about 300 children were cared for there each year. For a long time, the Anna Freud Centre was financed exclusively by donations. With the appointment of new directors in 2003 (Peter Fonagy, Mary Target, and Linda Mayes – the latter two stepping down a few years later), the AFC turned its attention to innovative areas of work, training and research in Mentalization-Based Treatment.

Anna Freud's child psychoanalytic training programme – widely considered the gold standard –closed its admissions in 2003, and the last candidate completed the training in 2009.

The discontinuation of child analytic training at the Anna Freud Centre has drastically changed psychoanalytic work. In 1965, for example 70 to 80 children came per day to the Anna Freud Centre (then the Hampstead Clinic), five times per week, for their intensive child psychoanalysis (Sandler, 1965). In 2016, there was only one psychoanalytic intensive case (three sessions per week) and a few non-intensive treatments (one session per week). What will remain of the psychoanalytic work with infants, toddlers and school-age children at the AFNCCF (the new 'Centre of Excellence') and the form of this work, is currently under review and it faces an uncertain future. The move to a purpose-built facility close to King's Cross station is the culmination of the new direction, initiated in 2003, that emphasizes research and not psychoanalytic treatment. The new building offers numerous rooms for research, teaching, training and further education, but no 'Toddler Hut' for the therapeutic parent–toddler groups and only a few therapy rooms. This evidences the priorities and restructuring of the AFNCCF. …

The Anna Freud Centre's pre-clinical course [observation of babies, toddlers and preschool children, theory courses on child development and psychoanalysis, and a research component] became a master's programme in psychoanalytic developmental psychology [MSc, Psychoanalytic Developmental Psychology]. In addition, students could undertake a 4–5-year training in child psychoanalysis and conduct, an independent research project which culminated in a doctorate in Psychoanalytic Child and Adolescent Psychotherapy [DPsych]. It was hoped that this academic title would help the foreign students to gain accreditation and employment in their home countries.... The Master's in Psychoanalytic Developmental Psychology (MSc in PDP) continues to develop, and two more master's programmes have even been established. The MSc in PDP is linked to the British Psychotherapy Foundation [BPF], which trains child and adolescent psychotherapists in the tradition of the so-called Middle Group (including Winnicott and Balint). When the Anna Freud Centre discontinued its training programme (2003), the BPF approached the Anna Freud Centre. Since then, candidates in child analysis can complete the clinical training at the BPF, while the research part takes place at University College London [AFC-UCL].

(Inge Pretorius with Alexander Frohn, interview, 2018,
transl. I. Pretorius, amended for this edition)

The houses in Maresfield Gardens (except the Sigmund Freud Museum, which is not under the auspices of the Anna Freud Centre) were sold in 2019, and the AFNCCF moved to central London, to the Kantor Centre of Excellence.

Notes

1 In Vienna, her name was Josefine Stross (1901–1995). She was a childhood friend of Marianna Kris, specialized in pediatrics and was involved in the famous Marienthal study on the effects of unemployment. She did her training analysis with Richard Sterba and joined the Vienna Psychoanalytic Association as a member in 1937. She accompanied the Freud family to London and looked after the medical needs of Sigmund and Anna Freud. She was responsible for the medical care of the children in the War Nurseries; afterwards, she led the Well Baby Clinic together with Anna Freud and Dorothy Burlingham, a department of the Hampstead Clinic, until her retirement in 1983. In her private practice, she mainly cared for refugees but also had a post in a children's hospital in the East End of London.
2 Her maiden name was Usher, and she was born in London on 27 March, 1919. She left grammar school at the age of 14 because she had to support her mother financially (her father died when she was six years old). After several temporary jobs she attended evening classes at the Workers' Education Association, and learned rather by chance about the possibility of going to college, where young adults could study. So she went to WEA College in Birmingham, which was for her the key to the spiritual world, and in the first

week (1940) she met her future husband Jimmy (James) Robertson. As a conscientious objector, he went to London to help during the devastation and chaos of the blitz; Joyce followed him in 1941. She had learned that Anna Freud was looking for more carers and was pleased to be chosen by her as a trainee. 'While courting Joyce, James met Freud and she appointed him as boilerman, handyman and fire watcher. By the end of the war he was qualified as a social worker. Joyce and James married in 1941' (Lindsay, 2013) Joyce Robertson received £1 that week for her help at the children's home. They were given food at the War Nursery so that they could just survive on it. Joyce Robertson worked with the youngest children, whom she was able to soothe very well, and soon became an expert on mother–child relationship issues. Interviewed by Dorothy Burlingham and Anna Freud, she was included in the training courses and later also conducted child therapies, but she never really completed it. She herself described herself as an 'honorary psychoanalyst'.

After her two daughters were a little older, Joyce Robertson worked with Anna Freud again from 1957, first in the Well Baby Clinic and then for a short time in the nursery school, which Anna Freud had built up. In 1965 she moved to the Tavistock Clinic and helped with the attachment–separation research of John Bowlby.

3   The Foster Parents' Plan for War Children, Inc. provided the *Questionnaire for the Personnel of all Colonies* (one of the 'Colonies' was the Hampstead Nursery), which everyone had to fill in and sign when they were recruited. From this it can be seen that James Robertson was born on 22 March, 1911 in Rutherglen, Scotland. He states that he came from a 'working class family on Clydeside for generations'; 'father and three brothers engineers'. He was in the Scout movement for over twelve years, in the Boys Club for two years, and finally in the adult education movement for several years. Between the ages of 14 and 27 he worked as a clerk in a steel factory, the last five years of which he was secretary of the workers' welfare department, in charge of the sick and medical aid programmes and responsible for the records of 1,400 employees and their promotions, dismissals, etc. He left the company in 1940 when it began manufacturing wartime munitions. He used the time to study for a college degree at Fircroft College, Bournville, near Birmingham. He also attended a course for two semesters at Woodbrooke, an associated Quaker college, to prepare for the reconstruction of war-ravaged areas, following the example of the Quaker units in the First World War. As a result of the war, he had to end another college position and later hoped to continue working in adult education (questionnaire signed by James Robertson on 14 May, 1941).

In August 1940 he arrived in London, where he first joined the First Pacific Service Unit. In the early stages of the Blitzkrieg, he provided first-aid and rescue work; later he was transferred to London's East End where conditions were chaotic. He helped to set up new volunteer rest centres in Bethnal Green and spent most nights doing social work in the emergency shelters of the underground tunnels, evacuating, reassuring and moving furniture out of bombed houses, and looking after unaccompanied children during the evacuation. James Robertson was not paid by Anna Freud but received five shillings from a Pacific association. The Robertson couple became famous worldwide for their films about the separation reactions of young children (Robertson & Robertson, 1989).

4   The 45-year-old Claire Nettl had already worked for more than ten years as a nurse, not only in Vienna, but also for two years at the psychoanalytic clinic in Berlin and five years at a 'private nursery for problem children' before she was employed at the Babies Rest Centre in 1941 for two pounds and ten shillings a week. This was the pay received by the experienced staff, while the trainees were paid five shillings a week and even less (cf. Questionnaire for the Personnel of all Colonies, 8 January, 1941).

In the reference that Anna Freud gave to Claire Nettl, she emphasized, 'Sister Nettl further possesses special knowledge of the training and handling of mentally backward or disturbed children and has very good results with several cases of this case whom the

Nursery had to receive, and who were given into her special care. Sister Nettl further possesses a very thorough knowledge of Dietetics for babies and young children. Her thorough training, her specialized knowledge, and her great experience make her a fit person for any position of responsibility in hospital work, children's work, or relief work' (Work reference from Anna Feud, 15 June, 1945).

5 Dr Liselotte Frankl (1910–1988) was one of the scientific research assistants with Charlotte Bühler, who began her analysis in Vienna with Ernst Kris and continued it in London. In London she also studied medicine and worked as a psychiatrist at the East London Child Guidance Clinic. She was responsible for medical and psychiatric care at the Hampstead Child Therapy Clinic. She became a member and teaching analyst of the BPaS.

1

Alice Goldberger (15.8.1897– 22.2.1986) – Mother of the Lingfield House Children

Alice Goldberger was born in Berlin on 15 August, 1897. Little is known about her family, as she never spoke – even to her friends – about her origins. Based on clues from her friend Elisabeth Moshagen, an artist with whom Alice Goldberger had trained as a youth leader, it can be assumed that her mother had committed suicide. Her brother Max, his wife, and their daughter were murdered in Auschwitz.[1] Gertrud Dann, who worked with Alice Goldberger for a long time, recalled in an interview that she had noticed that Alice Goldberger never talked about her childhood or adolescence, and she said: 'I think she must have had a difficult youth' (Dann, interview, 20 November, 1996).

From 1903 until completing the first grade of a secondary school in 1914, she went to schools in Charlottenburg, then to the kindergarten and nursery training school in Goethestrasse 22 in Charlottenburg, from which she graduated in April 1916 with a state examination for kindergarten and after-school care teachers. In 1930, she also acquired her youth leader's certificate there. From 1916 to 1917, she worked as a trainee at the youth home in Charlottenburg, Grunewald parish, from 1917 to 1919 in a war children's home, and from 1919 to 1920 as an after-school carer in a national foundation for war casualties. She led children's transports to Switzerland, and from 16 February, 1922 to 1923 she worked as a kindergarten teacher at the Mossestift orphanage in the Berlin-Charlottenburg district and was appointed as a civil servant on 1 January, 1926. From 16 February, 1923 to 30 September, 1930, she worked as a kindergarten teacher in a transitional home for orphans and from 1 October, 1930 until 1933 as headmistress at the municipal shelter in Charlottenburg, Sophie-Charlotte-Strasse 113.

> The last task was particularly difficult work, which, as far as I know, Ms. G. carried out with good skill and psychological aptitude. I think there can be little doubt that Ms. G. would have been promoted to the position of head of a day-care centre if she had not been dismissed by the National Socialists at the time [...]

to which the head welfare officer, Ms Koschwitz, attests in 1954 (compensation file E 18). 'At the end of March 31, 1934, she was retired on the basis of §3 of the Law for the Restoration of the Professional Civil Service (BBG)' (file 21 WGA 395/55).

DOI: 10.4324/9781003403906-2

Manna Friedmann (interview, 19 March, 2000) recalled that Alice Goldberger had talked a lot about her work at the shelter. She loved working there, had been 'cherished' and had 'adopted the homeless'.

Berlin's rise to become the capital of the Reich was accompanied by an extraordinary increase in population. Berlin became the largest city of tenements in the world and drove many into homelessness (Scheffler, 1990, p. 158). The situation worsened with the First World War and the Great Depression. Eva von Budritzki describes the 1924 shelter reform within which welfare work became necessary because the circle of visitors to the mass shelter had changed considerably compared to earlier times, whereby the resulting tasks also took on a changed character.

> The general public's perception of the visitors to the 'Obdach' [transl.: *shelter*] no longer corresponds to reality. The young lad full of wanderlust, the elderly vagabond or tramp, or the degenerate work-shy city elements only make up a part of the occupants of the 'Obdach'. The majority, on the other hand, is made up of completely different elements. Here the extraordinary economic difficulties and social changes of the war and post-war period take effect, which confronted many circles with the necessity to change their occupation and way of life and brought many into an unforeseen plight that they could not overcome by their own efforts, the main factors of which are housing and unemployment.
> (Budritzki, 1929, p. 70)

The municipal family home and shelter in Berlin-Charlottenburg was an institution adminstered by the district welfare office, Charlottenburg, and consisted of various sections: Night shelter for men and women, common rooms for homeless families who were allowed to live there for a maximum of four weeks (W 1911, Archive for Social Welfare 1921/1922, p. 14).

From 1933 until her emigration in 1939, Alice Goldberger was employed by the Jewish community and ran the Jewish day-care centre at Grolmannstrasse 59/60. She was responsible for 50 small children and 80 schoolchildren and was assisted by six assistants as well as kitchen and domestic staff (file 21 WGA 395/55). The nursery was located on the ground floor and a kindergarten on the first floor. It was one of the many establishments in private houses or flats that had been abandoned by Jews (Schonig, 1996, p. 160).

She herself states that she was involved in training schoolgirls in the youth hostel and was head of the specialist group for youth leaders, kindergarten teachers and after-school care workers (compensation file E 9). Until her emigration, Alice Goldberger lived in Berlin-Charlottenburg, Wielandstrasse 33, Garden House 3 c/o Fränkel. As part of the reparations (file number 21–3567/55) of 27 May, 1955, she applied for compensation in the amount of 997.44 DM, for the value of her assets, which she had been forced to leave behind at the Berlin Stadtbank. Starting on 5 August, 1950, she received the assurance that she would receive a pension as a former kindergarten teacher of the 'Städtisches Obdach' [transl.: state shelter],

Berlin-Charlottenburg, in the amount of RM75 per month from September 1939. At the time her address was Weir Courtney Hostel, Lingfield, Surrey.

Early days in England

On 27 August, 1939, equipped with a 'Domestic Permit' she could emigrate to Hindhead, Surrey, c/o Mrs Wolff, on the last ship from Germany – an area where she was later to live for a long time. Emmy Wolff (1890–1969) who worked with her at Stoatley Rough, Haselmere, a German–English school set up to prepare German refugee children for English schooling, which was 3.5 miles from Hindhead. Anneliese Schnurmann (interview, 24 November, 1996) reported that she had met Alice Goldberger while working as a domestic servant in Stoatley Rough.

When entering England, every German citizen had to appear before a tribunal to prove, based on certificates, assessments and other documents, as well as a personal interview, that he or she was friendly to the country. Persons classified as 'Enemy Aliens' were sent to a reception camp, from which further checks were made as to their eligibility to enter the country. It remains unclear why Alice Goldberger was classified as an 'Enemy Alien' at the hearing that almost all Jews with a German passport had to undergo. Perhaps the fact that she was a civil servant (revoked), or Anneliese Schnurmann's assumption (interview, 24 November, 1996), whose own classification was 'Friendly Alien', is correct: that Alice Goldberger defended herself badly:

> So, you know what, she was in the same tribunal with me, where the presiding judge joked with me and immediately declared me a 'Friendly Alien'. And he put her in the department, and she was interned on the Isle of Man. So, none of us ever understood that. I wonder if she behaved very clumsily. Whether her references weren't very good? I mean, I had better ones, it's true, because I knew the right people. So, it wasn't me at all, but because of the friends I had. That's how she ended up in the camp on the Isle of Man, where she set up a kindergarten on her own initiative.

Anneliese Schnurmann remembers another scene with Alice Goldberger at the very beginning of her time working in the War Nurseries: 'Funny, I don't remember that exactly. Anyway, I was a guest there, treated with distinction, and the unfortunate Alice was the domestic, the one who was treated badly'. Another memory of hers about Alice Goldberger (Schnurmann, interview, 24 November, 1996):

> I was always late for everything! I always got up too late. I raced out to get the bus from up there, down here to the clinic and Alice would run after me. Touchingly, with a cup of cocoa. Which I then drank. She was a very touching person. But she couldn't fight back! But at least she was so capable that she set up a kindergarten on the Isle of Man.

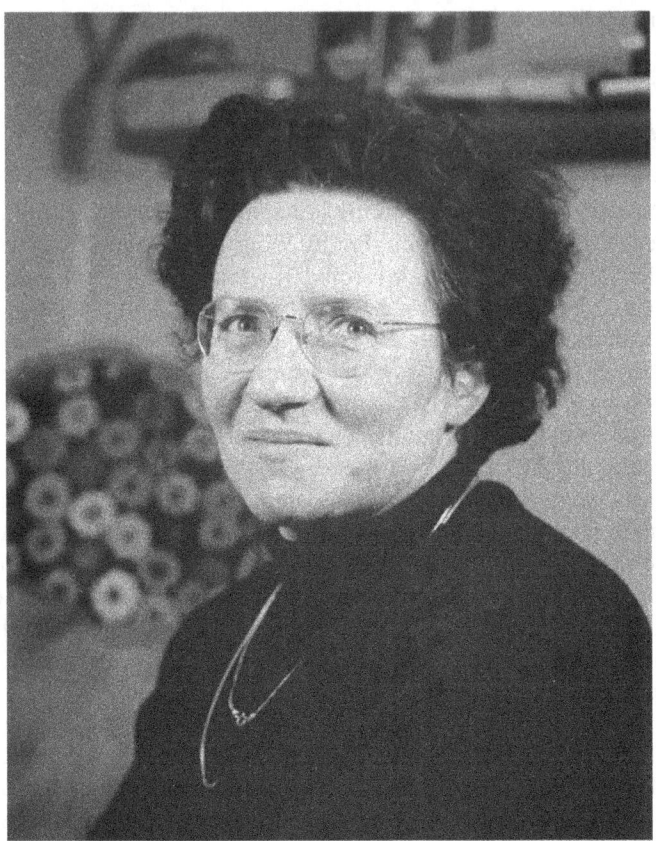

Alice Goldberger 1951 (credit: Gertrud Dann and US Holocaust Memorial Museum, Alice Goldberger Collection)

In her practical, hands-on way, full of imagination, optimism, and in possession of a good sense of humour, she immediately began to engage with the children present there. Everything that could be found – such as egg crates – was converted into playgrounds. She had the women collect the wool caught in the barbed wire surrounding the fields of grazing sheep, because the tufts could be used in all kinds of ways. According to Manna Friedmann, Alice Goldberger instructed parents how to make their own toys and other equipment. The high esteem in which Alice Goldberger was held by the internees was demonstrated by the fact that the women gave her a farewell gift of their own made from the scraps of wool they had collected and knitted.

When Anna Freud learned about her initiative in the daily newspaper, she immediately decided she was just the person she needed for her residential wartime nursery, which at the time, had to be evacuated to the countryside. As she was trying to get her nephew Ernst Halberstadt and the housekeeper Paula Fichtl, who were also interned on the Isle of Man, she met Alice Goldberger there. Through her interventions she was released earlier. 'Alice liked to recall her first meeting with Miss Freud. Asked what salary she expected, Alice replied that on the Isle of Man she was paid sixpence per week, to which Miss Freud replied: "I think we shall not pay you less"' (Friedmann, 1986, p. 313).

Anna Freud gave her the management of the Country House in New Barn, Essex, where the children from the London War Nurseries had been brought due to the bombing. She is described by those who knew her as an outstanding and respected woman. She had infinite patience and great intuition in dealing with children. Anna Freud often told Manna Friedmann the story of how a little boy asked a helper to carry him up the stairs, to which the helper replied: 'You're such a big boy already, you can do it all by yourself'. Alice Goldberger, who was nearby, gently replied: 'If it was your boy, wouldn't you carry him up?' (Friedmann, 1986, p. 313)

She is also characterized as a 'doer' who liked to get things done quickly. Nevertheless, she also had a 'disorganized almost "chaotic"' side, could sometimes plan poorly, and annoyed Gertrud Dann (interview, 14 July, 1996), who worked with her, by the fact that when she was in the middle of a job she would suddenly hear Alice Goldberger's voice in the house, asking her to do this or that immediately:

I think with her it was more [–] insecurity. She was quite insecure. And she had to show that she was the boss. [–] She was downstairs in a room and one of the staff and I were upstairs cleaning up. [–] and [in a very high voice]: 'Gertruuuud! Gertruud! Come down here.' 'What, now?' 'Yes, right now, please.' What was it? She asked me to address the envelopes or something completely unimportant. And it had to be now. She could drive me mad with things like that. I know I've done it a hundred times [–] that a hundred times I pretended I didn't hear her. With bad conscience, but [–] when it's such little things. I could just as well have addressed the envelopes three hours later.

From Gertrud Dann's point of view, Alice would never have been able to run a household on her own:

She would never have known what she had bought and then bought the same things again. She was completely disorganized. But she was a very good judge of character and had an infinite amount of patience. [–] I am very patient. I can put up with quite a lot. Unlike [–] in the past. And I knew that she had many great qualities. She also celebrated every birthday differently, always had good ideas. 'You've got an active mind.' And that was true too. But she could [–] could really drive you to frenzy.

(Dann, interview, 14 July, 1996)

Windermere

After the end of the war and the dissolution of the War Nurseries, Alice Goldberger, together with Oscar Friedmann, was commissioned to put together a team to take in the expected 1,000 young Holocaust survivors. While Alice was standing on the airfield at Crosby-on-Eden, near Carlisle, not thinking that it was her 48th birthday, memories of the children she had left behind in Berlin came to her.

> She saw their faces clearly. Their eyes, looking out to the playground forbidden to Jews, haunted her. Self-reproach filled her and abated only with the pledge to care for these child survivors with all her heart. This time she would not leave (Moskovitz, 1983, p. 5).

Alice Goldberger reported (Moskovitz, 1983, p. 5f): 'Plane after plane of youth arrived, mostly boys, but very few girls'. She later recalled:

> They had a grey, aged look which made it difficult to tell how old they were. We were relieved by their happiness on arrival. They joked, they laughed, they asked us whether they would be able to go to school. We welcomed each and when asked their age, most said they were between thirteen and fifteen, but it was hard to tell. (Later, we realized that even those who were over sixteen would not admit to it because they would not have been allowed to enter the country as part of this special children's airlift if they were older.)

They were accompanied by Edith Lauer, who herself had been imprisoned in Theresienstadt and had received permission to help as a social worker in the children's ward. She reported on the chaotic conditions during the train journey from Theresienstadt to Prague and how about 50 children and youths were crowded together on the hard floors of the bombers for more than 14 hours until they finally landed in Crosby-on-Eden. Alice Goldberger

> began to worry after so many planes of youths arrived that there would be no small children. I thought about the dolls and bears in each of the beds and what a joke that would be to these adolescents when they got to their beds in Windermere. Finally, the last two planes arrived with less than twenty young children in them.
>
> (Moskovitz, 1983, p. 5f).

Among them were six small children between the ages of three and four, who had lived in a group together in Theresienstadt. They were much too small for their age and stood out due to their tremendous attachment to each other. If they were separated, they supported each other against the adults who wanted to take care of them (Moskovitz, 1983). Alice Goldberger and Oscar Friedmann realized how important it was for these small children to be divided into a small, permanent group as quickly as possible or to find suitable adoptive parents, and that Windermere, with its many young people, was unsuitable for them. On 15 October, 1945, after several years in Theresienstadt, a month of waiting in Prague and two months in the Windermere reception camp, they were taken – accompanied by Alice Goldberger – to the Bulldogs Bank cottage, which Lady Rebekah (Betty) Clarke had provided. Sophie and

Gertrud Dann took over for a year to look after this group of young children. About these Anna Freud, together with Sophie Dann, reported in detail in her essay 'An experiment in group upbringing' (1951) (cf. chapter 2).

Bela Rosenthal, born in 1942 in Berlin, was separated from her parents at three years old when they were deported to Auschwitz and Theresienstadt. Her father was murdered in Auschwitz and her mother died of TB in Theresienstadt, where Rosenthal remained until its liberation. Her earliest memories were 'snatches of the plane. Very dark. Very noisy. Very scary. Nobody told us anything. We were on the last plane that left from Prague'. Zdenka Husserl recalled: 'We sat on the laps of grown-ups. There was a bucket to be sick in and to be used as a toilet'.

In a 1948 interview with the magazine *John Bull*, Alice Goldberger reported:

> On the night the first children arrived in 1945 they were full of hostility, fear and distrust. When they caught sight of food they rushed to it, snatching bits from each other's plates and stuffing their pockets with uneaten pieces. These they later hid under their pillows fearing that they would get no more. When the staff tried to undress them for bed, pandemonium broke out. They had decided that this fairyland was a trick, as soon as the lights were turned out the SS men would come and kill them in their beds. Some of the children were difficult to understand because they spoke a mixture of several languages picked up in the various camps through which they passed.
>
> (Bateson, 2004)

Gilbert (1996, p. 286 f.) describes in his book *The Boys*, which became the basis for the 2020 film of the same name, how the children and young people hoarded food, because they could not imagine having food at any time from now on. The remaining smaller children between the ages of four and ten years of age were able to find a home in December 1945 in Weir Courtney, Lingfield, Surrey, on the out-skirts of London. Sir Benjamin Drage, owner of a large furniture store and head of the West London Synagogue, had made a large part of his country estate available to these children free of charge and had moved his wife and daughter into a smaller part of the house (Moskovitz, 1983).[2]

Alice Goldberger volunteered to be a house mother (1945–1952). She was as-sisted by Manna Friedmann and Sophie Wutsch, among others. The children came to a house lit with candles for the first night of Hanukkah, which commemorates the re-dedication of the second temple in Jerusalem in the second century BC. Many later recalled their amazement when they arrived at night at the house to see the many windows lit up with candlelight.

The initial group of children living in Weir Courtney, Lingfield, often called the 'Lingfield (House) children', consisted of 18 children. Fifteen were part of the original group who came to Britain in 1945 and 1946, and three of the children had a surviving parent and were more recent arrivals (National Holocaust Centre and Museum, n.d.). The home also received donations at this time from the American Planned Parenthood for war children.

Zdenka Husserl (Husserlová) remembers how the children, who could only converse in different languages (Czech, Hungarian, Yiddish, Polish, French, Italian, German) were encouraged to learn English, and how Alice Goldberger insisted on this, as she believed the children should look towards the future and not be reminded of their heavy history (Memory of Nations, n.d.). We know from Holocaust research, that this was a common practice and that many children did not know of their parents' suffering. It was also common for the children not to be informed by their adoptive parents about their origins or were given a different first name by their 'new parents', which suited the adoptive parents better. In the film by Beatrice Schwehm (1999) about three of these former Bulldogs Bank Children, Bela Rosenthal tells how she was 'given' the name Joanna (Rubens), which she did not like at all. The carers spoke German among themselves and thought the children would not understand them that way. But Zdenka Husserl remembers that many children did understand a lot.

Other smaller children who were able to survive the war in hiding joined them eight months later. A total of 24 children were under the care of Alice Goldberger and her team in Weir Courtney (Moskovitz, 1983). In the short term, the six young children from Theresienstadt were transferred to Weir Courtney after the dissolution of Bulldogs Bank in 1947, five of whom were quickly adopted.

The children lived in Weir Courtney from 1945 until they were moved to 42 The Grove, Isleworth, London, in December 1948, where some of the children were able to attend secondary schools. All of them completed their schooling and education and were introduced to Jewish culture even more intensively. After the children were either reunited with family members or adopted, the house in Isleworth was closed at the end of 1957, and a flat at 159 West End Lane, Hampstead, London NW6 was found for Alice Goldberger and Sophie Wutsch, providing accommodation for the remaining four children and serving as a home, in a real family sense, where all the children could always return when they needed help and advice. Alice Goldberger continued to care for her foster family until her own death in February 1986 (Bateson, 2004).

Later, Alice Goldberger had this flat divided and rented out the second part to Zdenka Husserl, one of the girls rescued from Theresienstadt. Her flat remained the contact point for the children, who were scattered all over the world. Whoever came to London could stay with her. Sophie Wutsch cooked for the 'former children' who came to London on Friday evenings and weekends. Alice Goldberger's and Sophie Wutsch's strong point was to give support to children who were without parents or who had been badly parented. Alice had also been the one who had made it possible for all these children to have contact with each other to this day (Friedmann, interview, 23 April, 1997). Full of love and gratitude, the children, who later lived in different places in the world, called themselves the Lingfield House Children.

The main goal of the care was to give these traumatized children a sense of security and confidence and to provide a replacement for those who were homeless. Through daily routine, they were integrated into everyday life in a practical way.

They helped in the garden and were responsible for the animals assigned to them, such as chickens, rabbits, dogs, and cats. They used to paint, do handicrafts, and make music. For example, a large tablecloth was made from a bed sheet, on which the children and some of the visitors embroidered motifs from everyday life in Lingfield, such as celebrating birthdays, peeling apples, making music, and taking care of animals.

Alice Goldberger succeeded in persuading the members of the West London Synagogue to provide additional stimulation for the children through regular donations. The 'Aunties' visited children in Weir Courtney, took them on visits to London, to the cinema, to concerts and cultural events, so that they could experience other worlds. But the children didn't want to stay with the Aunties in London; their home – their family – were Alice Goldberger and Sophie Wutsch, who cooked so wonderfully for them.

The report from Lingfield House for the year 1950 gives an impression of the improvement in the situation after five years:

> In 1945 our aim was to provide a home for some of the Jewish children from the concentration camps. It seemed too much to hope that these children could reach maturity unscathed by the horrors they had witnessed and suffered... although they still require the greatest understanding and patience, most of them are now indistinguishable from normal children. Only one child, a girl now 15, proved to be a hopeless case and had to be transferred to a mental home where she is regularly visited by the matron.

According to the 1952 House Report, 26 children had left Lingfield House by then: of those six had been adopted, four had gone to Israel, nine had been reunited with a parent or relative, five were working in London, one was working in Canada, and one child had died.

Alice Goldberger remained a mother figure for all her 'family' of refugee children.

At Easter 1949, Oscar Friedmann, whose nickname was 'Ginger', went with two of the young people he was looking after to Weir Courtney to see the group there (and, no doubt, Manna Friedmann as well).

> There was an atmosphere of peace and plenty at Lingfield, and it drew as weekend visitors some of the older teenage boys who were settled in hostels in town – Wolf Blomfeld, Ben Helfgot, (Yeszhek) Jerczy Herszberg, Hofo Gryn, and Henry Green. Alice called them 'Our Boys', and they provided welcome older male companionship to the young children. (Moskovitz, 1983, p. 15; Herszberg, 1979)

It turned out that Wolf Blomfeld had already known Alice Goldberger from her work in Berlin. He came to Britain as a child refugee in March 1939, when he had just turned ten. When aged about 16, Wolf had been recommended by Dr Katz, a rabbi who taught history and Hebrew, to read Sigmund Freud's *Psychopathology of*

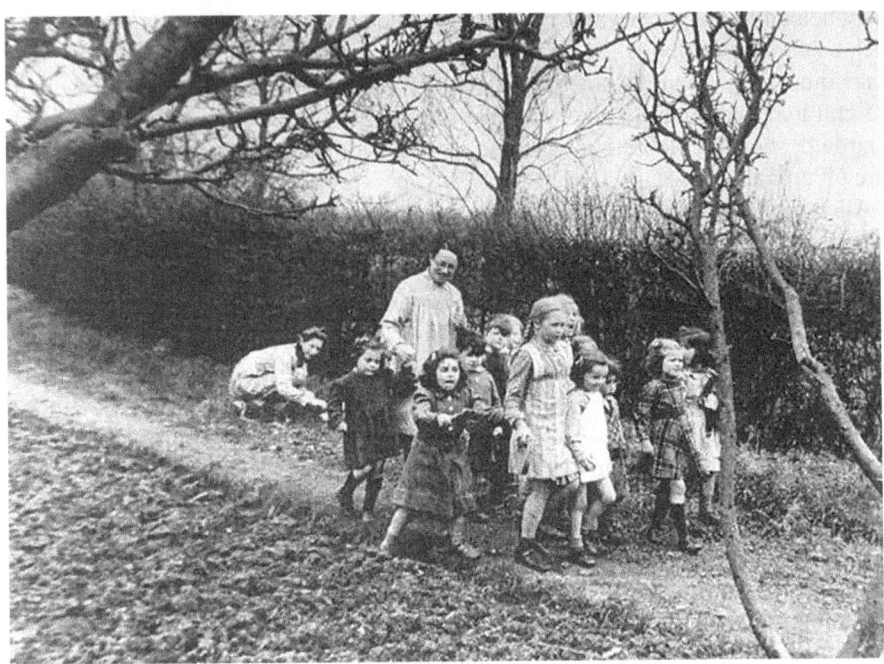

Alice Goldberger on a walk with children at Weir Courtney (credit: US Holocaust Memorial Museum)

Everyday Life, which ignited an interest in social work. In his testimony. he speaks of the reason for going to Lingfield House, as well as his journey to England, and his life there since leaving his father behind.

> It was a very good introduction to psychoanalysis. It was then that I decided to do social work. One way of getting into social work was to do residential work, so it was arranged for me to go to Lingfield House to work at a home for children who had been in concentration camps. Alice Goldberger ran the home. Alice was one of the most important people in my life. I knew her in Berlin as a young child, because she ran the 'Hort' I attended every day after school. [...] Alice was crucial in my development, both in Germany and in England. I don't think she is recognised enough for her achievements. In 1949 when I went along to Lingfield House, I didn't know that Alice worked there; it was fantastic to see her again. I was maybe four or five years older than the oldest children in the home. The gap between us was quite narrow. It's strange because I never felt lucky next to these children, even though if my father hadn't put me on that train, I may have ended up as one of these children instead. I know I was lucky. I am forever grateful to my father for his foresight.

I am still in touch with the Lingfield House children. When I go to Israel I always see one of the girls that I looked after, who is now a grandmother. It feels important to me to still know people that I knew back then. (Holocaust Memorial Day Trust, n.d.)

In Model (1986, p. 315) there are some reminiscences of Wolf Blomfield, by then a social worker trainer and psychotherapist himself, about his time in Lingfield.

It was here that he became aware of her gift for making everyone feel needed and special and of her attentiveness in the smallest matters that helped to transform Lingfield House from an institution into a home for many of the children. In Alice's last years, Wolf has been one of the people who visited her regularly and conveyed to us his happiness in being able to show the care for her that she all her life had shown for others.

Manna Friedmann writes that Weir Courtney was also the home of Alice Goldberger, Sophie Wutsch and, of course, herself. She held Alice Goldberger in very high esteem; she could empathise with her, and read her well, and Alice in turn relied completely on Manna Friedmann.

Gertrud Dann describes her relationship with Alice Goldberger: 'I was only friends with her on the outside, but on the inside [–] I appreciated her a lot, but she wasn't my type. I think she thought I was her friend. I have never had any longing for her' (Dann, interview, 14 July, 1996).

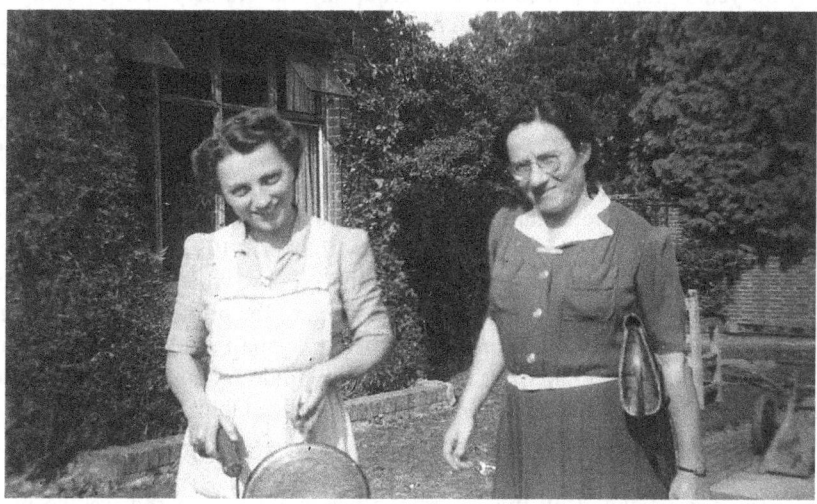

Manna Friedmann and Alice Goldberger in Weir Courtney (credit: Manna Friedmann and US Holocaust Memorial Museum, Alice Goldberger Collection)

Alice Goldberger knew about Manna Friedmann's loyal attitude towards her, but she was always in danger of having to fight with her for the love of the children. In the evenings she regularly went to all the children to wish them goodnight. Manna Friedmann often pointed out to her that there was no reason to be jealous. Alice Goldberger, for example, found it hard to bear the fact that Judith Sherman had taken Manna Friedmann so specially to her heart. Manna Friedmann felt that Alice Goldberger, who no longer had anyone in her family and was completely on her own, also needed the children for herself – to a greater extent than Manna had done for herself.

> Alice was very possessive, in a sense that she wanted someone to be firmly bound to her, to herself, to claim someone as her own, wanted to be the only one who was really liked by the children. And she was. The children all appreciated her wonderfully.
>
> (Friedmann, interview, 23 July, 1997)

While Manna Friedmann was mainly concerned with the children of latency age, as well as those in adolescence – she found this the easiest time – Alice Goldberger, and also Gertrud Dann, found it much more difficult to work with children of this age.

Work as a child therapist

Alice Goldberger gained British citizenship on 1 October, 1947. Also in 1947, then already 50 years old, she joined the first group of War Nursery staff to complete their training as 'child experts' (analytical child therapists). For over two years, according to Manna Friedmann's memoirs, she travelled to London three times a week for training analysis with Liselotte Frankl. In Manna Friedmann's perception, the psychoanalytic training had collapsed Alice Goldberg's – up until that point – good defences, so that she often returned 'disturbed' and depressed. If she had previously had immediate and very good access to the children, after the psychoanalytical training she became insecure, especially towards herself. 'She lost somehow faith in herself' (Friedmann, interview, 23 April, 1997). She was not academic and struggled a great deal with the regular reports, which, in order to meet Anna Freud's standards, they had to be almost ready for print. Alice Goldberger could hardly live up to this standard. Nevertheless, Anna Freud valued her work. She was particularly good at working with blind children and Anna Freud often assigned very difficult children to her for analysis. Alice Goldberger revered, even idolized, Anna Freud to a high degree.

> One was overwhelmed by this enormous personality – yet she was so modest in her appearance. She was not an overwhelming person. But Alice was completely infatuated. And Anna Freud held Alice in high esteem [–]. Alice Goldberger loved flowers and knick-knacks; so, there was a toy train set, things

that had to be especially well guarded. She loved Yardley lavender water, which everything around her smelled of.

(Friedmann, interview, 23 April, 1997)

In the memoirs of Manna Friedmann, Alice Goldberger was someone with little 'compulsive' elements; for example, she always had new telephone directories and never found a number she needed. She was even more dependent on having good helpers by her side – such as the Dann sisters. Instead of a clear yes or no, which she found very difficult to say, there was often a 'no-yes' (Friedmann, interview, 26 November, 1996).

Retirement and the end of life

There is a letter from Manna Friedmann dated 7 February, 1977 (in the author's possession) addressed to Dr Jack Crawshaw, James Television. 306 Euston Road London NW1, in which she refers to the 80th birthday of Alice Goldberger on 15 August, 1977.

Dear Sir,

I am writing to you on behalf of Miss Alice Goldberger of 159, West-End Lane London N. W. 6. who will have her 80th birthday on August 15th, 1977.

Miss Goldberger, "ALICE" as she is called by everyone, has been living a life dedicated to the Welfare and the rehabilitation of children in need. Her friends and colleagues feel it would be wonderful for her if you could consider her as a "Candidate" for your Programme "THIS IS YOUR LIFE", since she herself is an enthusiastic viewer of that programme.

Here, briefly, are the outlines of her life-story. Alice is Jewish and was born in Berlin, Germany. She became a teacher and Youth-Welfare-Worker. When Hitler came to power Alice was the State-employed Head of the Berlin "OB-DACH", a kind of Workhouse for deprived and underprivileged families.

Shortly before the outbreak of World-War Two she came to England on a Domestic Permit, and when war did break out she was interned on the Isle of man, an "Enemy Alien".

There she organized a Nursery-School for the children of the Internees, her work was greatly appreciated by the Officer in charge of the Internment Camp.

She was released from there to be one of the workers in charge of the WAR-TIME NURSERIES under the auspices of Anna Freud.

In 1945, when 700–800 children and young adults were liberated from the Concentration-Camps in Germany and were graciously admitted to this Country for their rehabilitation, Alice, who had lost her own family in the Camps, once again was summoned to play her part. She was one of the caretakers in charge of the "WINDERMERE RECEPTION CENTRE" and eventually she was appointed Superintendent of a home for the youngest of all survivors, 24 children, their ages ranging from 4 to 17 years. This Home, a beautiful Country-House in

Lingfield Surrey, "WEIR COURTNEY" was loaned to the Refugee-children by Benjamin Drage, and it was maintained by the West-London Synagogue. Here, for the first time, these children experienced the meaning of living in a free world in the care of "ALICE" and her devoted team, who like the children benefitted from her guidance and wisdom. Until the present-day Alice has remained in close contact with "her children" and her children's children.

Her private flat in West-Hampstead, which she shares with her former co-worker and friend Sophie, is also "home" for every one of her children, who frequently visit her. Many have settled in other Countries, Australia, U.S.A., and Israel. They all write, they all come. Alice has remained their "Life-Line".

During the past 20 years Alice has been continuing to live her life in the Service of children in need. As a member of the Staff of the Hampstead Child Therapy Clinic, under the Directorship of Anna Freud, where she trained as a Child Therapist, she became increasingly interested in helping blind children as well as those who care for them.

Should you find Alice a suitable personality for your programme and should you need further information I shall be happy to provide it.

In anticipation of a favourable reply,

Yours truly
Manna Friedmann
(Mrs. Manna Friedmann, one of her co-workers and friends)

Her letter was successful and, on 25 October, 1978, the story of Alice Goldberger's life was broadcast on British television on the programme *This Is Your Life*, hosted by Eamonn Andrews.

The idea was said to have come from Zdenka Husserl, with whom she had a particularly close relationship, but it was Manna Friedmann who brought it to life. The programme was a gift of remembrance and thanksgiving from all the children in Alice Goldberger's care, whom she saw – to her complete surprise – during the television show. Jerczy Herszberg, who was present at the party afterwards, recalled: 'There were some very emotional scenes. People who had not seen each other for over thirty years, and could not even speak the same language, embraced each other and seemed to have a mutual understanding' (Herszberg, 1979).

Jackie Young, one of the adopted children from Theresienstadt, had not been invited. His wife referred him to the programme by chance, and he was stunned to recognize Alice Goldberger. Since the age of twelve, when he had learnt from classmates that he had been adopted – which his adoptive parents vehemently denied – he had harboured this suspicion. He received confirmation when he had to present documents for his wedding. In a moving report about his lifelong search for his biological parents, he states that he learnt he had been taken to Theresienstadt at the age of three and a half months, separated from his mother, while she was being murdered in a camp in Minsk. On the one hand, he could understand why his adoptive parents had kept the truth from him, believing that this was the best thing for everyone; on the other hand, one also senses his despair that Alice Goldberger, who lived nearby and kept in touch with the adoptive mother, did not 'take his side' (Whitehouse, 2020). Although especially Anna Freud and her colleagues had thought so much about the reactions to separation in children, they denied these findings at the same time. Almost as if in a collective repression, such mechanisms can be demonstrated even among psychoanalysts. The author remembers how Gertrud Dann reported about Jackie and how complicated the situation was for all concerned. He had also sought out Gertrud Dann after the television programme in the hope to learn more about his past. In the end Alice Goldberger identified herself with the adoptive parents, especially since the couple had agreed to the adoption only on the condition that it remained secret. She, in turn, had the task of placing as many of the children as possible into adoption.

Alice Goldberger spent the last years of her life with Sophie Wutsch, who was Catholic, in a Jewish retirement home. Sophie Wutsch was admitted there 'because they knew how great she was' and because she had done so much for Jewish children (Dann, interview 20 November, 1996). Alice Goldberger, who would not have had needed to move to the home with Sophie Wutsch, had promised not to leave her alone. 'It was a good home, but they were all so terribly old, sick people'. Manna Friedmann still visited her there regularly (Friedmann, interview, 23 April, 1997).

Alice Goldberger died in London on 22 February, 1986. On 14 May, 1986, a memorial service was held in her memory at the Anna Freud Centre, where a recording of the programme *This Is Your Life* was shown again. Elizabeth Model (1986, p. 315) writes:

> Younger colleagues, to whom the War Nurseries and concentration camps were hitherto historical facts, found themselves involved and moved by this unique record. Older colleagues were again reminded of Alice's steadfastness and self-effacing care and of the place she held in so many hearts.
>
> Following the film, John Parkinson, who, as a conscientious objector, had been sent to work as a handyman and gardener at New Barn, the country house branch of the Hampstead War Nurseries, recalled Alice's period as superintendent there. While giving everyone involved the feeling that they were essential to the smooth running of the Nursery, Alice's primary concern was always the children's well-being, and she created an atmosphere of stability but also of liveliness and fun.

The family of surviving Lingfield children that Alice Goldberger and her co-workers had created, continues to exist. Thus write Zdenka Husserl, Joanna Millan (Bela Rosenthal) and Rachel Oppenheimer (2009, p. 4):

> Sunday 21 June 2009. It was a sunny day when we 'Lingfielders' – children from Lingfield House – were reunited in the wonderful setting of The Holocaust Centre/Beth Shalom in Nottinghamshire. It was a very moving occasion as we had not met like this for nearly 12 years. The 'children' came from as far afield as the USA, Israel, Portugal, and Belgium – a truly international gathering. [...] We were also given an opportunity to gather round the rose bush planted in memory of Alice Goldberger.

Notes

1 Max Goldberger, born on 13 June, 1894 in Berlin, Charlottenburg, Leibnizstraße 47 (deported on 16 June, 1943 to Theresienstadt, from there transported to Auschwitz on 23 October, 1944, Transport I/96 Et719), his wife Lilli Goldberger, née Arendt (21 July, 1905 in Königsberg, East Prussia), and their daughter Ruth Gertrud Goldberger (born 15 November, 1937 Berlin) (Transport I/96, No. 13433 on 17 June, 1942 from Berlin to Theresienstadt and from there Transport En, Nos. 867 and 866 on 4 October, 1944 to Auschwitz, where they were murdered) (Yad Vashem, n.d.)

   In Moskovitz (1983, p. xv), who was able to interview Alice Goldberger, one finds the following statement about the death of her brother and his family: 'The Nazis did not even let them die together, they took Max first to what they said was a labour camp, but it was Auschwitz. Then three days later his wife and little girl were told they could join him. [...] Couldn't they at least have let them die together?'

2 Benjamin Drage (1878–1952) was one of the founding members of the Golders Green Synagogue in London and was a member of the Council of the West London Synagogue. He was knighted in 1932 for his many charitable works. In 1930, Drage purchased Weir Courtney as a weekend and holiday home. At the outbreak of the war, the house housed several evacuees, and between 1942 and 1943 it was also used as a wartime kindergarten nursery. At the end of the Second World War, Mr and Mrs Drage provided Weir Courtney to the Central British Fund for Jewish Relief and Rehabilitation (CBF) for the accommodation of young Holocaust survivors. The house was sold to the Sheraton family in 1949 (Exploring Surrey's Past, 2017).

Sources

Interviews with Manna Friedmann: 23 April, 1997; 26 November, 1996; 12 July, 1996; 19 April, 2000.

Interviews with Anneliese Schnurmann: 24 November, 1996; 26 April, 1997; 8 June, 1997.

Interviews with Gertrud Dann: 14 July, 1996; 20 November, 1996.

Compensation files 21 WGA 395/55.

Compensation files E 4, 58782, 75372.

Compensation file E 35, 58782.

Compensation file E 18, 9.

Compensation file 2 WGA 2788/50.

Reparation, file number 21–3567/55.

Oberfinanzpräsident Köln, file number 05210-L 106-V 269.

W 1911, Archive for Social Welfare 1921/1922.

2

Sophie (3.3.1900–18.12.1993) and Gertrud Dann (27.5.1908–2.4.1998) – Home for the Children from Theresienstadt

Family home in Augsburg

Sophie and Gertrud Dann's father, Albert Dann (1868–1960), a businessman, synagogue commissioner and benefactor of the city of Augsburg, came from a traditional Jewish Frankfurt family. He was a descendant of the Levite Rabbi Joseph von Mantua, who came to Frankfurt around 1530 (Römer, 1998, p. 7). Their mother, Fanny Dann, née Kitzinger (1876–1910), came from a banking family in Fürth. Albert Dann had moved to Augsburg in 1897 to manage a wholesale business for haberdashery and manufactured goods, 'Gebrüder Heymann' which was founded by the three brothers Benno, Eduard, and Sigmund in Augsburg. Sigmund Heymann was married to Albert Dann's sister, Clemy. He took over the company after the early death of his brothers and after he also died young, it was continued by Albert Dann.

When Sophie, the eldest of the five Dann daughters, was born on 3 March, 1900, a nurse looked after mother and baby, and subsequently her grandmother, Ida Kitzinger, often visited from Fürth to help with the rapidly growing flock of children. One and a half years later, Sophie's sister Thea was born, followed by Elisabeth on 15 October, 1906, Gertrud on 27 May, 1908, and Lotte on 23 December, 1912. Sophie Dann was the first grandchild of both sets of grandparents.

The Dann family was a respected family in Augsburg who initially lived at Obere Maximilianstrasse 35, where Sophie and Thea were born. The foundations of the house are said – according to Gertrud Dann (interview, 14 July, 1996) – to date back to Roman times. The family then moved to Völkstrasse 26, opposite their aunt Clemy Heymann, in 1905, after she had lost her husband – childless. Elisabeth and Gertrud were born there. After the death of Albert Dann's father, who had lived with his daughter-in-law ('Auntie Clemy'), she spent a lot of time with the Dann family until 1910, when the family moved out of Augsburg to Hochfeldstrasse 15.

At the age of 46, Albert Dann volunteered for the First World War and later took on many honorary tasks in the city of Augsburg, for which he received the title 'Kommerzienrat' [transl.: Counselor of Commerce]. His parents ran a hospitable house in which not only Martin Buber, but also, among others, the 'mother of dolls' Käthe Kruse went in and out. The family was very close; the children were happy

DOI: 10.4324/9781003403906-3

when they could visit their maternal grandmother Ida in Fürth, who, in addition to a city flat, owned a house with a large garden in the countryside. It was even more exciting when mother's aunt, Minna Dunkels, who lived in London, along with her maid, Malier, and the chauffeur, Crumplin, visited them in Augsburg in her Rolls Royce. After the death of her husband, Minna Dunkels lived surrounded by many servants in a flat directly opposite the royal residence of St. James Palace. Her maid was very popular with the Dann children, as she not only played with them but also told them secrets, such as that the aunt's jewels were hidden in the hems of her skirts and that it was she who gave the aunt her daily insulin injections (Römer, 1998, p. 75).

'Uncle Berthold' (Kitzinger), the brother of the girls' mother, was also very popular with the girls – not only because of his exquisite parcels with unusual food, toys or clothes, but because of his cheerful manner. For business reasons, the bachelor was often in South Africa but lived in England. He died of lung cancer on 22 December, 1922. Fritz Kitzinger, another brother of their mother, was a professor of law in London. There was a close relationship between the family of their mother's other brother who lived in Munich and the Dann family in Augsburg. They visited each other, where the 'educational, museum or theatre visits' in Munich, which the eldest brother, 'Uncle Wilhelm', often prescribed, were less popular than the boisterous games the cousins played with each other.

Gertrud Dann characterized herself as a child as,

> [...] a disgusting woman! I was absolutely naughty. People used to say, 'She's just nervous.' But I was simply naughty. Insubordinate, unruly, terribly aggressive. And I knew I was loathsome [–], I knew I was an obnoxious brat. Until I became terribly remorseful, and I thought, if I don't have children of my own, then I want to raise and oversee other people's awful children.
>
> (G. Dann, interview, 14 July, 1996)

In her memories, she said her mother could only leave the house in the mornings when she was at school, because she was always arguing with her sisters. At the age of two she had already been nicknamed 'the little witch' (Dann, interview, 14 July, 1996).

> Sophie was a model pupil. I don't know what she was like at home. No, I can't say. Thea, who died so young, must have been quite marvellous. Terribly sensitive, very attuned to others. I still have a few essays she wrote as a ten-year-old girl. And she was certainly always well-behaved. They didn't fight either, Sophie and Thea. Whereas Elishibber [Elisabeth] and I not only argued, but also fought. Lotte was brought up by her four sisters. She suffered. [Laughs.] She tells how disgusting we were to her, but she was our favourite sister. She was such a sweet child. And Lotte and I were terrible eaters. Every meal a tragedy. [–] I'm sure I knew how to annoy the whole family. [–] With this non-eating.
>
> (G. Dann, interview, 14 July, 1996)

Gertrud's descriptions, but also those of her sister Lotte, are reminiscent of severe eating disorders. Regarding her youngest sister, Lotte Treves, Gertrud Dann
remarked (G. Dann, interview, 14 July, 1996):

> She [Lotte] had been so terribly ill. There was no hope at all, and she couldn't
> eat. And in February daddy got radishes in a hotel. And she [saw] the radishes
> and: 'Oh, radishes!' And with that she could eat again, and she recovered.

In the memoirs of Lotte Treves (Römer, 1998, p. 146 f.) one reads that at that
time, after a ruptured appendix, she had only narrowly survived and after five op-
erations, she was nursed in hospital for three months. Her already existing eating
problems intensified. While in the hospital, her desire to study medicine arose. All
five sisters went to the Stetten Institute in Augsburg, a Protestant secondary school.
Elisabeth was the only one who later transferred to a grammar school and was one
of the first girls in Augsburg to graduate from high school. She studied one term of
philosophy at the University of Munich, but mainly learned Hebrew in order to be
able to realize her wish to study Jewish theology. Her family managed to talk her
out of studying religion. So that, after two terms in Berlin, which she enjoyed, she
went to Kings College in London in the summer of 1928. It was in London that
Elisabeth met her future husband Siegfried (Shlomo) Stern, a lawyer. Elisabeth first
worked as a teacher in England and Sweden. In the meantime, her fiancé had been
imprisoned in Germany for critical remarks about Goebbels and was released with
an order to leave the country within three weeks. He went to Palestine, to where
Elisabeth followed him 1937 and married him there.

Sophie was reserved throughout her life, even very shy in childhood (Dann,
interview, 14 July, 1996). At primary school, she was the only Jewish child in her
class. If her classmates were in Catholic classes in the morning, her classes started
later. Precise as she was all her life, she was plagued by the fear that she might be
late for class, so that she often had to wait outside the school for a long time until
the Catholic religious education lessons were over. When Thea entered school and
had several Jewish classmates, they all received private religious instruction at the
Dann's home.

During the interview with Gertrud Dann (14 July, 1996), she said that she was
ill and was nursed by 12-year-old Sophie during the time that her youngest sister Lotte was born two days before Christmas in 1912. Sophie was asked by her
mother to take Gertrud's temperature regularly; she was to write down how often
she sneezed and coughed, what she ate, etc. It was at that time that Sophie had the
thought to become a nurse. Gertrud woke up one night to the sound of a baby crying and thought, 'What kind of idiots would take a baby out on the street on such a
cold night?' She could not imagine at all that the shouting and crying was coming
from her own house. Sophie had an inkling of the impending birth, however, because her mother had previously delegated tasks to her, and she had a feeling that
the impending birth also frightened her mother. So, she was told to take care of the
sisters' Christmas plates (G. Dann, as cited in Römer, 1998, p. 71).

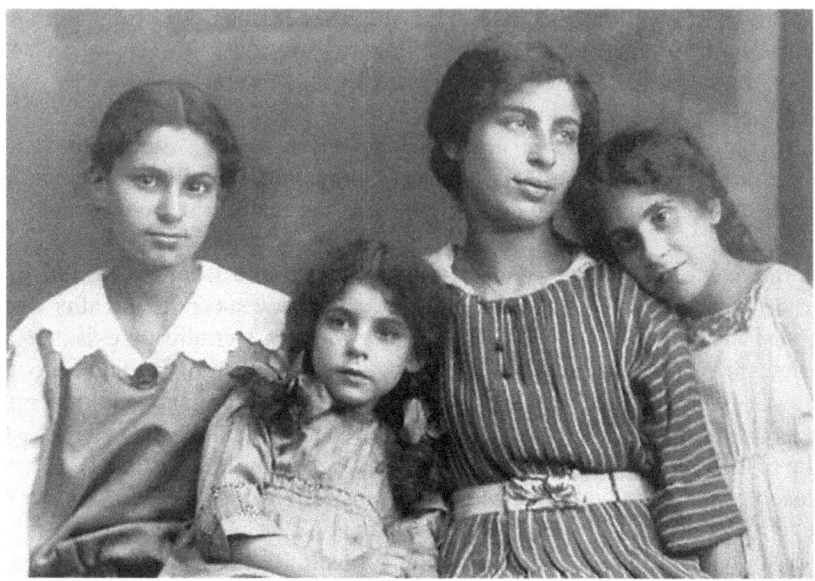

The siblings (left to right) Elisabeth, Lotte, Sophie, and Gertrud, 1919 (credit: Gertrud Dann)

Her sister Elisabeth writes in her memoirs:

> The next morning, we found out about Lotte's birth. I could not imagine how the parents knew that the child would arrive just when it did, and the room was ready just in time. We were allowed to tiptoe into the room and see the baby: a lovely little girl with red cheeks and a head full of dark curls. We loved her too much and often tormented her with our love.
>
> (E. Dann, as cited in Römer, 1998, p. 71)

The question of whether her father – as Gertrud Dann reported it to me – had been completely 'indifferent' to again not having male child, remains open (G. Dann, interview, 20 November, 1996). In any case he was later very pleased when his grandson, Claudio Treves (the son of Lotte), visited him in England after the early death of his father, Paulo.

The close birth order of the Dann sisters brought its own dynamics. This is how Elisabeth remembers it:

> Actually, I should have started school before Lotte was born, but it was decided to make me wait another year, and for good reason: I was smart and strong, very proud of both, and I loved to show off to Gertrud. She was not strong, but full of energy, which I lacked. Mother said that if I came to school two more years before her, my imagination would know no bounds. Mother was right, for in later years I used to tease Gertrud until she flew into a rage; then our endless

wars began, so that for years mother did not leave the house when the two of us were home in the afternoon.

(E. Dann, as cited in Römer, 1998, p. 71 f.)

From the sisters' accounts, one can see how terrible the sudden death of their 17-year-old sister Thea was. She suffered from asthma and died in the winter of 1918 after an operation in an unheated operating theatre. Four years earlier, she had undergone blind bowel surgery. It was assumed that her pain was caused by adhesions that needed to be removed. 'I think I was too stupid. I didn't really understand it until much later. I saw how my mother was suffering, and Sophie' (G. Dann, interview, 18 September, 1997). Sophie and Thea

had grown up together, gone to school together a year apart, joined the Wandervogel together and, despite being so fundamentally different, they were the very best of friends. Sophie was blonde, Thea had dark hair and the most soulful black eyes I've ever seen.

(E. Stern, as cited in Römer, 1998, p. 72)

On later trips to Germany, Sophie and Gertrud Dann regularly visited Thea's grave, where a large chestnut tree now stands, grown from a chestnut that had been planted on her grave. In 1985, Gertrud took a chestnut from Augsburg to England during a visit there (Dann, interview, 18 September, 1997).

Gertrud Dann, who was otherwise full of respect, was amused by a quirk of her sister Sophie. As a teenager, Sophie was impressed that Victoria Luise of Prussia, married to Duke Ernst August of Brunswick and Lüneburg, was able to live with her baby Friederike for a while with the cousin of one of her maids in Augsburg after the abdication of her father, the emperor. The cousin, an insurance agent of Albert Dann, turned to him with concern. Sophie collected baby linen and food to take to the young mother with her friend. Sophie's preference for closeness to nobility remained in any case. This is how she describes it:

I had my first royal handshake in 1908, when Thea and I presented our homemade baskets of reed grass to Prince Regent Luitpold of Bavaria and received a silver and a chocolate coin each in return. When I nursed Princess Maria Bonaparte [Princess George of Greece], who was ill in Miss Freud's house, there were no handshakes, but there was the first five-pound note in my life.

(S. Dann, as cited in Römer, 1998, p. 56)

Sophie also tells how she and Gertrud were invited to the opening of the Freud Museum in London:

Gertrud and I received an invitation to the opening of the Freud Museum together with a letter saying that Buckingham Palace had asked those who had known Anna Freud for any length of time should be introduced to the Princess Alexandra. This meant: our hats from Augsburg, from Mrs. Grossner's shop in

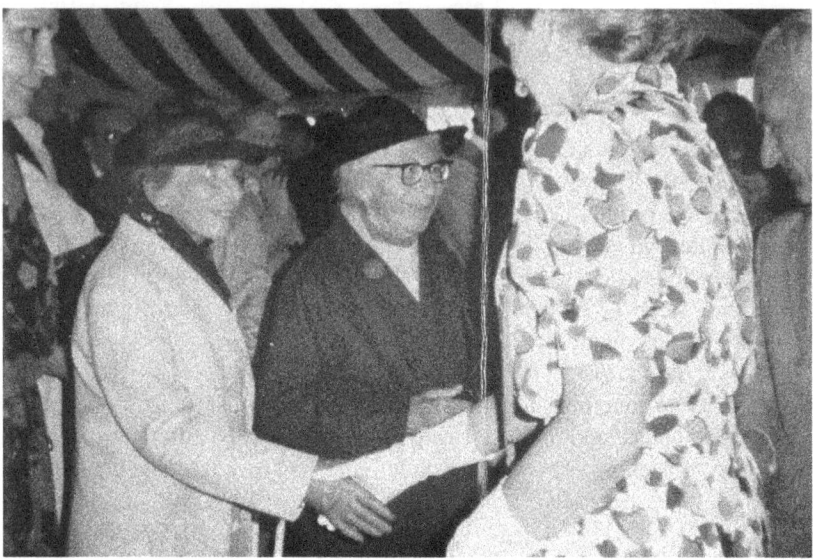

Sophie and Gertrud Dann at the opening of the Freud Museum (credit: Gertrud Dann and the Anna Freud Centre)

1938, gloves and court curtsies. It was a wonderful celebration. Only eight people were present. The princess was lovely and very kind to us.

(S. Dann, as cited in Römer, 1998, p. 56)

Gertrud Dann (interview, 14 July, 1996) told me how Sophie came out of hospital in 1988 after a severe stroke:

When she came back, she was wonderful, actually like before. [–] Interesting, really, you always think of something. So, the first few days she was unconscious and [–] then very soon she said: 'We must be careful not to confuse Prince Charles' money with ours.' The royal family played a big part in her head. That was, I think, the first real sentence [she spoke after her stroke].

Back to Augsburg times

After completing her educator training, Sophie helped at an orphanage in Munich, where her aunt Elisabeth Kitzinger (married to Wilhelm Kitzinger, one of her mother's brothers) was the headmistress, until she was old enough to start training as an infant nurse. It was the deprived time of inflation, when many – including Sophie – went hungry, and she was grateful when someone gave her something. During her subsequent training as a visiting nurse in Nuremberg, she was able to visit her uncle Gabriel Kitzinger's family in Fürth and find support there. After

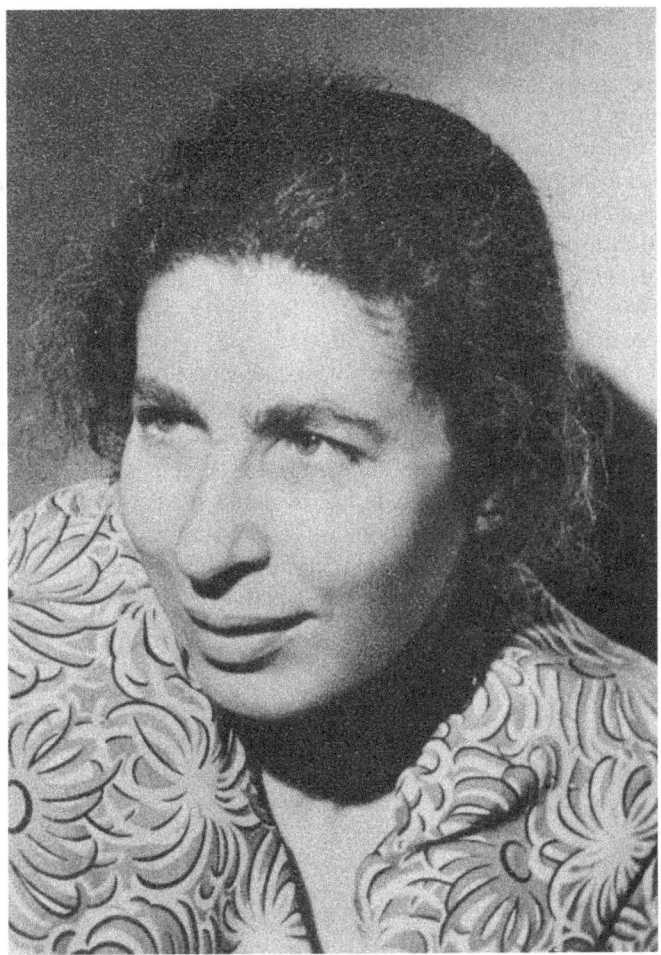

Sophie Dann in her early days in England (credit: Gertrud Dann)

her training as a general nurse at the municipal hospital in Augsburg, Elisabeth Kitzinger wanted Sophie to take over the management of the orphanage in Munich. It was with great misgivings that she finally agreed, as she was afraid of the responsibility – including bookkeeping, but also working with older children. She became seriously ill, had to stop working and after a one-year recovery period she underwent an operation on her thyroid gland. In 1930, she found fulfilment in the task of founding a mothers' school on behalf of the Augsburg Women's Association and giving courses for young women, mothers, and the unemployed, as well as social workers. In addition, as managing director of the home care association, she was responsible for the organization and accounting of approximately 80 domestic helpers. She loved this work, which came to an end in 1933 with the exclusion of the Jewish community from welfare life. From 1934 to April 1939, she worked as a nurse and welfare worker and, for a while, took over the organization of welfare work for the approximately 1,000 Jewish members of Augsburg, supported by former superiors and friends, and finally gave maternity school courses for Jewish girls who had to emigrate. It was hoped that this would lead to better working conditions. Hostilities grew, Aryan staff were no longer allowed to work in Jewish households and beloved employees had to quit.

In addition to her work, Sophie Dann took care of her aunt Clemy, who was seriously ill with diabetes (her legs had been amputated). She received her daily injections from Sophie. Clemy Heymann died shortly before Sophie and Gertrud's parents were able to escape to Palestine.

Gertrud Dann was talked out of her wish to become a dancer, or at least a gymnastics teacher, because she was too delicate. From autumn 1926 to spring 1928 she attended a kindergarten seminar in Dresden-Hellerau, run according to anthroposophical principles. Apart from the gymnastics lessons and folk dances, she felt very unwell there and, according to her own statements, completed the training with mediocre results (Dann, interview, 20 November, 1996). In Augsburg she learnt infant care and worked in various children's homes between 1929 and 1932. She remembers how unpleasant the work was in a Jewish Orthodox children's home 1931 in Hamburg-Blankenese, as the nurses were very unfriendly with one another, worked against each other and complained about each other. 'They were

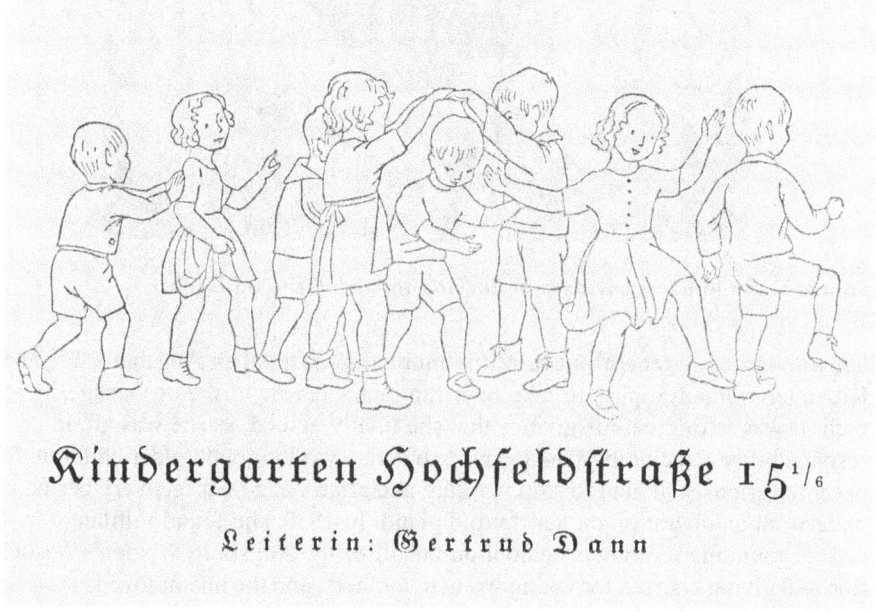

Poster of Gertrud Dann's kindergarten in Augsburg (credit: Gertrud Dann)

only there for four weeks. Four weeks of Berlin children, four weeks of Kassel children' (Dann, interview, 14 January, 1996). She took over a kindergarten with 10–12 children of all denominations from a colleague in Augsburg and ran it in her parents' home.

As of 1934, however, Gertrud Dann was no longer allowed to look after Aryan children in her kindergarten and had to move into an annex of the synagogue. Soon, there were no longer enough Jewish children, as many Jewish families emigrated, so from 1937 to 1939 she worked at the Jewish Children's Home in Munich, which had been founded and run by her aunt and where Sophie had also worked. 'And my aunt was always afraid that people might think she favoured her nieces, and she was especially strict with us. Much stricter than with the other staff' (G. Dann, interview, 20 November, 1996).

In the meantime, business at the Heymann company was in decline. When Lotte graduated from high school and wanted to study medicine, she moved to Munich and lived in a room together with her sister Elisabeth, who had in the meantime completed her teacher's examination and was teaching in a secondary school. When Elisabeth went to England in autumn 1933, Lotte moved to Turin with Elisabeth's friend, who had already passed her medical exams. She wanted to repeat her MD there, in order for her exams to be recognized in the British Empire. Lotte Dann kept her head above water by teaching German lessons and doing translations after her father was no longer allowed to transfer money to her.

After Albert Dann was briefly imprisoned following the destruction of the synagogue in November 1938, Albert and Fanny Dann accepted the offer of their daughter Elisabeth, who had meanwhile managed to escape to Palestine with her husband Shlomo, to flee there as well. This was only possible through the friendly relationship between Fanny Dann's brother Wilhelm and the British consul in Munich.

During a stopover in Italy, the parents were able to meet their daughter Lotte who had in the meantime passed her medical exams, in Milan on 20 March, 1939, before they travelled by ship to Palestine. There, they initially lived cramped in the tiny two-room flat of their pregnant daughter Elisabeth until she managed to find a room for them. At first, they were supported by Sophie and Gertrud – after their flight to England – with £10 a month, which was the maximum amount that could be exported.

Sophie and Gertrud Dann decided to emigrate to England after their parents left. Sophie, who had arranged household jobs in England for some Jewish girls, was tipped off to place an advertisement in *The Times* in November 1938 by an Englishwoman, who then paid for it (as Jews were not allowed to transfer money abroad) and who also sifted through the job offers for her. The surplus offers meant that another seven more people were able to emigrate as well (unpublished memories of Sophie Dann, 1986, p. 9).

After the sale of their parents' house, Sophie and Gertrud lived with relatives for a while, but they still had to heat their old house in Augsburg until they emigrated, because the buyer did not know how to operate the heating. Aunt Minna had given

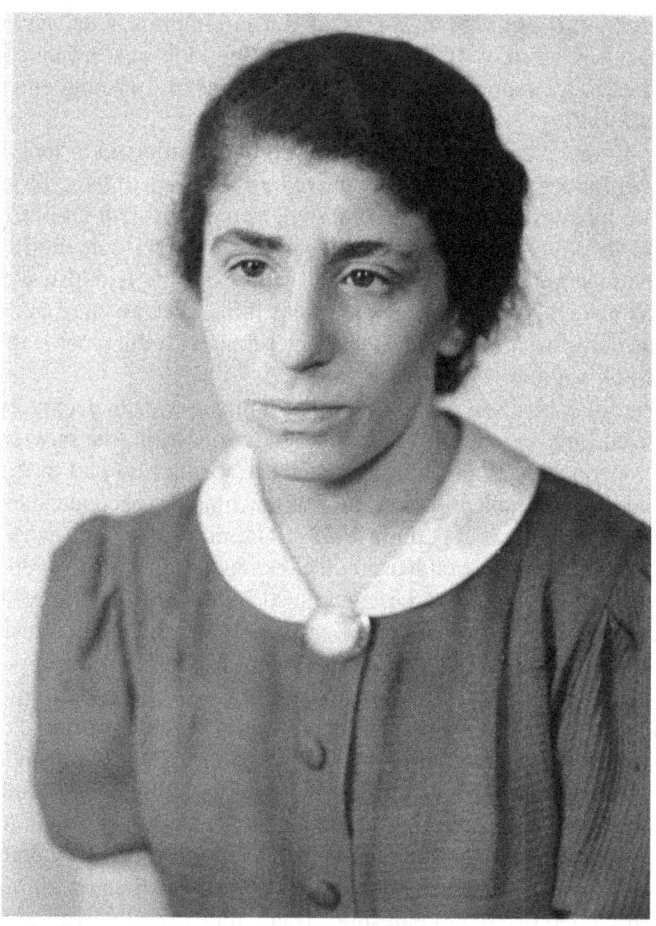

Gertrud Dann in Augsburg (credit: Gertrud Dann)

them a crash course on how to set and serve the table in England, and they were also given daily advice by telephone:

> Our last day in Germany was very sad. Due to very particular harassment, we were not allowed to board the train in Cologne, for which we were pre-registered, and had to wait for the evening train. It was a wet and cold 12 April, and we had no money except the precious ten marks that everyone was allowed to take with them. So, we sat by the Rhine all day and took turns going to the cathedral where it was a bit warmer. Fortunately, mother's relative Thekla Dünkelsbühler had given us sandwiches. Of course, we didn't have a cabin on the night boat [to England]. We sat somewhere very uncomfortable and slept very little. We slept on the train from Harwich to London until the ticket man woke us up. We were

told that in England we could travel first class with our second-class tickets. But the man shouted at us that we would have to pay extra. While we explained to him that we had absolutely no money, the city gentlemen sat around us reading the newspaper. The man took our tickets, and we were sure we'd be taken to jail when we arrived in London. But instead of the police, Miss Bruell, Aunt Minna's companion, was waiting for us, and in the elegant Armstrong Siddeley we were driven to our employers.

(G. Dann, as cited in Römer, 1998, p. 114)

Even if one had wealthy relatives in England, this did not mean that one received official permission to stay in England. For Gertrud and Sophie Dann, who in their childhood and youth were accustomed to being cared for by servants, the sudden role reversal was extremely difficult: 'I am sure we were the most inexperienced cook and maid in our position, just as our lady was the most [–] impatient employer. The lodger, the writer Laurens van der Post, helped us in many difficult situations (G. Dann, as cited in Römer, 1998, p. 114).

They also continued to receive daily support by telephone from their Aunt Minna, who gave them tips: for instance, that horseradish belongs with beef, etc. Gertrud Dann remembers how she and her sister ate the leftovers of the cold chicken in the kitchen after dinner and were indignantly told that they were to 'never eat in the kitchen what is served in the dining room' (G. Dann, as cited in Römer, 1998, p. 115). They were used to the servants at home eating the same food as the family. The influence of Aunt Minna, who had invited their employer to her home to make her understand the conditions under which Sophie and Gertrud Dann had previously lived, helped somewhat, so that, from then on, they did not have to receive visitors exclusively in the kitchen, for example. The situation was no better with other employers.

When their sister Lotte, who had in the meantime also managed to come from Italy to London, visited them, her sisters had to serve her as a guest:

Lotte never worked practically, only scientifically. She then got permission to do scientific work on healing wounds at Cambridge. She also met her husband there and they were married on 22 July '44 and were able to return to Italy before the war was over. He was a parliamentarian. His father was [a] great enemy of Mussolini, had a duel with him. The father had to flee; it was terrible, they went through a lot. They wrote a book 'What Mussolini Did to Us' [–] and in 1952 after eight years she had her son Paolo.

(G. Dann, interview, 14 July, 1996)

When Sophie Dann learnt in December 1940 that Anna Freud was looking for a nurse for her sick aunt, Minna Bernays, she first had to change her work permit to that of a nurse and her place of residence from Essex to London, which prevented her from starting work with Anna Freud immediately. The need for a nurse, however, came to nothing since Minna Bernays had been hospitalized in the meantime. Sophie and Gertrud had just started a new job with an elderly lady in Peterborough

(Sophie as nurse and companion and Gertrud as cook and housekeeper) when they received a telegram from Anna Freud telling them that they could work at the newly opened war children's home in Essex.

It was with a heavy heart that they had to decline the offer at this point. They felt obliged to find a replacement for their previous employer first. They did not want to leave the impression that Jewish employees were not reliable. They were finally hired in July 1941 when another Hampstead War Nursery Home opened at 5 Netherhall Gardens. Sophie Dann was responsible for the care of 18 babies from birth to about 18 months, for the mothers when they visited their children, the milk kitchen, and later for the sick children. 'It was ideal work: nursing, training young female students, and there was enough time to write reports and make up diagrams' (S. Dann, as cited in Römer, 1998, p. 43). There, Sophie Dann worked together with Anneliese Schnurmann.

For example, Sophie Dann kept an 'Air Raid Chart Hampstead Nursery', detailing when there were bombings and how the children reacted:

After the start of the flying bombs, we also took down the times of the alerts and again I drew a chart. It shows the attacks from 16.6.–15.7.1944. Actually, the first V1 bomb landed on 13.6.1944. As it was impossible to keep toddlers for hours on end in a shelter built as a dormitory, the children were evacuated to the Country House. But the 18 babies were in quarantine for whooping cough or had the illness already and had to stay in London until they were well. The chart shows how often the children had to be carried to the terrace to have the urgently needed fresh air and had to be rushed into the shelter again. [...] The household and the kitchen staff, everybody helped to bring the babies to safety.

(S. Dann, n.d., original English)

It was Anna Freud, who had already conducted direct observations in the Jackson Nursery and continued to do so in the War Nurseries, who instructed that this should be done (Midley, 2013; Pretorius, 2019, 2022). Gertrud Dann remembered that in the beginning she was annoyed, wondering what she was supposed to note, until Anna Freud told her, 'Write down what is getting your attention as being "particular", particular because a child behaves differently than you expect or behaves differently than before' (Dann, interview, 21 November, 1996).

Because of the bombing, the 50 children had to be accommodated in the house's safety bunker, where they slept at night. Three people were responsible for the many children at night. 'During air raids, one of them had to be on the roof with the fire marshal, and one with the night watch in the bunker' (S. Dann, as cited in Römer, 1998, p. 43). When Gertrud Dann showed me the photos of the cots, she explained:

The nets in front of the beds are there to keep the children from falling out of bed during the bombs. Miss Burlingham and Miss Freud knitted them. Made of horrible material, that made their fingers rough. The Hampstead Nurseries were three houses. First in Wedderburn Road where it started and then in Netherhall

Gardens as the number of children increased and the Country House was opened in the summer of 1941. Parents could come and visit their children once a month. The Country House had a sloping floor, and it was hard work. When it got so bad with the bombs, the little ones came out, too. [...] Sophie [Wutsch] was a cook and children's maid for the Misses Herzberg, who were the head of the household at Hampstead Nursery. Also from Vienna. And she emigrated with them. The strangest things come to mind. [...] Anna Freud said to Sophie Wutsch: 'We're going to have two sisters and they're trained infant nurses and you could learn from them.' 'What, two nurses? Well! They are against me then!' She was against us from the start. She could have learnt. 'No! The two sisters are against me, I won't do it.'

(G. Dann, interview, 14 July, 1996)

After the war came to a head in 1944, the children sometimes had to stay in the bunker for 24 hours or more, so they were taken to the countryside in New Barn, Essex (Kennedy, 2009). Sophie Dann stayed in London for the time being with 18 babies who either had whooping cough or had to remain in quarantine until they were also transferred to Essex after they recovered. She additionally cared for Dorothy Burlingham, who was ill with tuberculosis, and remained in London to continue caring for the children after their evacuation. After the end of the war, the Hampstead children's homes were closed and Gertrud's whereabouts were uncertain.

Gertrud proudly told me that she came up with the idea of the foldable bathtub.

I did that so you could see the primitive bathtubs. They were made of rubber. There was a war on, and it was so difficult to get anything. You put it near the washbasin and let it run in. And there was a bucket underneath where you let it run out again. That was a good idea. And when everyone had had a bath, you folded it up and away.

(G. Dann, interview, 14 July, 1996)

It was a pleasant atmosphere. I had two playpens. One with those who bit. Those were the biters. You had to watch out for them, and in the other one was the gentle, loving ones. You didn't have to watch out all the time. [–] Yes, and they pulled each other's hair, and who knows what else. That was the cheekiest one of all [pointing at a picture in her album]. She was on a slippery slope. A miserable rascal. The moment you put her on the potty, she was already up and away again. And once she got stuck, so I said, Loreen should be examined, she's probably going to be ill. She already had a high fever. It was only because she was sitting down that I noticed it. The children were let out into the fresh air as often as possible, even when it was snowing, even the little ones in their cots. Between air raids. [...]

And that's when Sophie had such a wonderful dream. James was a sweet child, always merry, always radiant, never crying or anything, he was always cheerful. And Sophie dreamt that the full moon [–] was crying. She saw the real full moon, but she knew [–] it was James. She thought that if the full moon was

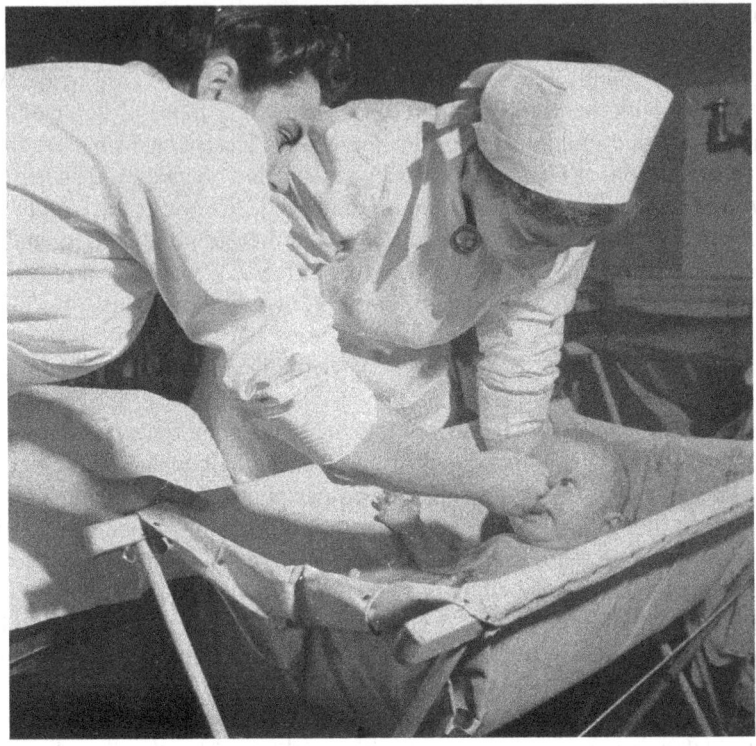

Hansi Kennedy (left) and Sophie Dann with the folding bathtub (credit: Gertrud Dann and the Anna Freud Centre)

crying, then he was hungry, then she would have to warm up the bottle for him. Number eight – that was his number – in her dream. And then she thought, he's still crying, he must be sick. And then she realized those were the sirens for the next air raid. That was the full moon in the sky [–] What a great dream. Sophie often had great dreams. I can't remember what it was, it must have been very beautiful – and she dreamt that the sky was full of violins. And she saw the constellations – she knew the constellations very well – as violins. All the violins were hanging down in the shape of Orion or Cassiopeia or whatever it was. She was quite delighted and said: 'I dreamt such a beautiful thing.'

(G. Dann, interview, 14 July, 1996)

Gertrud Dann, who had previously run her own kindergarten in Augsburg, was irritated by the different way of dealing with the infants and toddlers in Anna Freud's war children's homes. She remembers one of her first working days (Ludwig-Körner, 2012, 2017):

… and I realized that someone was watching me and that this someone did not like what I was doing. I thought that I just cannot do anything different. I fed that baby as any other baby and this someone then came up to me and said: 'I am Anna Freud.' I did not ask 'What actually did I do wrong?', but I was absolutely sure that something was wrong. Much later in a meeting, people talked about children's nutrition, and then it came up. It is totally wrong to hold children in such a way, to educate them, so that they should not touch the food. The children should be allowed to 'smack into' the spinach, into the porridge, that this does not matter, and one should not hold the babies in the way we had learned in baby-care. The baby holds the thumb and then one can [spoon]feed. Sophie said: 'But the spinach and the fresh overalls ...'. Then Anna Freud said: 'Does not matter. The fresh overalls – you can replace and wear another one, but the babies need to know what they eat.' And the 'Junior Toddlers' did eat really terribly. With the hands. [But] it did not take long, and then they learnt quite fast to eat with a spoon. And without drilling them. Then they, the children, learnt voluntarily. And when they wanted, one would help them. Yet very soon they wanted to eat alone. And it was very interesting – that's what Miss Burlingham wanted to try – if a child, about one and a half years old, was able to decide for himself what the right food would be for the child. Thus, there were ten or twelve Junior Toddlers, sitting in a circle, though in a way that each of them faced the back of the next one. Each had a small table, on that table was a board with, I think, about ten small bowls. In each bowl was something different. A piece of meat, a piece of chocolate, a piece of cake, a salad leaf, totally different and in the middle, there was an adult, who each time, when meat had been eaten, could add another piece into the bowl. We did this – don't know – perhaps three weeks. And then it was already absolutely clear that those dumplings had eaten the chocolate, the cake, the cookies, the others the meat, the piece of apple. That was quite interesting, but not yet necessarily proved. And then came the flying bombs, and one had to bring the children down into the cellar in the middle of the meals, and one had so much annoyed the children, and they were so furious that the meal was interrupted. There was no sense in starting this again. And Miss Burlingham sat always apart and was recording which child took meat or cheese. It was a very interesting experiment.

(G. Dann, interview, 14 July, 1996)

Time at Country House, New Barn during the war

Looking at her photo album, Gertrud Dann explained to me that the photo was of New Barn, Country House.

Yes, this is the big house [New Barn, Country House] and how [when] it started with the Flying Bombs, the Junior Toddlers and the babies were also evacuated. And that was terribly primitive, in this golden farmhouse. With a sloping floor. And downstairs in the laundry room a tap for cold water only. Yes, that was difficult. [–] And there were so many children. And when it started with the Flying Bombs and the London children were evacuated, the little ones, they took the farmhouse. It was maybe four minutes away, across the fields.

(G. Dann, interview, 14 July, 1996)

It was very hard. But it was cosy and nice, after all, you got the job done. And there was a fence around, but a lot of slats were gone. And when we arrived with the little Junior Toddlers [–] they immediately wanted to go through the slats, out [laughs] to where the cows and the calves and the pigs and the tractor were. And how are you supposed to get them back in, there must have been 10 or 12 of them. And shouting at them, and 'you're not allowed out' – doesn't help, of course! So, I sat down and made them stand in line, on their backs and somersault over my knees. That was great. That worked wonderfully. There they queued up properly and none of them ran out into the dangerous area. And then the fence was repaired very quickly. [Laughs.] It's funny how you remember stuff like that. Sloping floor, very uneven floor, and Alexandra [Dann's favourite child] had learnt there: 'up the stairs'. That was so wonderfully interesting.

(G. Dann, interview, 20 November, 1996)

Lady Clarke, married to Sir Ralph Stephenson Clarke, a Conservative member of parliament (1936–1955) for East Grinstead, was very committed to the mentally ill.

As Lady Clarke had for many years been involved in caring for the mentally ill in Sussex, Anna Freud invited her to attend the lectures she gave to us every Wednesday. These were excellent lectures, not only for us – many analysts also attended. Lady Clarke was the only outsider, and she was usually alone before the lectures. As an old social worker, I began to talk to her. I had no idea that her husband was one of the biggest landowners in England. Sometimes she invited me to her London home or her Hoathly Hill home in the country. But I never went. It was only when Anna Freud told her about my impending operation and invited me for a follow-up cure, I gratefully accepted.

(S. Dann, as cited in Römer, 1998, p. 45)

The Dann sisters reported on the six small children from Theresienstadt and the misgivings about sending these small three-year-old children with the older 10- to 12-year-olds to Weir Courtney. When Lady Clarke heard this, she suggested that she buy the detached house opposite her country house, Bulldogs Bank, and to offer it rent-free to the Jewish organization on the condition that the Dann sisters take care of the children from Theresienstadt. In addition, there was free support from their staff as well as fruit and vegetables from their garden. The Dann sisters were supported by Maureen Wolfison, who had already worked in Windermere, and Judith Gaulton.

From mid-October 1945 until September 1946, Sophie and Gertrud Dann cared for the Bulldogs Bank children. 'But it was such an important year – for the children and for us too. For me, it was certainly the most important work in my life. I think for Sophie too' (G. Dann, interview, 20 November, 1996).

Maureen Livingstone, a Scotswoman who worked at Windermere, remembers the shock of seeing the six little ones with their shaved heads for the first time in Crosby-on-Eden. Judith Prewitt, an Englishwoman, was another carer.

'All the children were terrified of feathers. When they had a pillow fight and whirled out feathers, they screamed in horror' (Gilbert, 1996, 285 f.; G. Dann, interview, 20 November, 1996). Gertrud Dann reports in Beatrice Schwehm's film (1999) that they could never explain their fear of feathers. 'You can annoy people a lot with feathers, but you can't hurt them'. On the other hand, the children's fear of dogs and black cars were completely understandable.

> These youngest concentration camp children were very, very difficult at first. They were sooo... They didn't know they could trust us. They were used to not being able to trust anyone. And then, as you noticed, they had more confidence in us, then things really started to look up.
>
> (G. Dann, interview, 14 July, 1996)

With regard to food, they worked off of the experiences from the Jackson nursery. 'The children had a buffet so they could choose what they wanted to eat. The interesting thing was that none of the little ones got an eating disorder either' (G. Dann, interview, 14 July, 1996).

Gertrud Dann, who already knew many children as a kindergarten teacher, was – like all those who cared for them – at first very irritated at this method.

From the Dann sisters' notes, Anna Freud (1951) – together with Sophie Dann – wrote 'An experiment in group upbringing', where she pointed out that the group had taken on surrogate parental functions. They had formed a strong bond with each other, caring and protective of the others in the group. They were far too small for their age, showed multiple developmental delays, sucked thumbs, and one little boy masturbated excessively. 'All were noisy, bit, spit, hit, and were easily upset' (Moskovitz, 1983, p. 8).

When they first met a small dog in Windermere (where they stayed for two months), they panicked, threw themselves on top of each other and knocked Alice Goldberger to the ground. They had only known threatening dogs from the concentration camp. The six small children from Theresienstadt are described in many places with changed names. They kept getting new names. Some of them had already been given names before they were admitted to Bulldogs Bank, or they received new names from their adoptive parents. Sarah Moskovitz (1983) interviewed them all as adults in 1979 and 1980. From the interviews one learns how they came to Theresienstadt, how they survived there, about their desperate search for their families and their further – often arduous – paths through life. Regrettably, their fate cannot be further discussed here, but there are several accounts preserved in writing and film.

The time in Weir Courtney – Lingfield

In June 1946, Sophie and Gertrud Dann were granted English citizenship. This ended their stateless period. After the dissolution of Bulldogs Bank in 1947, after just under a year, both worked for a short time in another home for refugee children

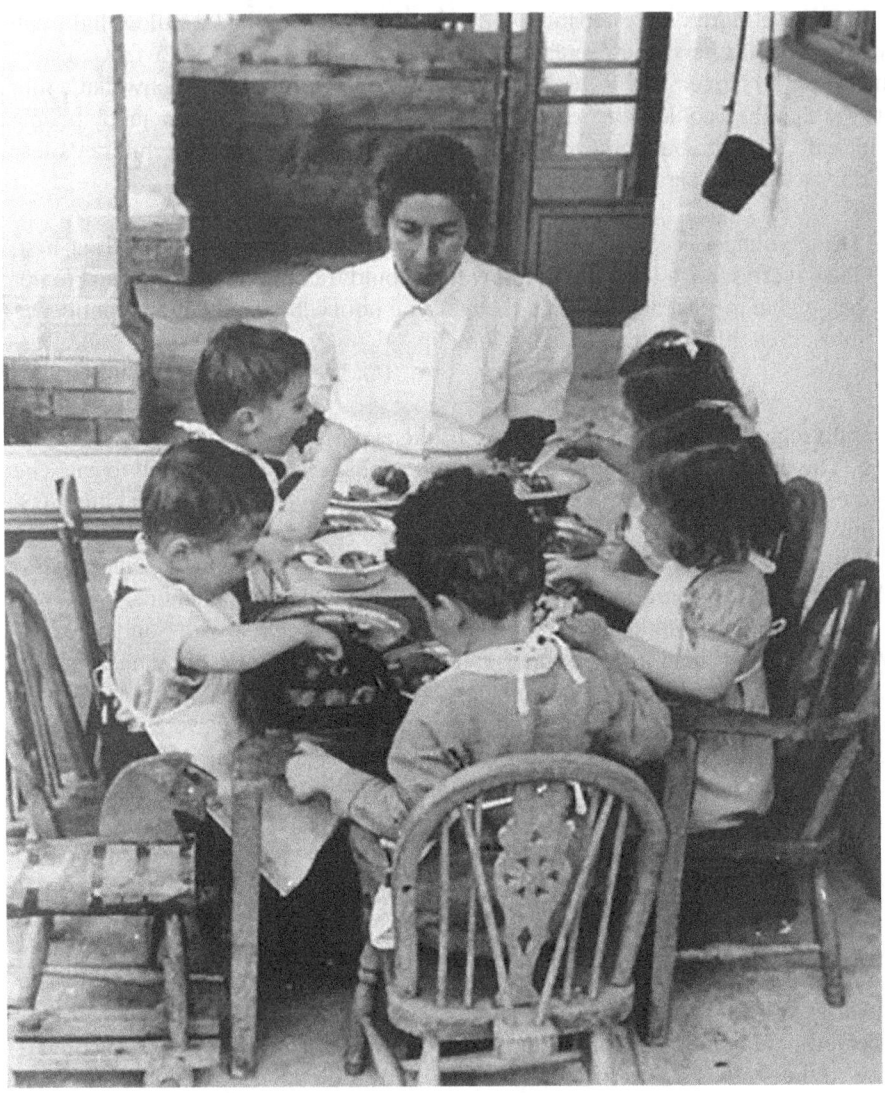

Sophie Dann with the children from Theresienstadt on the terrace in Bulldogs Bank, summer 1946. (Clockwise from lower left: Paul, Peter, Sophie Dann, Ruth, Mirjam, John) (credit: Gertrud Dann and the Anna Freud Centre)

in Pinner, which was run by the same organization. They could hardly stand the conditions there: children were beaten and abused; the staff was untrained. When typhus broke out and the home had to be closed, Gertrud was able to return at the end of 1948 to 'her' concentration camp children (G. Dann, as cited in Römer, 1998, p. 123). Five of the children from Theresienstadt had been adopted in the meantime, but this did not work out for 'Paul', as he kept returning to Lingfield House, where he lived with the older children (G. Dann, as cited in Römer, 1998, p. 125).

Each of the carers had their favourites, including Gertrud Dann. Looking at photos of the children, she exclaimed:

> Oh, that was my favourite. I liked that age terribly. There [in the photo], Alexandra had to sit separately, yes, such a sweet thing, Alexandra. A gentle, clever baby. One time, one of them had a terrible fit of rage, threw himself on the floor and hit his head really hard [...], yes, terrible. And she saw that and lay down next to him and did the same. But very gently and smiled at him sweetly and that's when he stopped. That was really impressive.
>
> (G. Dann, interview, 20 November, 1996)

Alexandra also visited Gertrud Dann later:

> It was so disappointing, very disappointing. Maybe she had become a journalist. I don't know any more. There wasn't anything any more. She was no longer my Alexandra. She was someone else. And she had probably shaved off all her hair, wore a silk scarf, but so tight that no hair could get out from under it.
>
> (G. Dann, interview, 20 November, 1996)

In old age, Gertrud Dann was visited once a month by Zdenka Husserl, 'subservient, overprotective', as Manna Friedmann reported (Friedmann, interview, 26 November, 1996). When Gertrud Dann was asked with whom she most liked to work, she answered:

> I have to think very hard about that. [–] Hmm, I think I liked them all, appreciated them all, but there were no real friendships like that, from within. No, family was much more important to me. I was very lucky to belong to a good family.
>
> (G. Dann, interview, 26 November, 1996)

Asked whether she had ever considered becoming a child therapist herself, Gertrud Dann replied:

> I had no idea about analysis at all, absolutely not. And one day Miss Burlingham was talking around the point. She had a great way of driving you into a corner. I noticed she wanted something from me and – I already suspected what – but didn't want to, and [left] the room. She kept following me, very tactfully. I couldn't escape her. She suggested I go into analysis, and I didn't feel like it. Not at all. I consulted with an acquaintance who was a psychologist and a doctor. And he said: 'Why dig down into the depths because of a bit of shyness? I think you'd better leave it alone.' That was exactly what I wanted. I said to Miss Burlingham, 'I'll think it over.' She knew... that meant no. She left me alone, but

[–] she was very upset. She didn't say so, but you can sense that. [-] I had a) no desire. I knew that a personal analysis would be necessary, which I did not like at all, and b) our financial situation was so miserable that it was out of the question. And Miss Burlingham said. 'We've always got some sources that can help you.' I said, 'No, thank you. Help others, but I don't want to do that.' The financial situation was really such that you had to consider 'If I write in small letters, I can get it all on a postcard.' – because postcards probably cost a penny and letters cost a penny-and-half. It was serious enough. It was a very welcome excuse.

(G. Dann, interview, 14 July, 1996)

She [Dorothy Burlingham] always looked very stern through her thick glasses. She was also strict, but not as strict as people thought. I liked her very much, but 'forbidding', a respectful person. Yes, but once you found you'd got through that strict layer – then she was very personable. I was in Walberswick a couple of times when her children were there from America, and it was extremely un-pleasant. The children and grandchildren were spoiled rotten. And you couldn't shout at them, they were Miss Burlingham's children. It was not pleasant!

(G. Dann, interview, 20 November, 1996)

When Dorothy Burlingham's children came to visit from the USA and the house was full of grandchildren, both sisters were often brought to Walberswick to help, until they withdrew from this unpleasant task for reasons of age.

In January 1948, the Dann sisters were finally able to move into a tiny uncomfort-able cottage, 2 Highcroft Cottage: 'The little white cottage where we lived for 41 years. It was a bit primitive, but we liked it so much. Very steep steps, which were difficult for our parents. They managed it all' (G. Dann, interview, 14 July, 1996).

The cottage was primitive but so cosy, so nice. The parents managed it so well, without any difficulties. There were many, many refugees, who didn't want to come to terms with their fate. Always: 'Now we live in a little flat, and when you think of the big house we had, that we had, etc.' And our parents never had that kind of attitude. They always said how good they had it.

(G. Dann, interview, 20 November, 1996)

In 1947 and 1948, the Dann sisters were visited by their parents, who decided to move permanently from Palestine to join them in Highcroft in September 1950. Manna Friedmann experienced the Dann parents as 'Jewish aristocrats'. They were German citizens of Jewish faith and would have spoken through the third person, as her mother had done.

Cautiously, I tried to find out (G. Dann, interview, 20 November, 1996) whether Sophie and Gertrud had ever thought of starting a family of their own:

No, the two men in my life I would have been interested in were married. So, it wasn't possible. [–] It would have been difficult, if one of us had married,

Sophie or me, it would have been very hard for the other. [–] If it had been an option for me, I would have felt [–] I would have had a terribly guilty conscience towards Sophie. And then there would have been a big conflict. Should I – shouldn't I? But it was out of the question. [–] And it was the same with Sophie. She had never really thought about it. [–] She was too strong a personality. If she had married, it would have been a sissy at best and wouldn't have suited her. She had many friends. Good friends. But I don't think she ever thought about getting married.

When I asked her, she replied: 'We didn't talk about it at all. It was taboo. You could guess what was going on with the other one, but [laughs] it was very funny. We were very close, but such personal things were not discussed'.

Wherever possible, Albert Dann supported his daughters in typing, which was especially difficult for Gertrud Dann in the beginning.

And Sophie was already typing at the time. I had nothing to do with it. I was in the home for the concentration camp children, the big ones. Which I didn't really like – I get along better with younger – much younger children. Working in Bulldogs Bank, that seemed like the right thing to do.

(G. Dann, interview, 20 November, 1996)

On her days off at Lingfield House, Gertrud returned to her parents and Sophie in Highcroft. As connections on public transportation were very poor, Albert Dann

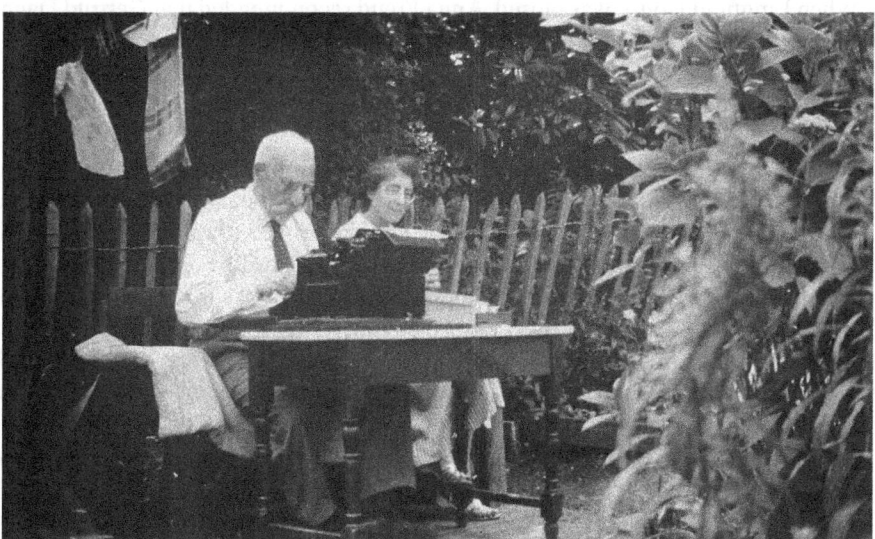

'Father Dann typing.' Albert Dann and Gertrud in Highcroft Cottage (credit: Gertrud Dann)

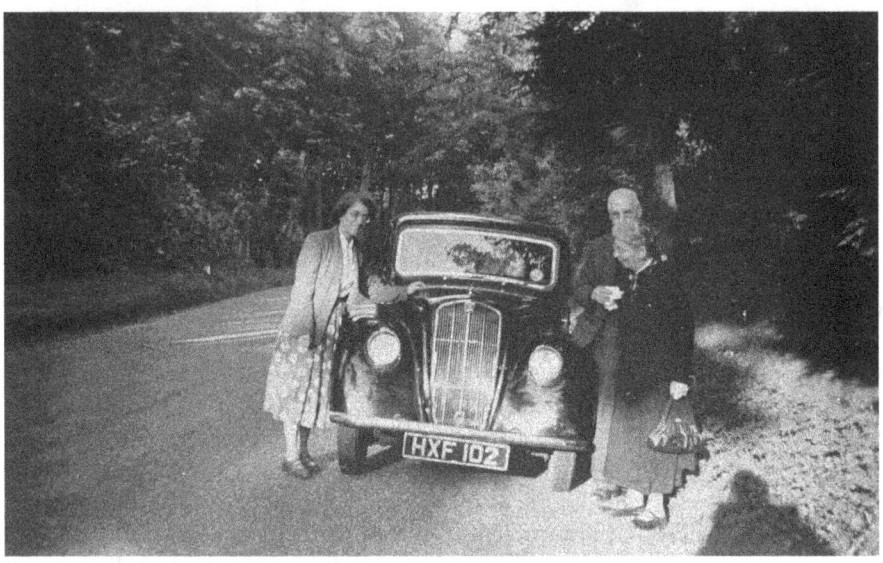

Gertrud Dann with her parents and their Morris, 1957 (credit: Gertrud Dann)

persuaded his daughter Gertrud to get a driving licence in 1955. This was preceded by lengthy and arduous claims for compensation for lost property, so that they could now afford a car.

When Lingfield House was closed, Anna Freud recommended that Gertrud Dann learn to type so that she could take over any library work that arose. She had previously been asked if she wanted to run the kindergarten, which was then being done by Manna Friedmann:

> But I felt that I was too old for children and that their noise made me nervous. In January 1958, I started working for the clinic library. One day Anna Freud asked me if I could do the index for Professor Freud's private library. This work had been started several times by different people, but it had never been finished. I was to start with the 'reference library'. They are the books that Professor Freud wrote. Every time I had time to leave the clinic library, I went across the street to Anna Freud's house and worked there. It was very slow going, and I was glad when Sophie came along after a while, and we could do the index for the books together. It was very interesting to handle all the valuable books, but I didn't like doing it at all. There were also many pieces from Freud's large archaeological collection lying around. One day I was about to get off the ladder when I noticed that one of the Egyptian gods had put his outstretched hand in the pocket of my jumper – one more little moment and all the little statues would have fallen. I was really relieved when this work was finished without anything happening.
>
> (G. Dann, as cited in Römer, 1998, 130 f.)

After working in the library for six months, she learned that she was to be re-lieved by Dorothy Burlingham's daughter-in-law, Mossik:

And I very much had the impression that she would now be trained in the work and then they wouldn't need me any more. [–] And she was very inse-cure; I wasn't so confident either. But she asked me for advice a lot and we got along very well together. No one was the boss of the other, but we went very well together. She then took over what I hated to do: a summary of a book, table of contents. That was a great help. And we created a very nice index by author and a subject index by sleep disorder, eating disorder, etc.... and a lot of times when I didn't know where stuff was supposed to go – on what list, she would look at it and say which list. I don't know how much knowledge she really had. She was treading water; we both were, but it went well. I don't think she had any analytical background but she was the daughter-in-law. [–] We worked together for about a year maybe; and well together, with no prob-lems. I didn't want to go in more than three times a week. And she then did the other days.

(G. Dann, interview, 20 November, 1996)

After the death of her mother, Sophie Dann helped out once a week with the index work in Freud's library, initially assisted by a young psychoanalyst. She stood on the ladder with Sophie to dictate the author, title, etc., until she fell silent because she had once again found an interesting passage in a book and delved into it. When she stopped doing this work, Sophie and Gertrud worked together.

Anna Freud liked to draw on the practical experience of Sophie Dann in par-ticular, which was also used in a series of publications (e.g., Freud & Dann, 1951); however, Sophie also published her experiences independently – for example, on how the children from Theresienstadt, who had grown up with different languages, acquired the English language (S. Dann, 1960).

Sophie Dann was often called upon to act as nurse for Anna Freud or for the grandchildren of Lady Betty Clarke. When Alice Goldberger was to be surprised on her 81st birthday with the presence of all the Lingfield children, Gertrud Dann had been asked to take part, as she had been involved for over nine years. In retro-spect, she was glad to have agreed after some hesitation. Later they found out that several doctors were present, as it was feared that one of the people present might collapse:

When one of the former children, who is now a physiotherapist in Israel, heard this, he said: 'No doctor was needed for Alice. She dealt with us. She can handle anything!' Wherever I went in the next few days, I was stopped because so many people in shops, in the bus, on the train, in a concert, they recognized me.

(G. Dann, as cited in Römer, 1998, p. 130)

I learnt from Hansi Kennedy that the two Dann sisters received little pay for their work and, therefore, only a tiny pension. It is likely that they lived off their parents' money.

Gertrud and Sophie also always wore worn-out clothes; they were insanely thrifty, an exaggerated thriftiness. Gertrud was the ugly duckling. Sophie was also physically larger. Sophie adored Anna Freud, was almost devoted. [...]
     They have a very – she might not tell you this – but they got a very small pension. They were two of the few who get a very small pension. They needed it. And when I went to Anna Freud in later years and said: 'We have to pay the employees more, we pay them far too little.' Then she would say, 'Oh, everything would be much easier without money.' [Laughs.] Because, how can you not ask a patient for money when you have to pay the staff? That's right. [...] Yes, that's what I thought too. It's a pity. [Laughs.] But she never, never, never paid herself. Not in the war, not after the war, not in the War Nursery, never. Nothing. [...] But then of course she expected other people to do that.
                                                                    (Kennedy, interview, 11 July, 1996)

The Dann family had many ties, which helped them to get over difficult strokes of fate. In 1958, the husband of the youngest Dann sister, Lotte, Paolo Treves, died unexpectedly in Italy at the age of 50. Sophie came to help with her six-year-old son. In 1959, the husband of their sister Elisabeth died just as unexpectedly in Israel, and a year later Albert Dann died, in September 1960. Lotte Treves also worked as a translator with Amnesty International. In August 1969, when she visited her mother and sisters in Hoathly with her son Claudio, Elisabeth Stern was also visiting, and Fanny Dann fell ill with pneumonia and died. 'A great consolation for us was that we were all together and the four of us were able to nurse mother' (L. Treves, as cited in Römer, 1998, p. 221).
     In the summer of 1987 Lotte Treves underwent hip replacement in London and then joined her sisters in good health to look after Gertrud Dann, who had had a fall in her home in October 1987 and had to stay in hospital for a long time. It was then Elisabeth who took care of Sophie and Gertrud until the beginning of 1988. Elisabeth and Lotte had just barely arrived in their home countries when Sophie fell seriously ill at the end of January 1988. This was the beginning of the commuting period for Elisabeth from Israel and Lotte from Italy, as Sophie kept falling seriously ill.
     The time had come long before when Gertrud had to realize that she would not be able to resume her interrupted library work in London. 'Although this was a sad idea, I suddenly got quite cheerful at the thought that now, by leaving so abruptly, I had avoided the usual, greatly disliked, farewell party' (Gertrud Dann, memories of life, 1986). She could not escape it after all, and on 26 May, 1988, the two sisters were given a thank you party for their 47 years of work at the Anna Freud Centre.
     When Sophie Dann had a stroke in 1988 and fell down the stairs in her cottage, suffering a hip fracture, Gertrud rushed up worriedly. Sophie answered Gertrud Dann's question: '"Did you hurt yourself?" with "You're not wearing slippers.

Go upstairs at once and put on slippers!" Very, very – cannot say surprising – but very strange after all' (G. Dann, interview, 20 November, 1996).

She has always felt responsible. And very typical of her: how she was in the hospital after the first very difficult [operation], when she was out again and sitting in the chair, she said, 'That's very good. Now I can supervise.' That was so typical of her. [–] She was always responsible. Sophie always felt responsible for others. And sometimes you could decide for yourself. But she didn't like that.

(G. Dann, interview, 20 November, 1996)

As Gertrud Dann pondered how hard it must have been for her sister, now that she had become dependent on others, her sister Lotte reminded her:

'That's true, but you also have to remember that she loved to be served.' That's true, in general, in her whole life; she liked it very much when someone did something for her. It was very pleasant for me to think that she liked it that way. Whenever I walked with her in the wheelchair, I thought it must be terrible for her. But it probably wasn't.

(G. Dann, interview, 20 November, 1996)

The five-week hospital stay had to be followed by a move to the nursing home at Horncastle House, Sharpthorne, Sussex, a mile from her cottage. Gertrud Dann followed her sister there on 2 January, 1989, after the cottage had been sold. The sisters were pleased that much of the furniture and household goods rescued from Augsburg could now be returned to Israel, to Elisabeth's eldest granddaughter who had just married. 'Thus in the end every single item found a useful purpose and a good home' (Gertrud Dann, Addendum Life Memories, p. 4). In the nursing home, Sophie's wish was to live in the great hall with others:

And she was down there in the hall, at the back in the corner; had a cosy corner for herself with furniture that was placed in such a way that she was quite isolated. And I think she felt comfortable as far as possible. And I went down every morning at eight, and in the evening, I said goodnight to her. And when she was ready – in the morning between ten and half past ten – I was with her downstairs in the room where we had lunch. And as soon as the weather was reasonably nice, we went out into the garden. And in the afternoon, again at three o'clock, she was usually finished. And the great thing was that I could hear the lift coming up and I opened the door. Sometimes she would say: 'Gertrud, are you there too?' Quite astonished.

(G. Dann, interview, 20 November, 1996)

Sophie Dann's 90th birthday was celebrated quietly in the nursing home, where she died on 18 December, 1993, at the age of 93. Her death must have been very difficult for Gertrud, who had always lived with her family. In an interview on 14

July, 1996, she said in retrospect: 'I have experienced many things. And it was not always easy. We had a good basis at home. We all had good support.'

At the end of her memoirs, Gertrud Dann writes (1986–1992, p. 5):

> I want to end in a similar way as Elisheva ended her story: To thank our dear parents for their wonderful example, coping with all situations with dignity and courage, for bringing us up with warmth and understanding and for teaching us to be tolerant, considerate and helpful and to appreciate the value of belonging to a good family.

How close not only the familial bond in the Dann family remained, but also that the work of Sophie and Gertrud Dann with the children they cared for, was posthumously evident when their niece, Shula Levital, met with Jackie Young and Joanna Millan – two of the former Theresienstadt children – in June 2017 and this event was published in the Anna Freud Centre (AFNCCF) *General News* (McGourty, 2017).

Sources

Interviews with Gertrud Dann: 14 July, 1996; 15 July, 1996; 20 November, 1996; 21 November, 1996; 18 September, 1997.
Interviews with Manna Friedmann: 12 July, 1996; 21 November, 1996; 26 November, 1996; 23 April, 1997; 5 June, 1997; 19 September, 1997; 28 June, 1998; 19 March, 2000.
Interviews with Hansi Kennedy: 11 July, 1996; 23 April, 1997; 5 June, 1997.
Gertrud Dann: 1986–1992 (supplement to her memoirs from 1986).
Memoirs of Gertrud Dann (October 1986).
Memoirs of Sophie Dann (October 1986).

Publications by Sophie Dann

Dann, S. (n.d.), Air raid Chart Hampstead Nurseries and Sleeping Chart.
Dann, S. (1960). Beobachtungen an Kleinkindern bei der Anpassung an eine neue Sprache [Observations on young children adapting to a new language]. *Schule und Psychologie*, 375–381.
Dann, S. (1978). Zum 3. Reich in Augsburg [On the 3rd Reich in Augsburg]. *Augsburger Blätter*, Heft I, 26.
Dann, S. (1979). Juden in Augsburg [Jews in Augsburg]. *Augsburger Blätter*, Heft 1, 11–18.
Dann, S. (1981). Tagebuchnotizen der Fürsorgeschwester der Jüdischen Gemeinde [Diary notes of the welfare nurse of the Jewish community]. *Augsburger Blätter*, Heft 3, 14–18; 81–85.
Freud, A. & Dann, S. (1951). An Experiment in Group Upbringing. *Psychoanalytic Study of the Child*, 6, 127–168.
Freud, A., Burlingham, D., Dann S. (1971). *Heimatlose Kinder. Zur Anwendung psychoanalytischen Wissens auf die Kindererziehung* [Homeless children. On the application of psychoanalytic knowledge to child rearing]. Frankfurt a.M., Fischer, pp. 165–217.
Hellman, I., Dann, S., Dann, G. (1942). Annual Report of a Residential War Nursery: a thank-you letter. Anna Freud Centre Archives, London (unpublished).

3

Manna (Marta) Friedmann (8.1.1915–16.11.2013) – Surviving to Ensuring the Survival of Others

Both parents of Marta Friedmann (later nicknamed Manna) came from Polish rab-binical families and retained their Polish citizenship after emigrating from Galicia to Cologne in 1908. Her mother, Auguste (Gusta) Weindling, née Horowitz (born in 1886, presumably perished in a concentration camp in 1941 or 1942 – the date is not certain) was from Biala (Bielitz), a place that was sometimes Polish, then Austrian again, and, as such, she spoke excellent German. She was one of the few girls in her area who was sent to school:

> In her day, girls in Poland were not sent to school, only the boys. The girls had to help at home. But her mother still thought it was important and sent her to a convent school. That was something quite extraordinary in those days. And I remember my mother telling me what a wonderful school it was, this convent and how happy the children were there, how they could attend school. All the Christian children said, 'Praised be Jesus Christ' and the sisters answered, 'Forever and ever, Amen.' But the Jewish children said, 'Good morning' and the sisters said, 'Greetings to God my child!' They were so close together and there was no hatred at all.
>
> (Friedmann, interview, 5 June, 1997)

Nathan Weindling (1882–1940), Manna Friedmann's father, came from Krakow. Both his parents were devout Jews, and his father was a prayer leader in the Jewish community in Cologne. His brothers had a small clothing shop and Nathan Wein-dling travelled the country as a salesman for this textile company trying to gain cus-tomers, an often laborious and not always successful job. But he managed to feed his ever-growing family. 'We were never hungry' (Friedmann, interview, 12 July, 1996).

Manna Friedmann, the second oldest of seven children, was born in Cologne on 8 January, 1915. Her brother Salo, who was more than four years older, had the same birthday as his grandfather (7 November, 1910), who died six months before his birth. One of Manna Friedmann's first memories concerns the First World War.

> I remember the First World War and I remember the end of the First World War in 1918, when I was three years old. [–] I have a very clear memory of how air

DOI: 10.4324/9781003403906-4

raids were carried out at night and how my father wrapped me in a blanket and took me into the cellar. That is what I remember. And that there was a woman who had a dog and she said, 'As long as we're all right'. Mrs Holland was her name; but I don't know if that was the story that was told – there was so much talk about it afterwards. She used to say: 'Wenn et uns nur jut jeht' [transl.: If

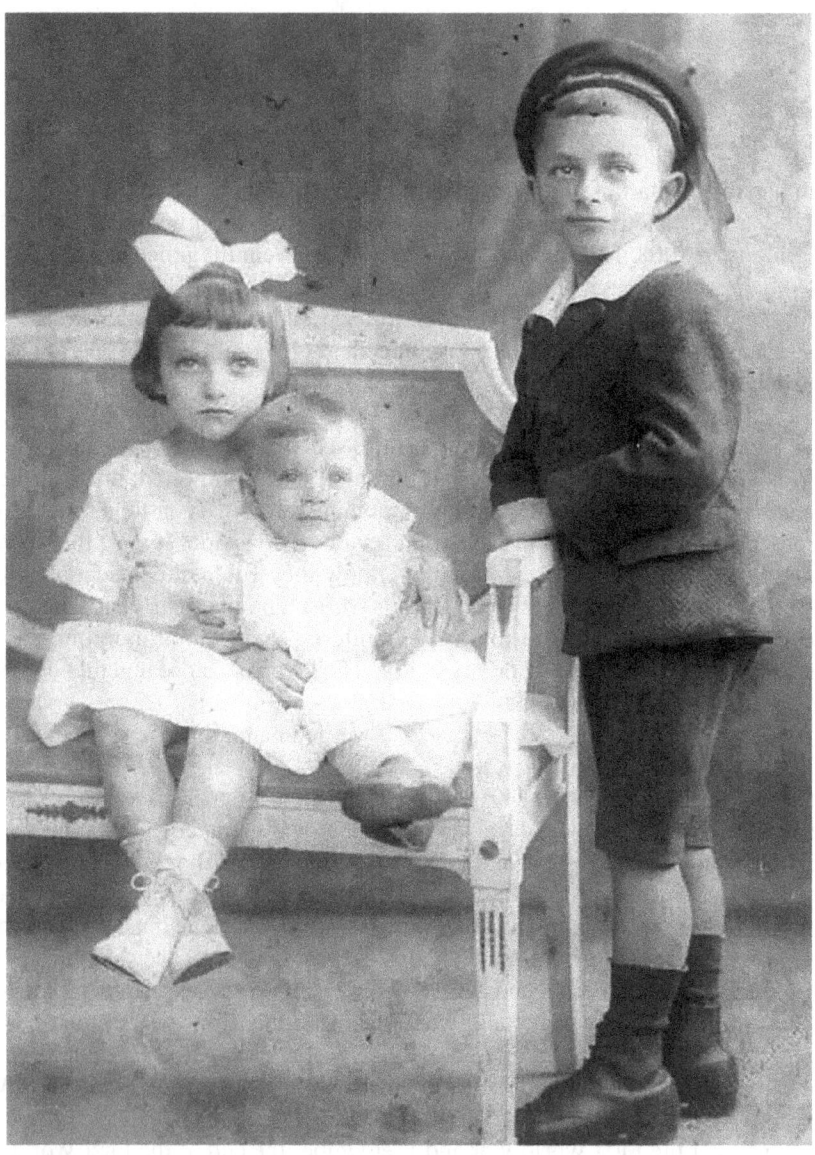

Manna Friedmann, aged six years, Albert, aged two years, Salo, aged ten years. (Credit: Manna Friedmann)

only we are well], yes, the dog and her, that's the main thing, isn't it. [–] And I remember another incident. There were still air raids, and it was on a Saturday afternoon. My brother was bored, and our mother said: 'Go to the synagogue, daddy is there too'. And then he left, and very shortly afterwards there was an air raid. And mother was of course beside herself. I remember that, but shortly after that he came home. And of course, she was happy to see him. 'How, how did you get here?' 'Yes', he said, 'when the air raid came, I thought you were going to worry. I went from one house to another until I came back home here'. But it says something about the community, about our family.

(Friedmann, interview, 23 April, 1997)

Four years later her brother Albert was born, and two years later (21 June, 1921) her only sister Dora, who was followed by Paul, called Poldi, in 1923. When the fraternal twins David and Julius (Jodi) were born in 1925, ten-year-old Manna, who had just been enrolled in the fifth grade at the Jewish grammar school 'Jawne' in Cologne, walked around the old town of Cologne and joyfully announced to everyone:[1]

'We have twins, we have twins.' My mother was not very happy. But [...] I thought that was something wonderful. Julius weighed three and a half and David, the second born, only two and a half pounds. But he developed wonderfully. It was a miracle in those days! My mother was a fantastic woman.

(Friedmann, interview, 23 April, 1997)

As a matter of course, Manna Friedmann took over the mothering duties for one of the twins. When she went to school in the morning she said – in role reversal – to her mother: 'Mother, watch out for David.' As she was already very good at needlework at the time, she did not have to do the usual

silly things that school children learn at school. My teacher, Miss Dahl, always said: 'You can do whatever you want'. What did I do in my needlework class? I knitted and crocheted for the twins. That means my mother knitted for the bigger one (twin) and I knitted for the smaller one.

(Friedmann, interview, 12 July, 1996)

David became like her own child. Through him she learned at an early age what it means to be a mother.

I have always planned not to have children because I saw how hard it was. We were a wonderful family, but I saw how hard it was to raise seven children in Germany on a small income. My mother, of course, couldn't work in town; she was fully occupied with work at home. So, I thought, well, when I grow up, I'll have an orphanage. When I was a child, I always wanted to do that. I will have a children's home, I don't want to have children myself, and then I can do everything that children should have. Because there was a lot I didn't have as a child.

(Friedmann, interview, 12 July, 1996)

At that time, the family lived in a small flat at Dasselstrasse 8 in Cologne.

And I was a very lively child. Seven children in a small flat, when could I write my school assignments? I had to wait until all the children were in bed, in the kitchen. There was no luxury and yet, strangely enough, I have only good memories from home. There was a lot of singing and laughing. My mother loved to sing, and we all loved to tell jokes.

(Friedmann, interview, 12 July, 1996)

Manna Friedmann remembers how she, a very studious child, refused to go to the school retreat in the countryside, because she knew that her father could not afford the expenses. Her position at school was financed by donations from the Jewish community. When she once again decided not to go on such an excursion, the teacher interpreted her refusal correctly and convinced her that there were other children who were also poor and who were financed by a fund. This empathetic manner of the teacher was in stark contrast to the Jewish welfare officer, from whom Manna had to get additional support. The condescending way this welfare worker treated her was one of the reasons why she later became a social worker herself. She wanted to have an impact such that people were not humiliated when in need.

At the age of 16, after the tenth grade, she left school. 'I was not as eager to continue my academic work as my brother' (Friedmann, interview, 12 July, 1996). She wanted to become a kindergarten teacher, but her mother refused. 'My mother had the final say on this; my father did not interfere' (Friedmann, interview, 19 March, 2000). Manna's parents would have preferred for her to learn a commercial profession. 'Then you're just a maid; that's a nanny after all' (Friedmann, interview, 12 July, 1996). But she insisted on at least being around children, so she applied to a large Jewish children's home in Cologne for an office job that bored her terribly. This administrative work did not suit her. Without telling her parents, she went to the director of the children's home and asked him to be assigned to the baby department. She loved the work, for which there was almost no payment, as it was a so-called 'internship'. It didn't bother her either that she had to start work at seven in the morning, especially as she lived nearby with her parents.

One day I was called by the director of the children's home, thinking, 'what I have done'. 'Yes,' he says, 'your brother just called and asked me: How come my sister has to start at seven o'clock in an office? Or is this the instruction of one of your subordinates?' That's how he put it. 'But your sister works in the baby ward, and now she's going into the larger ward,' and so on and so forth. And so, I got scolded at home at first, but I stayed there for the time being. [–] I went through all the wards there. Baby ward, schoolchildren's ward and larger children's ward.

(Friedmann, interview, 12 July, 1996)

Although Manna Friedmann did not receive a degree for this work (from 1931–1933), she did receive professional training to look after children. On the recommendation of her headmaster, Dr Klibansky, she met a Cologne family whose children she looked after, starting on 27 March, 1931.

This was a very well-known and famous family in Cologne, the family of Professor Kisch.[2] He was a heart specialist who worked in the Cologne Lindenburg [University Hospital]. And his wife was an oratorio singer. And they had two small children – Charlotte was four and Rifka two years old. And they turned to Dr Klibansky and said: 'Why don't you recommend a student who has finished school, someone you know, who will visit our children only in the afternoon and look after them? Well, it's not a big job, because the woman is sometimes travelling and has her studies.' And he recommended me there.

When the third child, son Arnold, was born in 1933, Manna Friedmann moved entirely into the Kisch family home.

And then I was sooo in love with this family, really devoted. Through this family I entered a completely different world. I like being the second in command, just like Alice Goldberger, i.e. I like being in the second row. This has always been my position – even when I was raising my younger brothers as a surrogate mother. And there I was with them until 1938; until they emigrated to America. It was a big house on Käsenstrasse, which I visited recently. It still exists. And this family also wanted to take me to America, because of course I was very important for the children. They could hardly function without me. After 1933, the permission for non-Jewish domestic workers to work in a Jewish household was revoked. Thus, suddenly Maria, the maid, and the cook, all had to leave. There was still a young couple who were responsible for the house and the garden, and suddenly everyone was gone. And I would sometimes get up at three o'clock in the morning – nobody asked me to – to scrub the porch, which was white marble, because the professor, who was then also no longer allowed to work in Lindenburg, started seeing his private patients in the house. And everything had to be in order. So, I was really a housekeeper for everything in the fullest sense of the word and enjoyed every minute there. I loved the family so much. [...] But when the family emigrated – he got his immigration permit to America [1938] as an exception because he had his job at the university, and he could only take his closest family with him. [Mrs Kisch lovingly introduced her to the guests as 'house daughter' or 'this is my eldest'.]

(Friedmann, interview, 19 March, 2000)

In the journal *'45 Aid Society* (2007) Manna Friedmann wrote about her time in Cologne:

In the evening of November 9th, 1938, 'Kristallnacht,' while the synagogue in the Roonstrasse was on fire and the books from the Jewish Library were burning in front of it, I took the three children in a taxi to a friend of Professor

K, and Ruth K.A. in the suburb of Köln. We arrived at the house of Professor Statts. Our host opened the door and led us into his study. From above his
writing-desk a large picture of Hitler in uniform and swastika looked down on
us. The professor turned the picture round and on its back was the picture of
a friend, Professor K., the children's father. 'Don't worry' our host whispered,
'all this nonsense will soon be over. We are keeping our daughter Elisabeth
out of the Hitler Youth as long as possible.' (All schoolchildren had to be in
uniform with swastika.)

The following morning, I took the children home. When we arrived, a
Gestapo official was there questioning the mother about the coin collection, the
family's hobby, but he soon left. At last, while hiding with a Christian friend,
Professor K., received his papers for the family's emigration to the USA and, in
December 1938 they left for America. The 'Lift' with their belongings was still
in the house guarded by a friend, Dora Loeb,[3] and myself.

(Friedmann, 2007, p. 36)

The family then tried to get a travel permit for Manna Friedmann from America.
She was eventually given an affidavit (it had been stated that she had a teacher's
certification). When she went to the American embassy in Karlsruhe at the beginning of 1939, she was ambivalent about whether she should leave the country.
Although the years with this family were highly important for Manna Friedmann,
she also had an internal conflict, because she knew that her parents would have
preferred her to at least finish her training as a kindergarten teacher and work in
this profession instead. She suddenly understood that she was about to become the
house-daughter of this family for life. When the man at the agency asked whether
she was a teacher, as she had no papers with her, she answered truthfully. She was
so relieved that she did not have to leave for America and was able to express her
regrets in letters to the Kisch family.

Well, I kind of slipped into it. It was good for a while, and I was captivated by
this family. It was a fantastic family. I am still in touch with the children today,
they are in Israel now. Little Arnold, who was very attached to me, called me
'Mumo'. He longed for me especially. It had been very difficult for the children
and for the mother at the beginning. Now she had to do everything, the household, cook.

(Friedmann, interview, 19 March, 2000)

Throughout her life she was reminded of this family also by her name, Manna,
which was given to her by the children. She later kept it in England, partly because
the English pronunciation of Marta sounded terrible to her ears. 'And when I came
to Israel, there I am back to my name Marta. But at the [Hampstead] clinic I am
known only as Manna Friedmann. In the whole clinic, my husband also called me
Manna' (Friedmann, interview 12 July, 1996).

Deportation and emigration

Despite many warning signs, Manna Friedmann, and her family – like so many – did not recognize the growing danger of National Socialism. She remembers when she was in a sanatorium:

> And it was around autumn. It was a wonderful children's home in Kreuznach on the Nahe River, near Bingen. And there we went for a walk through the forest, and I remembered how the leaves fell here. I walked through these falling leaves as often happens now. Suddenly I saw myself walking there in those autumn leaves, and then I remembered the song we were singing then, and that we didn't even know what we were singing. It was the song, 'When we walk side by side and sing the old songs and the woods sound again, we feel it must succeed. The new time is moving with us, the new time is moving with us.' That was the new time of which we sang enthusiastically, that it was coming. We did not know what we were singing. Yes, that was the Horst Wessel song.[4] Yes, he was such a handsome, likeable young man, wasn't he? Who all, all the children were looking at, God, this is a fabulous human being. How was that possible?
>
> (Friedmann, interview, 19 March, 2000)

On 28 and 29 October, 1938, in the so-called 'Polish Action', over 17,000 Polish Jews were expelled from the German Reich to Poland in barely two days. Deported overnight, they had to vacate their homes and lost all their belongings. At least 600 Jewish citizens were deported from Dortmund and Cologne to Sbondschin in Poland. These were people with a Polish passport, but who had been living in Germany for many years. Since the Polish government wanted to declare these passports expired, the Nazi German government took advantage of this to inhumanely send these people to Poland. Within a few hours, all affected people were to gather at certain assembly points and were then deported from Cologne-Deutz. Manna Friedmann's parents and brothers Albert, Paul, Julius and David were part of this first group of Polish Jews. Salo Weindling, the eldest, hid in time, as he did not want to separate from his fiancée. Together with her, he managed to escape to England.

This 'Polish Action' was the reason for the assassination of the Delegation Counsellor of the German Embassy in Paris, Ernst vom Rath, by a 17-year-old Polish Jew, Herschel Grynszpan (pronounced 'Grünspan'), on 9 November, 1938. This in turn was exploited by the National Socialists to create the horrible pogrom which claimed the lives of many Jewish people on 10 November, 1938, and destroyed almost all synagogues and a large proportion of Jewish shops and private homes. 'Immediately after this action, Klibansky made every effort to move his entire school to England if possible' (Corbach, 1990, p. 150). Further deportations of thousands of Jews followed in the coming years.

> And since we were not German citizens, rather, foreigners with Polish relatives, all Poles were collected and sent to Poland on 28 October, 1938, without

warning [–] In general, a terrible, sad memory of the separation, because I stayed behind to dissolve the orphanage, and it was my intention to follow later. Why, why did I not go? Why wasn't I picked up?

(Friedmann, interview, 12 July, 1996)

Manna Friedmann was with the Kisch family when she heard about the deportation. Her own family lived at Fleischmengergasse 41 in 1938.

It was on 28 October, that was a Friday evening, they were gathered at Cologne Central Station. I cannot erase the date. They were not particularly frightened. You didn't know. [-] They didn't have to go to a camp. They thought they were Poles. We had people in Poland, they were doing quite well, so we're going to Poland. We don't have to stay in Germany. It was on a Friday evening that they were picked up. The Orthodox Jews, my family was one of them, didn't go on the Sabbath, and that was the start of the Sabbath. And there I was in a dilemma. If I walk to the main station now, I might not find them. Then I sinned and took a taxi and went there and saw them. I went there with a bottle of wine and the one hundred marks I had. And I gave it to them, and the youngest said: 'Marta, come with us.' And I said: 'I'll sort out the flat and then I'll come along.' I had every intention of coming. That's why I didn't feel guilty about staying behind or not going, didn't I? Later I thought that my mother didn't have to go either, because in Cologne it was like that, in Cologne the police were very good, actually, friendly towards the Jews. [...] But my mother wouldn't have let her husband and the four boys go alone, because she didn't know where to go. We saw Hitler come in '33; we didn't want to believe that it was possible. Otherwise, we could have got out earlier. People ask: Why did you sit there for so long? Yes, well, you know that; everything is always easier in hindsight. And then they reached the border, and then they wouldn't let the Poles in. And the Germans didn't let them back in. So, they settled in Bentschen – a no man's land with a large no man's camp. And they were housed there; they didn't have enough food. Thousands of people in a small camp who couldn't get in and couldn't get out. (Friedmann, interview 23 April, 1997)

Until 1942 they still received letters from time to time. The last one was written by her 19-year-old brother Albert, who was already a teacher and prayer leader at that time:

'Great luck! I got a job in a Jewish children's recreation home outside Warsaw. And not only me, but my mother can go with me and the three younger brothers.' And we were happy! He had sent a picture, a photograph, with the children still in it and my mother. In the meantime (1940) my father had died of an illness in this camp; I think it was cancer. And, of course, it was a very sad story with these children. We heard that they were no longer alive, we don't even know where they died – I think in Warsaw. They were sent to Warsaw afterwards. So, I tore up the picture. I thought, if they're no longer alive, I can't look at the picture any more. So, I said, then I don't need a picture any more either. The picture is in here [points to her heart], anyway. But today I'm sorry, because in all museums and so on you're always searching. And that was a picture of these four brothers with their mother. Fabulous people. The youngest were 15, 17 and 19 at the time, and that was a wonderful letter. And that was the last letter. So, we think that they probably died there in Otwock or Warsaw, or somewhere. We don't know where or what. And then I couldn't have this picture any more. Although I still have the other family pictures of these children, when they were little. I couldn't and didn't want to give them away. But I couldn't look at them. No, I thought: 'If they're not alive, I don't need another picture. I have no idea where they even died. But we know that they didn't get out. They were not among the survivors.

(Friedmann, interview, 12 July, 1996)

Manna reported that, unlike the girl she mentored at Weir Courtney, Judith Sherman, she had never felt guilty about having survived.

I never had that. Because I had no intention of saving myself, I would have gone with them. It was by chance that I thought: Well, let me clean up first and then I'll join you. [–] So, when these surviving children came, it was like a resurrection, so to speak, these children who had lost their lives, I threw myself into this work and the children threw themselves at me! And it was all gone! That is, it wasn't gone, of course. But it was like a buried layer.

(Friedmann, interview, 12 July, 1996)

It was impossible for her to talk about it with her older brother. Manna Friedmann had never made any enquiries about the whereabouts of her family, nor did she know whether her brother Salo had.

I know it's so painful for him, and that's why I don't ask him. No, I was recently in America again and I didn't ask him. I asked my sister-in-law if he had ever spoken to her about it. They've been married for sixty years now, so it's an old relationship. And she said: 'No'. And she doesn't know what happened to her parents either, and she asked me, 'Do you want to know?' 'Yes, I actually want to know, at least, where [–] they are buried! So many people know that.' And that's when she said, 'No, I don't even want to know that. It's, it's nothing to do with knowing – that's just worse!' So, I didn't ask him. The only thing I did [–] I was in Israel, and I didn't even tell him, and I gave all the names in the Holocaust Museum Yad Vashem. I went there because I have the feeling that somehow the names must at least be immortalized. There is no gravestone, you wouldn't know where. I wrote down all the names of my siblings and my parents there. And that is recorded in the computer, so that somewhere, at least their existence is known [–] that they were once there. But I haven't even told my brother yet, because he'll probably say, 'What did you do that for?' [Laughing.] He's quite autocratic. [Quietly.] But I wanted to do that. Yes. I can't even [–] I can't even talk about it with my brother. He can't talk about it. I can much easier [–], I don't find it so difficult to talk about it. He can't talk about it.

(Friedmann, interview, 23 April, 1997)

After Dr Salo Weindling died in the USA in September 1999 – Manna Friedmann was just visiting – and then, in December 1999, also his wife, who had already been living in a nursing home for a long time, their daughter Helen Cohen found a stack of correspondence from his family after their deportation. In this way, Manna received letters from her mother and brothers from the concentration camp. Her nephew Eran Wolkowski still managed to talk to his Uncle Salo about this time. On this occasion, Manna Friedmann learned for the first time that her brother Paul had written to his eldest brother in London from the Bentschen camp, asking him to get him out of there. However, this was probably not feasible for Salo Weindling, especially as the World War broke out shortly afterwards. He also feared difficulties because, as a Polish citizen, he had taken advantage of German scholarships (for school and university). Now Manna Friedmann could see more clearly that it was his guilt that made her unable to talk to him about the past. She now also felt guilt, because she had lived with the Kisch family and had only gone to the collection centre to see her family. She had not known about the danger of what was happening (Friedmann, interview, 19 March, 2000).

Manna describes how they, in Cologne, had felt like German Jews, but nevertheless, to a certain extent, also like outsiders and felt the effects of anti-Semitism at an early stage from other children.

We lived in an area where there were many working-class families, and you walked past and the children would call out: [she sings]: 'Jüd, jüd, jüd – schepp, schepp, schepp – steck die Nas' in den Wasserschepp. Wenn der Jüd gestorben ist, kommt er in die Eierkist.' [Jew, Jew, Jew – skewed, skewed, skewed – stick your nose in the water shed. When the Jew dies, he'll go into the egg crate]. That was sung to us, and we played together with these children in the afternoon. They didn't really understand it, did they? Well, for us the whole misery was not as traumatic as for these Germans, who suddenly [–] suddenly they did not belong. We always felt more like guests here. We liked it very much, and we felt good, in and of itself. But there was a difference. So that this youth, in which I grew up, was also somehow inspired by learning the Jewish scriptures [–] and the longing for Palestine or for the Jewish state. Yes, so we all belonged to the Zionist movement. Of course, that was very good, because there we felt we had a goal. We will achieve that one day. And if you have such an ideal, that is very, very good, growing up. So, it was always our intention that if we could immigrate to Palestine, then we would go there. We would be welcome there. [...] That made it easier; but we didn't know that there would be a border there. That they would not let us in. After all, this was a British mandate, which had to take care of the Arabs, the Palestinians who lived there, and be on good terms with them, so that it was all a difficult, very ambivalent story. And apart from one other young person, our parents were so against it. They were not Zionists; we children were Zionists. And when we talked about wanting to go to Israel back then it was Palestine, well, there was crying and moaning, so we didn't do it.

(Friedmann, interview, 23 April, 1997)

Manna, like her younger sister Dora, was eager to emigrate to Palestine.

Her father then turned to Professor Kisch and asked him to influence her, as she now listened to him more than to her father. It was Manna Friedmann who brought Jewish thinking into this family, including ideas about the state of Israel (Friedmann, interview 9 March, 2000). Her sister Dora took part in preparations in Germany for kibbutz life in Israel. Since their parents had been deported in the meantime, the eldest brother Salo, as guardian of the 17-/18-year-old sister, received a letter from Dora saying that she wanted to leave for Palestine illegally and that he should give his consent: 'And my brother refused to give it to her because he knew that the ships were not seaworthy. She then did it anyway' (Friedmann, interview, 23 April, 1997).

Eran Wolkowski, Dora's son, reports that his mother sailed with her youth group across the Danube to the Black Sea and made it to the port of Haifa in Palestine on another ship. They were arrested by the British police and taken, together with many other illegal immigrants (2,000 men and women), to a special large ship, SS *Patria*, for deportation. The local Jewish underground military organization (*Hagana*) attempted to stop the deportation to a camp in Cyprus and attached a bomb to the bottom of the ship. Dora Weindling, who was unable to swim, was rescued by a Chinese member of the ship's crew (Wolkowski, email 8 November, 2020).

Manna's eldest brother, Salo Weindling, had studied philology at the University of Cologne and was about to submit his dissertation in Bonn when he was told by his supervisor that this was no longer possible. Like his fiancée, he taught elementary school German and history in Essen, for which both had won prizes. Salo Weindling was offered a position in England by the Refugee Committee; he would have preferred to stay in Germany but managed to escape in July 1939. In August 1939, Salo Weindling married his fiancée Karola (Carol) Heumann. Initially, Weindling was in the military in England, where the couple lived for ten years, but there they earned too little and, finally, they emigrated to the USA. Although they had to sit all their exams again, this was not difficult for Salo Weindling in particular. 'He was always brilliant' (Friedmann, interview, 19 March, 2000). He was given a professorship in German, history, and philology at a college where he was able to set up the German department and produce all the materials himself – a job he valued highly. He was fluent in six languages; his fine feeling for language also enabled him to translate works by Dante, Shakespeare, Petrarch, and Omar Khayyam into German. Active until the end of his life, he taught non-Jewish Americans (Jehovah's Witnesses) who wanted to read the Psalms in the original Hebrew.

Manna Friedmann regularly visited her brother and his wife in the United States. After sustaining a broken pelvis due to a fall, her sister-in-law had to move into a nursing home where her husband visited her every day. When Manna Friedmann was visiting them, her sister-in-law – with the support of a nurse – lived at home again for a few weeks. On the one hand, Manna enjoyed these last family ties; on the other hand, used to taking care of others, she had to be very careful to continue her own life, neither brother nor sister-in-law having future expectations to fulfil. After her brother died in October 1999, Manna Friedmann flew even more frequently to the United States to care for her sister-in-law.

> I'm always afraid I won't get away again. Because I am so much [laughs] here. [–] And now I am alone and have time. And [laughing] my health is good. So, so to speak, I am available, right? [–] But my brother is not someone who has expectations and who would somehow make me feel [–] you must do that, and you don't do that. On the contrary! It is my own feeling. They are the only ones left of the family now.
>
> (Friedmann, interview, 5 June, 1997)

Her first period in England

While her brother was already in London, Manna Friedmann, still rather unconcerned, was waiting for a 'domestic permit' in England to be able to work with a family.

> In and of itself, Cologne, where I grew up, was a friendly environment, so it was hardly possible to believe that they would do that. I received a letter from some authority. If you have not left the country by [–] I think [–] 31 July, we will deport you. And I didn't take that seriously either [...] And then I thought, this can't be true! My parents were originally from Poland, and we had never taken German citizenship. So somehow we were foreigners in their eyes, although we were all born in Germany. [–] Maybe that was it? But at the same time that it was happening, a policeman saw me coming back to the Kisch house late at night in Käsenstrasse [–] one wasn't concerned – that was 1939! Then he said to me: 'What are you still doing here!' And I said: 'I live here!' He said: 'Get out of here!' But in a friendly way. Well, it was so different in Germany. My brother had already received a summons. We knew that those who were not German citizens would be deported. It was called deportation. [...] I had to wait for a domestic permit. Families had to offer a job, so that the state would not be burdened with this. And I did not have such a permit. And my brother called every evening. 'Have you got that permit yet?' 'No, not yet!' So, I finally got it. Not from a family, but from the Jewish committee at the Bloomsbury house. They had some permits without [needing] families, so to speak.
>
> (Friedmann, interview, 23 April, 1997)

When she left Germany in July 1939, her path led her via Antwerp, where her mother's relatives lived. She would have preferred to stay there, especially as her relatives urged her to stay with them. She was not at all aware of the seriousness of the situation. She was not interested in politics at the time, and it was inconceivable to her that people are willing to do terrible things to other people.

> Hatred was foreign to me. People had already heard and were spreading rumours, but one did not know what was coming. Antwerp was not yet under German occupation. And (her relatives in Antwerp) who said: 'You're not normal! A domestic worker in England? You stay here, we will find you a good groom,' as was the custom with Jews, 'maybe a diamond dealer.' And then I got a telegram from my brother, who was already here in London: 'Come at once!' So, I thought, there must be a reason for that. So, I came straight here to London – they were beside themselves. Because he saw what was coming. And I arrived around July 1939 before the war broke out. They didn't believe it here at all. They knew, through America, that a lot of things were going to happen there.
>
> (Friedmann, interview, 23 April, 1997)

According to her niece, Hannah Helen Cohen (personal communication, 2 April, 2023):

> When she dallied in Antwerp, my father frantically sent her a telegram telling her to get out NOW. He told her that if the border control asked why she spent the time she did in Antwerp she was to tell them that she had been ill. When she did use that excuse the police slyly noted: so, another sick one. It worked though, and she sailed for the UK.

Her Polish citizenship proved to be an advantage in England.

> We were 'friendly aliens', not 'enemy aliens' and so we had no difficulties here at all. I remember coming to the police with my Polish passport and he said: 'Where were you born?' I said in Cologne. He said: 'Why do you have a Polish passport?' It was hard to explain. And he said to me: 'But you look as if you have the world's worry on your shoulders, don't worry! Nothing is going to happen to you here.' He was so nice. This was my first experience here with the British police.
>
> (Friedmann, interview, 23 April, 1997)

In 1939, with a domestic permit from the Home Office, she went to Golders Green:

> To a very nice Jewish family who had been here in England for many years. They had three sons aged 12 to 17. Charming boys they were. When I got there, people said: 'Yes, well, we've never had anyone like you here as a maid. But in

our house the maid eats in the kitchen. I said, 'That's good for me, yes; I don't mind.' I was glad I was alive; that's a good condition after all. [Laughing.] But before I knew what was happening to me, the three boys said: 'Well, we're eating in the kitchen with Marta'. And so, I was asked to come in. 'Well, we didn't know her and so on.' But I didn't really mind.

(Friedmann, interview, 23 April, 1997)

She stayed with this family for barely a year, who were very disappointed and angry when she found distant relatives of hers in London. They told her, 'As a foreigner, you are not allowed to change jobs because you are obliged to stay with us for a year. So, every time I had to fight to get away and go somewhere else' (Friedmann, interview, 23 April, 1997).

She first heard of the existence of these distant relatives (three unmarried cousins of her father), who lived in Hendon, London, when she was in Antwerp before leaving for England. They had come to England through a Jewish aid organization after they had lost their mother in the First World War and their father had been taken prisoner of war (though they were later reunited). Enthusiastic about having found a family member, they persuaded Manna Friedmann to give up her work as a domestic helper and to live with them instead.

You don't have to be a maid here. You will be our fourth sister; we will adopt you. And they were quite beside themselves that we had never approached them; they might have been able to help us with the immigration to England [...] And they had done very well in life; they had all studied and worked. The eldest one was particularly capable. She became a director in a large, well-known grain company, Luis Dreyfuss, as the only woman among many men. They had a very good life and a very pretty cottage in Hendon. They were three very capable women who worked there, but it was not my milieu. I always wanted to go to Israel. I had a different attitude. They were very English. But after the first year I thought, this is not for me. It was very comfortable and all that, but that was nothing. Besides, we had different ideological attitudes. But it took me a year to get myself out of there without really hurting people, because they were so friendly and so good to me that I didn't want to rebuff them.

(Friedmann, interview, 23 April, 1997)

Manna Friedmann stayed with these relatives for a total of two years. 'Of course, they wanted me to stay with them, but they understood, I had to return to working with children, and from there I went to Birmingham' (Friedmann, interview, 23 April, 1997). At the time, her brother Salo and his family also lived near Birmingham, in Stratford-Upon-Avon. According to her niece, Hannah Helen Cohen (personal communication, 3 April, 2023):

When my mother became pregnant with me in London, the Blitz was in full force and my parents spent nights in the underground stations. On one of these occasions, a Rabbi saw my father reading a Hebrew Bible and suggested that my father take my pregnant mother out of London, suggesting Wales or Stratford-Upon-Avon. They chose the latter, and I was born on March 9, 1941. Because my aunt was relatively close by in Birmingham, she came very frequently (probably over Shabbat) to our place and thus began the profound connection we had until she died. My father was a boys' grammar school teacher and was drafted into the British Army only what would [turn out to] be late in the War. While he was in the Army we lived in Manchester for some time. The presence of my aunt, who had an excellent relationship with my mother, must have been a great comfort as there was no one else to turn to. After the War ended, we moved to Northampton and my father continued to teach – this time in Northampton. Auntie never stopped being an integral part of our lives, and in the summers, we visited at Weir Courtney. When she would come to visit, she would leave her shoes by the door, and when I spied them, I would shout with joy. She then would say in a sing-song voice: 'I'm going to tickle your toes tra-la-la.'

In Birmingham, Manna Friedmann was able to work in a kindergarten where the children went home on weekends. The parents were engaged in war labour and worked in factories. There she received further training to become a nursery nurse, but she was immediately hired as her special abilities were quickly recognized. She was then in a position to guide future kindergarten teachers. After she had passed the examination a year later, she was given a management position in the Public Health Department and was responsible for a large day nursery with over 60 children. In total, she worked in Birmingham from 1942 to 1946.

When, in 1945, between 800 and 1,000 children and young people – survivors of the concentration camps – arrived in England, there was an appeal in the newspaper that volunteers were needed to look after them. Manna Friedmann knew immediately that she wanted to take over the care of these children, as it was a way for her to be able to share in the fate of her siblings. She enquired and found out that she had to get to know Anna Freud, who was responsible for the selection of the staff. After meeting Anna Freud in 1945 in Mansfield Gardens, who wanted to hire Manna Friedmann immediately, she was so impressed that she first went in the wrong direction. Anna Freud suggested to her:

> I know where you would fit in. Alice Goldberger has just taken over this group, the youngest – that is twenty-four children, aged three to fifteen. She desperately needs good help, who can lead the group if she is not there.
>
> (Friedmann, interview, 12 July, 1996)

It was another year before Manna Friedmann could start there, because she couldn't give up her own work in Birmingham so soon. 'And in 1946 I packed my things, hadn't met Alice, hadn't seen the place, hadn't seen anything, and went there' (Friedmann, interview, 12 July, 1996). About her work there she said:

> I think these were my happiest years. This was something very special. First, it was in the countryside in a wonderful old house with a beautiful garden – a

paradise for children. Weir Courtney was the name of this wonderful, this wonderful residence donated for those children. [...] And we had those children, who needed to be rehabilitated and whom one could make so happy, because they were used to nothing. [...] and that was the most wonderful work, because they were just filling you up with gratitude and they were therapeutic for me. I know when I arrived there [–] I arrived there with my violin and I looked through the window and saw these six-year-old children with shorn hair, who danced, and there I stood outside and started crying. It was a fantastic workplace [–] And there were many helpers, many. People almost sought to work there as volunteers. And sure, we got a salary. It was not very much, but we got money. [...] Hence, it was a fabulous healing through this work and through this spirit with these children. You see, all this time, I was here in England and worked with the children, with the survivors. And that was for me naturally like a therapy, since I knew that my siblings were no longer alive.

(Friedmann, interview, 12 July, 1996, published in
English prior to this edition)

In one of her memories from that time, Alice Goldberger said to her:

There is a girl [Judith Sherman] outside under the tree who refuses to come in. She is so depressed; feelings of guilt that she has stayed alive. Her whole family – she has a younger sister [Mirjam] here. See if you can get her in! She won't take off her dress. She arrived here yesterday.' She was still wearing a lice-ridden dress. Her hair was full of lice, she was ashamed, didn't want it to be combed. And somehow, I managed to get her in. And she let me wash her and the dress. And I sewed her a new dress – I sew dresses too. And she became very much mine; my special one. You had to be careful because the other children got jealous, of course. As I said, we had a fabulous teacher in this home. She got this one and another one to go to the grammar school in Croydon, although at first with much younger children. But she worked hard and got her A-levels here in England.

(Friedmann, interview, 12 July, 1996)

Manna Friedmann had a very close relationship with Judith Sherman and her family for over 60 years (United States Holocaust Memorial Museum, n.d.). Judith Sherman came from Kurima in Czechoslovakia. From Auschwitz she was sent to Ravensbrück in 1944, where she was liberated by Russian soldiers during the death march. In 1946, she came to England with her younger sister Mirjam, who, at age 6–7 years old, before being sent to the camps, was hidden with a family in Czechoslovakia. She remembers how she was seriously ill with diphtheria and overheard the foster parents discussing whether to give her up; however, both (the foster mother as well as the foster father) remembered they had promised Mirjam's biological parents that they would take care of this child until the end. It must be considered, however, how this family had put itself in mortal danger, especially as they had children of their own. When Judith was released from the camp, she went to see her sister at the foster family, as she knew where she had been hidden.

Manna Friedmann reported on Judith:

> Not a day goes by when she takes a shower [-] where she does not see in front of her the place where she was in the camp [–] where she could wash herself. And she had a choice, either to stay lice-ridden or to go to the mortuary, where the dead were laid out. There was a cold [–] a cold tap, where she could wash herself. And she says, to this day, every time she [–] she thinks: 'God [–] how well I'm doing.' So, it's probably things [–] But you probably must [have to] work at it a lot to digest those memories and be finished with them. But now she has a man who was not in the camp, to whom she has never spoken about the camps. And when you [–] ask her [why, she says]: [–] 'I don't want him to be sorry for me.' A fabulous man, who is also a psychotherapist. [It was the same] for the children. She didn't want the kids to feel [–] to feel that 'God we have to be good to our mother.' They have great relationships with the children, so normal; they would never think that she had experienced this. [...] And there are still things today [–] The second generation, that somehow still knows about it [–] is affected by this [–]. And these children are all [–] like siblings, these children are close among themselves. They are all like one [–] perhaps closer than siblings can be in many families. They are all connected.
>
> (Friedmann, interview, 12 July, 1996)

When Manna Friedmann was asked about the fact that she herself lost almost all her siblings in the Holocaust, she replied: 'That is exactly what I meant. They have absolutely taken the place of my own brothers and sister, and it was a good [–] a replacement as good as possible' (Friedmann, interview, 12 July, 1996).

Anna Freud and Dorothy Burlingham visited this orphanage regularly. 'And then we sometimes performed little children's concerts, and that was always a big day when Anna Freud came' (Friedmann, interview, 12 July, 1996).

Manna Friedmann's brother Salo, his wife Carol and their then six-year-old daughter Helen visited Manna Friedmann in Lingfield and gave the twenty-four homeless children an impression of what family can be.

On 23 November, 2013, Judith Sherman, one of the Lingfield House children, wrote a moving obituary to Manna Friedmann, describing how the 24 'Lingfield Children' arrived destroyed and were lovingly brought back to life by Manna. How they, who could only communicate in different languages (Czech, Yiddish, German, Italian, Polish), had to learn English. Manna was like the 'biblical manna' for them, who introduced them to music with her violin or harmonica, brought them back to life with folk dances, minuets, games. They woke up to the sounds of *Kleine Nachtmusik* [transl.: little night music; a composition by Mozart]; the gong lured them to breakfast. She adorned their shorn and regrowing hair with combs and bows.

In Weir Courtney, after a year of individual care by Gertrud and Sophie Dann, the remaining 'Bulldogs Bank children' who had not been adopted were integrated.

The change of group was difficult in that the older children, who had become a group of their own, experienced the Bulldogs Bank children as intruders.

> It's like having an unloved sibling and now six at once. [...] After a year these children came to us in this wonderful home. And Gertrud was then the one who was responsible, because the children knew Gertrud. And they were, they didn't feel very well with us. And our children did not like them very much at the beginning. Because they were small, they disturbed us, but we treated them well. Yes [–] and they continued to behave as a group, and that was the enemy. But the idea was to have these youngest adopted as well as possible. So very often people came to Weir Courtney in Lingfield, Surrey, who would have been interested in adopting children. Not only the youngest, but also the older ones. But they didn't want to. The older ones didn't. [There were] only a few, one or two, where the adoption worked out, but the little ones were all adopted.
>
> (Friedmann, interview, 12 July, 1996)

Manna Friedmann and Alice Goldberger got along very well and quickly became friends: 'When I went there, she [Alice Goldberger] said: "You have to commit for at least two years", because I wanted to go to Israel.' Manna Friedmann stayed for three years, 'because it became so insanely difficult for me to leave the children again. But I am still in very close contact with these children, with most of them, to this day' (Friedmann, interview, 12 July, 1996).

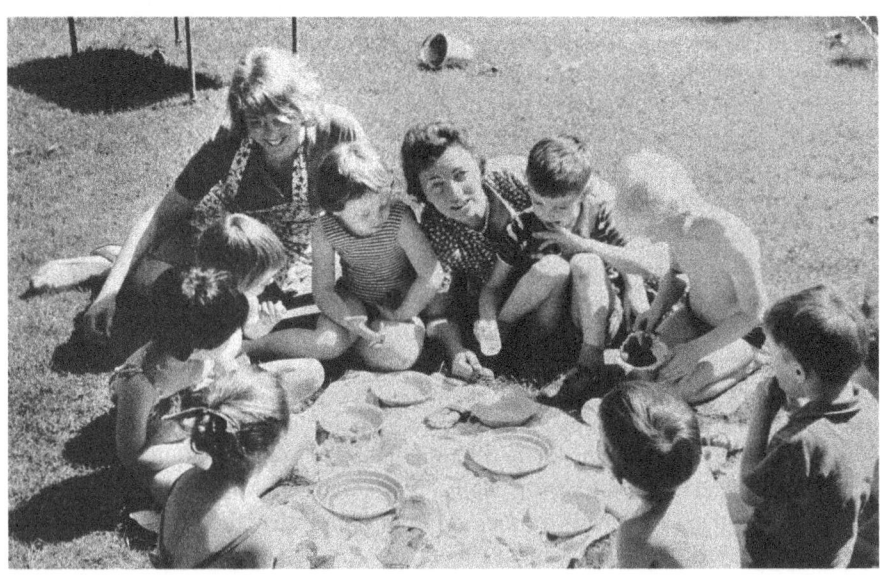

Manna Friedmann (centre) with children at a picnic (credit: Manna Friedmann and AFC)

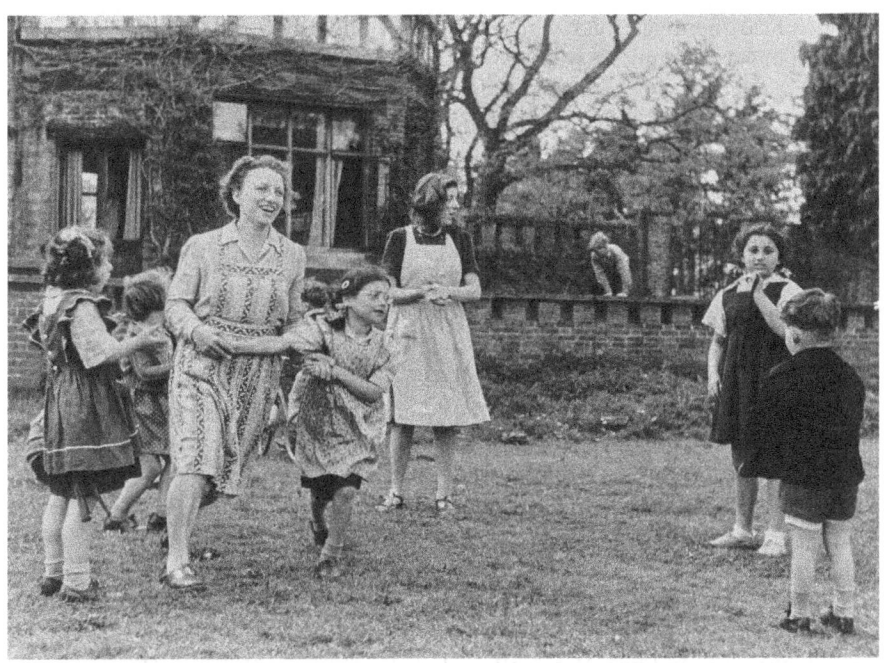

Manna dancing with children in the garden at Weir Courtney (credit: Manna Friedmann and AFC)

Her time in Palestine (1949–1955)

Before Manna Friedmann left for Israel in 1949, she helped Alice Goldberger and the children move to Isleworth, Middlesex. It was very difficult for her to say good-bye to the children, but she was also drawn to Israel to visit her sister, where she learnt how seriously ill she already was.

> I went to Israel after three years [in Weir Courtney] and stayed there for six years as a kindergarten teacher as well, studying social work. And also worked as a social worker. But I already had a relationship with a [–], my husband, who was an analyst, but who didn't want to go to Israel. [...]
>
> But I kept in touch with these children as I was leaving, and I wrote a report to these children every week about what I was doing and where I am. And Alice Goldberger collected [them] [–], but I didn't know that. When I came back, Alice Goldberger had two files like that with all my letters in dates. And so, I asked her to give them back to me because that was a story in a new country.
>
> (Friedmann, interview, 12 July, 1996)

Manna Friedmann later gave these letters to Judith Sherman's daughter. She had a lifelong close relationship with her and her family.

I'm in contact with them all the time. [–] She's like my daughter, you know? Another one of these children comes to me every year from Italy [-] to learn English and stays with me for about two to three months [Andra Bucci].

So, I've had children around me all my life and a lot of them. But not only that, but also relatives. Because when I came to Israel, I found my sister, who I hadn't seen for ten years, who had emigrated illegally to Palestine at that time on the ship *Patria*, and she had two little children. A two-year-old and a four-year-old. She herself was seriously ill with cancer. [–] She was 28 and died very early. I was there for a year, to be with the children [–], in a kibbutz that was. And so, I stayed in that kibbutz after she died, because she asked me not to leave the children, you know, and then I became the kibbutz aunt, so to speak. I was known there, that's the [laughs] Aunt Marta. These children are like my own, of course. And one of these two children is an artist, an artist, he's with me now [Eran Wolkowski]. He works on a newspaper, a national newspaper [–], [he] is the cartoonist. A fabulous guy, and he comes to visit me twice a year and he's here now. These are his works here, that's why the table looks so messy. He does the cartoons for the newspaper; he often sits here in the room and just paints the surroundings. Yes, well, as I said, so are my children. His sister with her husband, she was here with me four weeks ago for two. These children, who are related and the other children from the home, who are somehow like my own children. So, one of them says: 'You know, you have more children, than we who have children.'

(Friedmann, interview, 12 July, 1996)

Eran Wolkowski wrote in an email (11 November, 2020):

Yes, it was [a] difficult feeling without 'proper' parents around like 'normal' children. At the same time my father[5] wasn't popular in kibbutz, he was a kind of a bohemian, not totally devoted to the kibbutz dogma, so it was kind of easier to be accepted when he left. He wasn't very protective or active as a father. The departure of Marta was hard. (In the kibbutz she was called by everyone Doda Marta, which means in Hebrew Aunt Marta, this is what we called her too). She was very popular and gave us a strong backing. I felt very proud and in top spirits every time I was with her among kibbutz members. We used to wait desperately for her spring visits every year all through our childhood and later. In fact, my Father was aware of Marta's stronger ties with us and considered letting her adopt us and follow her to London. She had such plans (she told me many times), but her friend and future husband Oscar Friedmann talked her out of it.

In the conversations with Manna Friedmann, it became clear how difficult it had been for her to leave her sister's children behind; how torn she was between them and her love for Oscar Friedmann. At first, she worked in Ramle, a suburb of Tel Aviv, for two years as the director of a large kindergarten run by WIZO (Women's Zionist Organization in Israel). 1949 was the time of new immigration, and she was responsible for 50–60 children:

> That was a fabulous job. And so, I got involved in social welfare, because I took great care of these children where they came from, the families. A German pediatrician, who came there very often, suddenly saw a pretty well-run kindergarten and said: 'Well, what are you doing as a kindergarten teacher, you should be a social worker, that's what you do anyway.' And I said: 'Yes, but I won't do that without being trained. I don't want to be one of those, she's not trained, but she's all right.' And she said, 'If you want, I'll recommend you as a student, as a meteor student.' And so, I went to school for two years and studied there. But if I'm honest, I did it mainly to explore and learn the language even more, and I learnt a lot of Hebrew during my training. I had to learn and work there, and I learnt it well.
> (Friedmann, interview, 12 July, 1996)

After her exams she worked as a social worker in Tel Aviv, mainly with children who had to be placed in children's homes or kibbutzs. Torn between her work, which she loved, and her love for Oscar Friedmann (in England, he used the English version of his name), it was hard for her to decide. She was also afraid of becoming unemployed in England, while in Palestine she had a pensionable job as an employee of the city of Tel Aviv.

Her nephew Eran wrote (personal correspondence, 14 June, 2020) 'When we were children, she came over every year at the Easter holiday. It was a great thing for me and my sister as she became a mother for us.'

Her love for Oscar Friedmann

Oscar Friedmann (born Oskar but changed his name after emigrating to England and later published under the name Friedman) was born on 22 March, 1903, in Düsseldorf as the eldest son of a total of nine children. For a long time, he was the only son among many sisters. His early childhood is said to have been very beautiful and carefree, but it was suddenly completely changed by the death of his father when Oscar was ten years old. His father's brother decided that Oscar, his younger brother, and all the sisters should be taken to an orphanage. The conditions in the first home must have been terrible – even though he did not have to stay there for long. In the second orphanage he managed to establish a close relationship with the director of the orphanage, which lasted until the director's death, which was only a few years before Oscar Friedmann's.

These experiences not only accelerated his personal maturation but were the basis for his lifelong professional commitment to isolated or abandoned children and young people. His greatest concern was to preserve children's homes or, if they no longer existed, to create a new one for them.

Oscar Friedmann first worked as a teacher and then as a social worker in Düsseldorf before he became director of an institution for delinquent youths in Wolzig, Brandenburg, in 1932 (Hirsch, 1990). On 7 June, 1933, the District Administrator Lindig in Beeskow ordered a search of the correctional home in Wolzig. During the search, a sidearm and clubs were found in Friedmann's desk, which he had taken from the youths and kept there. Other weapons were found in their possession. Together with the youths he was taken to the concentration camp in Oranienburg, where he was maltreated. For the rest of his life, an ear injury as well as a slight hemiplegia of the face and weakness in his hands reminded him of this time. Fortunately, he was transferred from the camp to a prison, from which he was released in 1933. He voluntarily continued to look after the 60 delinquent youths who found this to be heroic and never forgot about it. As a result, he could only work under great personal restrictions. The young people lived in two rooms under constant surveillance, but nevertheless he managed to engage in constructive activities with them. In psychoanalysis with Ada Müller-Braunschweig in Berlin he tried to work through the psychological damage he suffered during this time (Ludwig-Körner, 1998, p. 177).

In 1934 he was offered the management of the Reichenheim orphanage in Berlin, which served the Jewish community and was later destroyed during the Second World War, but on condition that he was married. 'Many women always loved Oscar; he was idolized by women" (Friedmann, interview, 15 February, 1998). He consulted with his sister Marga (Male) whether he should give in to the urging of his friend Eva Huth (born 1906) to marry her. She also worked as a welfare worker in the Reichenheim orphanage. The marriage came about despite great misgivings with the agreement not to have children. After the birth of their daughter Barbara, the couple separated, only to reconcile later and their son Peter was born (Friedmann, interview, 15 February, 1998).

When he took a large group of Jewish children to England in 1938, he wanted to return to Germany at first, but after long discussions he was persuaded to stay in England. Thus, his first wife, the two children and his sister, who had taken care of the family, were saved. The children kept a close relationship with both parents.

Until 1945, Oscar Friedmann worked as a social worker and was one of the leading staff of Bloomsbury House in London. The Bloomsbury House Committee looked after children and young people rescued from concentration camps. Oscar Friedmann was the director of the Windermere Reception Centre and later became the director of Bloomsbury House and helped the Primrose Club, so that the many young people who had to live on their own after leaving Windermere or other centres had a place to go (Gilbert, 1996).

On 14 August, 1945, over 300 children and youths landed in Crosby-on-Eden, having been flown to England on various military planes and were then taken to a reception camp in Windermere. Leonard Montefiore and Oscar Friedmann were particularly concerned about these children. Friedmann realized that the right help for them would not be to shower them with gifts, but to find a suitable new home as quickly as possible. Seven hundred and thirty-two Jewish children and youths, most of them from Eastern Europe, were either taken in by him or passed on or referred to him. Donald Winnicott wrote in Oscar Friedmann's obituary: 'And he continued his policy of trying to give the children independence from a fixed attitude of "the world owes us something"' (Caldwell & Taylor, 2017, p. 535). Oscar Friedmann saw his task primarily in the psychological care of these children and young people. His good experiences in psychoanalysis with Ada Müller-Braunschweig had awakened his interest in psychoanalytic training, which he – being completely broke – could not immediately afford.

After his training as a psychoanalyst at the British Psycho-Analytical Institute (his analyst was Katja Levy) he had his own practice in London. Oscar Friedmann had been a Freudian but had also worked a lot with the 'Middle Group' (Friedmann, interview, 19 March, 2000). He also worked on a research project at the Hampstead Child Therapy Clinic: 'The simultaneous analysis of mother and child', published with Ilse Hellmann and Elizabeth Shepheard (Hellman et al., 1960). One analyst treated the mother, another the child, and another evaluated the weekly reports that had to be written about the treatment of all patients, which were regularly read by Anna Freud.

During his work as a social worker, he sometimes had to visit the children's home in Weir Courtney, where he met Manna Friedmann:

But he was really just the boss of the whole thing, so to speak, and I was the worker. And when he came to us, he often said: 'Yes, don't you ever come to London? Don't you have to consult with me? And anyway [–] don't you have any difficulties with the children?' And [laughing] that's when I said – very snootily, 'But I don't want to be one of those who stand in line until you have time for an interview!' Because it went around that everyone was chasing him. I believed that too. He denied it, 'That's not true at all! That's what they're saying about me, it's all not true.' But I think it was true after all. That's why I didn't really get my hopes up any more. It was such a game from my point of view; I enjoyed it. I could tell he was interested, but I didn't think it would ever happen. But it did happen! And it was good. But he was a fabulous person, of course. [...]

He knew that I was going to emigrate to Israel [–], so he said, 'Yes, well, now we part ways.' He was a colossally attractive person. But I never thought there were many after him. Because when I went to Palestine, even though they were no longer together – separated for twelve years – he was, but she [Friedmann's first wife] didn't want to give him a divorce. And for me, at that time, it was still an impossible situation to get involved in such a relationship. So, I couldn't. It was against my culture somehow. But then, when he came to visit me and I saw [–], I still wanted to get married, that is, I wanted to have a person for myself. I had taken care of so many people. But he came to visit me in Israel in 1952 and 1953, and the following year I came back to England. And then when he came and said, 'Well, I can't promise you marriage, because I can't get a divorce. But it depends on you whether you want to get involved.' And that's when I said yes. So, I returned to England in 1955 – only because of Oscar.

(Friedmann, interview, 21 November, 1996)

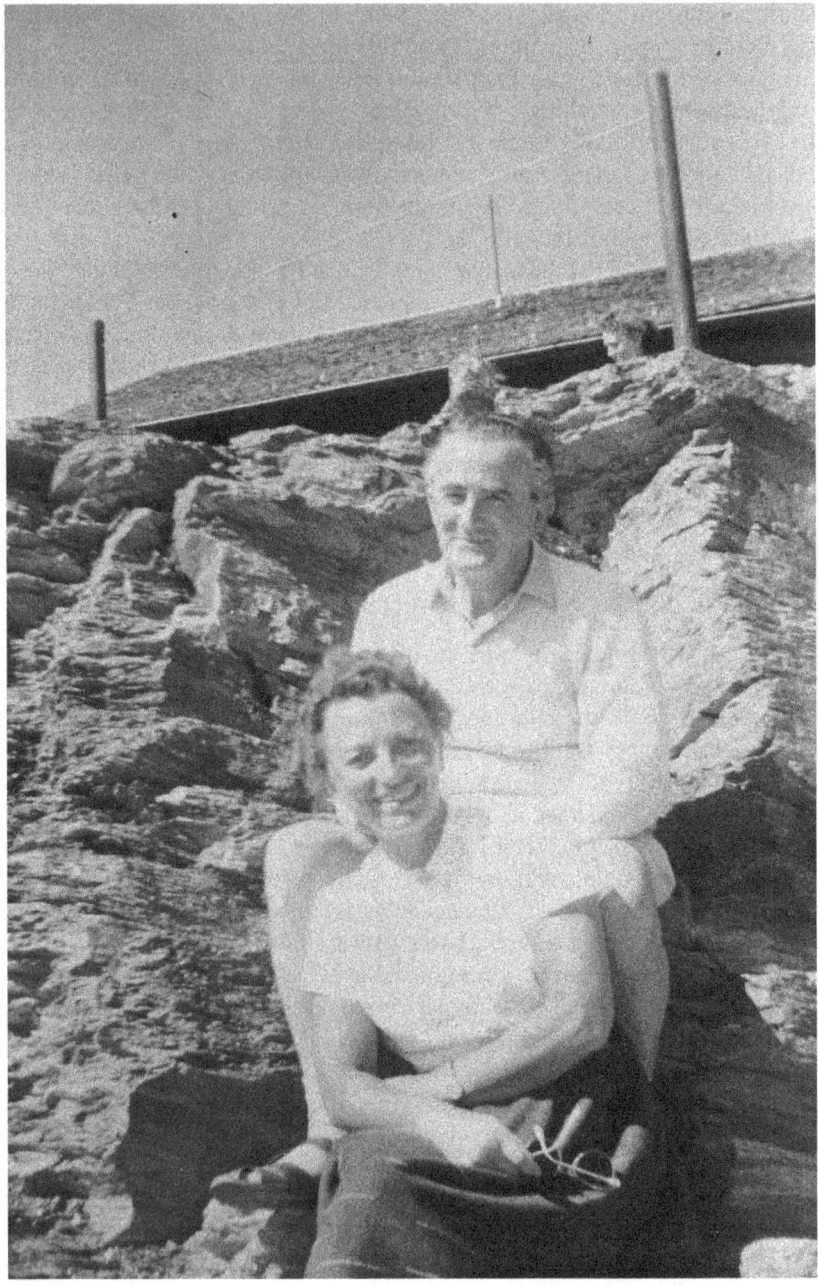

The married Friedmann couple during their holidays, 1957 (credit: Manna Friedmann)

After her return from Israel, Manna Friedmann moved in with her husband, who was living with his sister, who had previously run the household for him. Their address at the time was 30 Fitzjohns Avenue. It was the daughter, Barbara, who had persuaded her mother to finally agree to the divorce.

> Although his daughter once said to me, who also loved her father very much: 'I don't think you're the right woman for my father either. But you are better than my mother for him.' Because he was very interested in elegant women, and I am not an elegant woman.
>
> (Friedmann, interview, 19 March, 2000)

> So, in the beginning, for me, that was such an ideal. And we were discussing something, and I said: 'I don't agree with you about this at all!' And he replied: 'So, now we can get married! Now you are independent.' And then we got married. Otherwise, I would [–] I think [–] never have left Israel. It was just as difficult for me to part with Israel and the children there. Even though we are of course in frequent contact, these children, these two, nephew and niece.
>
> (Friedmann, interview, 26 November, 1996)

At the beginning of 1956, after more than twenty years, she met Professor Kisch again in London, where he attended a congress. She drove to their hotel; it was a Friday, and by then the family had become 'over-religious' and did not drive on

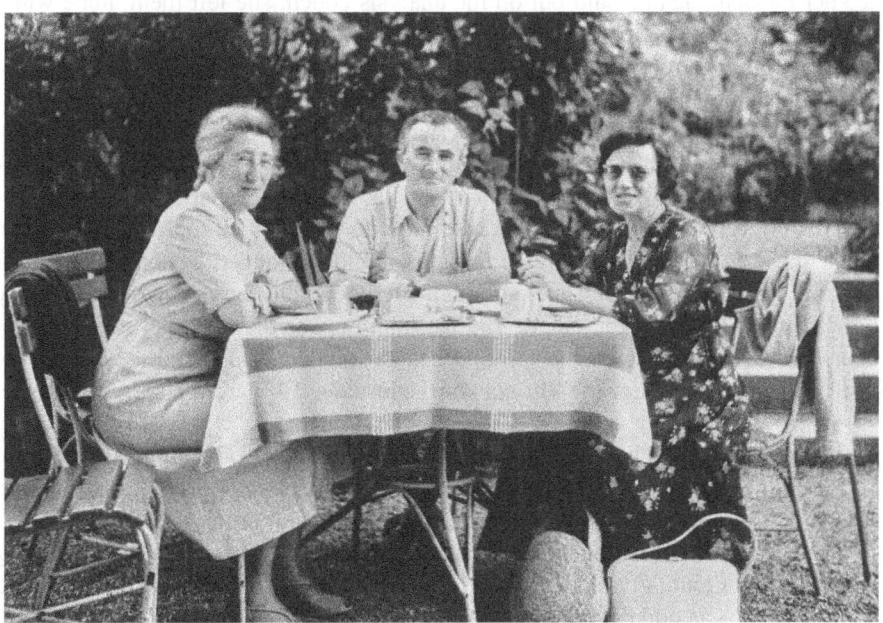

Oscar Friedmann, 1957, with his sister Male (Marga) left and Alice Goldberger, whom they had met in Bad Gastein on her 60th birthday (credit: Manna Friedmann)

Fridays. Manna told them that she lived with a man and wanted to introduce Oscar Friedmann to them. She then received a letter from Professor Kisch saying that he was furious that she was living with a (still) married man. It was a shock for her. As a result, she burned all correspondence with this family, including the photos from that time (Friedmann, interview, 19 March, 2000).

Oscar Friedmann and Manna Weindling were married on 27 December, 1956. Their happiness lasted only three and a half years. Lotte Kearney, who was first an assistant to Manna Friedmann at Hampstead Kindergarten before she also began her psycho-analytic training, was a friend of theirs and enjoyed playing bridge with Oscar Friedmann. She happened to be visiting them when Oscar Friedmann suddenly suffered a heart attack on 28 December, 1958, one day after their wedding anniversary, and died.

> And I always had the feeling, well [–] that it is my happiness now, my whole life is exactly the way I wanted it. Namely, I love caring for people. And here was this man whom I absolutely adored. And for him I would now, when he gets nice and old, I would be able to take care of him. He was twelve years older than me. And, well, that didn't work out either.
>
> (Friedmann, interview, 19 March, 2000)

After Oscar Friedmann's death, Manna Friedmann immediately informed his children and his first wife. Naturally, Manna gave in to Eva Friedmann's wish to see her husband again. Laid out on the analysis couch, she left them alone while she sat with friends in the next room. The divorced woman then, when she had said goodbye to her former husband and joined the others, took a blanket, and lovingly wrapped Manna in it.

After her husband's death, Manna Friedmann received an official letter from Germany informing her that, in addition to her own small pension, she would receive her husband's widow's pension from his former occupation. She first consulted a lawyer, as she believed that his first wife was entitled to this money. Even when she was officially told again that this money belonged to her, she found it difficult to calm her conscience, although she knew that the first wife had a very good pension of her own. 'So, by the fact that he was divorced [–] if he had not been divorced [the pension was mine]. Because it was such a short time, somehow, I felt it was not really for me' (Friedmann, interview, 19 March, 2000).

> Many people thought that I would probably go back to Israel, especially because the children were still there, but then I already had the memories of my husband and of that time and it was three and a half very important years for me, so I couldn't give that up easily. And besides that, I really, really enjoyed working with Anna Freud. I couldn't start all over again. It was already a new beginning here, then a second beginning in Israel, then the third new beginning. So, I visit Israel about every two years, and I still have many friends and colleagues from the past. And my nephew and my niece come to visit me.
>
> (Friedmann, interview, 26 November, 1996)

Work at Hampstead Nursery School

After returning to London from Israel and not yet having found work, Manna Friedmann, on Alice Goldberger's recommendation, went to Eva Hauser, who owned a
gallery for art and weaving and was looking for a weaver. "'But I am not a weaver."
Then she said: "But you will be able to do it!" So, I went there, and she hired me,
and I could do it. I mean, I started with very simple work and learned it slowly'
(Friedmann, interview, 26 November, 1996).

Only later did she learn that at the same time Anna Freud had also learnt to
weave there. Later, Manna Friedmann was able to help her with weaving. It was
also Alice Goldberger who advised her six months later to go to Anna Freud, who
at the time was planning to set up a kindergarten where training candidates for
child analysis would have the opportunity to meet 'normal' children.

> Anna Freud asked me in her interview: 'Have you ever thought of studying
> child analysis?' So, I said: 'No.' – 'Why not?' And then I told her: 'Because I
> prefer to work with the ego of the child rather than with the unconscious.' That's
> why. And she accepted that. No, I was never particularly interested in that. I
> wanted to know and learn a lot about it. But much more theoretically than thera-
> peutically applying it with children.
>
> (Friedmann, interview, 26 November, 1996)

Manna Friedmann (1988, p. 277) wrote about Anna Freud's idea to build a
kindergarten.

As is now well known, the purpose of such a Nursery for 'normal' children with,
in Anna Freud's words, 'no more than the developmental hazards' was threefold:

1. To offer students in training at the Clinic the opportunity to observe normal
   behaviour and development in children between two and a half and five years
   of age.
2. To bring together the two disciplines of education and analysis.
3. To offer a nursery service for a group of children.

When her husband heard about the possibility of her working at Hampstead Clinic
in the kindergarten, he did not like it very much:

> My husband, who had a good sense of humour, said: 'You, don't go there, they'll
> only ruin you' [laughing]. I said: 'Yes, good.' [–] And later, after I had worked
> there for a while, he said: 'You were such a lovely person. They have corrupted
> you.' [–] I knew too much already. I learnt about him too. Of course, of course!
> Every person is only human. [...]
>
>   But it turned out to be very good, because when he had to write his papers
> at the weekend, he dictated them to me, and I wrote them. So, I think it was a
> wonderful collaboration because we had common interests. That was the other
> nice thing about this connection.
>
> (Friedmann, interview, 23 April, 1997)

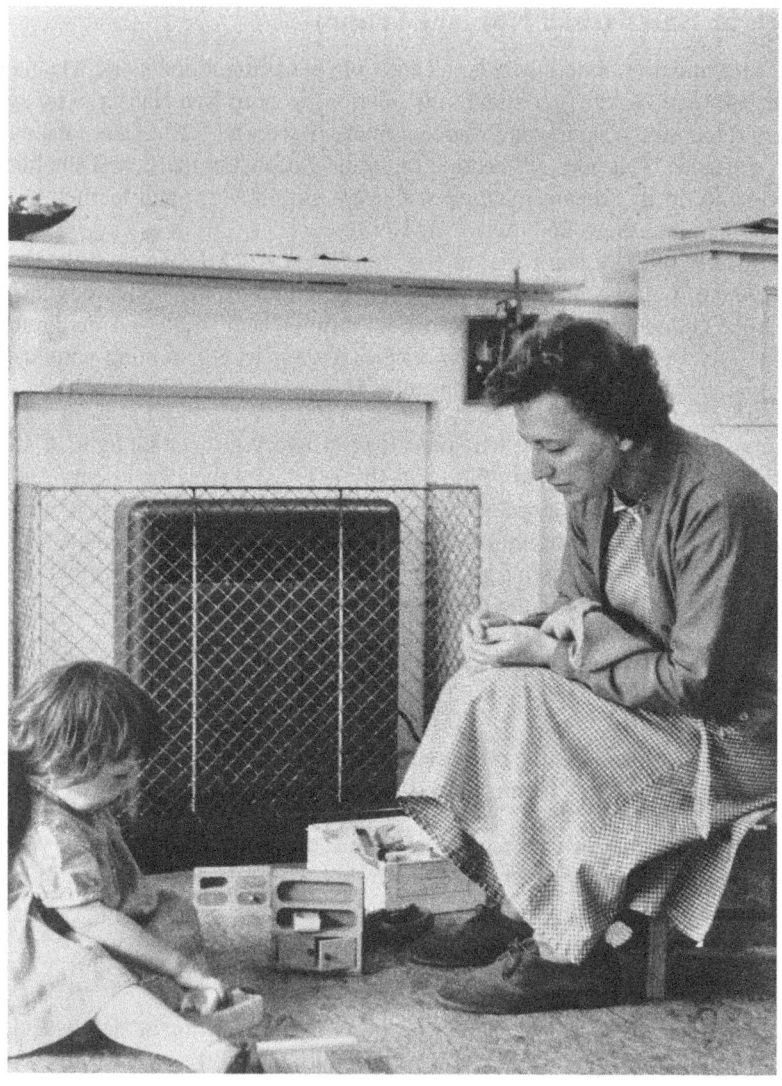

Manna Friedmann while working with a child at Hampstead Clinic (credit: Manna
Friedmann and AFC)

But they were wonderful years. Too short, unfortunately. Yes, it was a very, very
eventful and interesting time, which gave me colossal impulses to mature.
(Friedmann, interview, 26 November, 1996)

From 1957 until her retirement in 1978, she was head of Hampstead Kindergarten. When a kindergarten was to open in the basement of 12 Mansfield Gardens,

many structural changes were required. Anna Freud surprised Manna Friedmann with this proposal:

'There is a Montessori teacher in America who used to work with me in Vienna, Anni Hermann. She is now director of the kindergarten in New York in an agency. What if I asked her to come here for half a year to help build the buildings and the acquisitions and all that?' I have already been here in England. Would I approve of that? I was overjoyed and so Anni Hermann came, and we set up this nursery. Now it is even more beautiful than it was before.

(Friedmann, interview, 23 April, 1997)

She reported in another interview:

But one little thing, for example, how Anna Freud was still working at that time [–], or perhaps how something changed. There was such a big room, and the whole wall below was a blackboard, because this place was used for very disturbed children. There were autistic children who were being treated, so this place was needed. Now, when Anni Hermann and I looked at it [our reaction was], 'My God, we don't need that big room with a big blackboard'. Anna Freud thought: 'Why, it would be very good for the children to write there.' So, it took quite a long time before Anni Hermann was able to move it, only a small part, right by the window is a small part, that's what remains of the blackboard. 'But why [–], because the children will, if the walls are light, won't the children make it dirty?' 'No, they won't, because we will teach them that it is better in a nice room than in a dirty room.'

(Friedmann, interview, 12 July, 1996)

Anni Hermann also taught her Montessori education during this time.

I have no [–] I have no children myself. This was planned. Because it already [–] it was already too late by the time I got married. No, I just had time, you know? [–] By the way, we started [–] it was only a half-day programme [–] till noon. And these were children from the area, children from absolutely normal, and not just normal, but affluent [backgrounds]. [–] Anne-Marie Sandler's two children were in our kindergarten. So, in the beginning it was a private kindergarten with minimal costs, of course, because Anna Freud had the idea that it was necessary for people without money. But since we needed children for this kindergarten, everyone could [–] everybody could apply and we only took – at the beginning, Anna Freud said – eight children, because this must be a small group, this must be absolutely optimal. But eight children, how can you run a kindergarten with eight children? And then when I told her, but if one or two children are absent, are at home for some reason? And then a child asks: 'And where is the school?' So, we slowly brought it up to ten and then slowly to twelve. Anni Hermann stayed with me. [–] In six months, we completely renewed this place. [...]

When I started working here at the Anna Freud Nursery, a former colleague from Israel came to visit me. And she came to the kindergarten and stayed there for one or two hours. And she said to me afterwards: 'Aren't you ashamed, you call this work? It's a luxury. It's a gimmick.' But it wasn't such a gimmick. That is, instead of working with 50 children, it's nothing. But that's a different kind of work. At that time, we also had children from the employees. And that was not so good either; it was very difficult, because we had to report on the children as well.

(Friedmann, interview, 12 July, 1996)

For Anna Freud, there was one main rule in kindergarten: anything that is fun and does not harm oneself or others may be done. If the children had done something that was not allowed, they had to sit down on a bench, being told: 'I'll let you sit here so you can think about it'. Anna Freud suggested the name 'thinking bench' for this, but this was dropped because it did not seem sensible to combine thinking with punishment.

(Friedmann, interview, 19 March, 2000)

Anna Freud associated the kindergarten with a pedagogical idea. She needed children for training the students. Gertrud Dann remembered (interview, 11 November, 1996, published in English prior to this edition),

She needed children for the training of the students. There are often students with great academic education and a lot of theories of just about anything [–], but they've barely seen children. They have to learn that [–], and they enjoyed it very much, too. And it is still the same; even now, there's always people in the Anna Freud Houses.

Manna Friedmann (1988) and Hansi Kennedy (1978b) have described this in their publications.
During the daily work of Manna Friedmann, training candidates were often present:

They observed what and how I was working with the children. And how, for example, I was dealing with a child in a certain situation; did not interpret it, as you would perhaps be doing in a therapeutic session, but just being pedagogical.

(Friedmann, interview, 19 March, 2000,
published in English prior to this edition)

When Manna Friedmann was told by Anna Freud that she would be observing children, she asked her:

Well, what should we observe? Children, what is there in particular to observe? As I also had students, I had to tell them what to observe, too. Although we always had these meetings, where everything was carefully noted, and reports had to be written. And then she said – just like that – but that was her skill anyway, to just bring everything down to a simple point. It wasn't particularly academic. She could be academic with academics, very academic. With kinder-garteners she could speak a kindergartener's language. That was the great thing. And then she said: 'Just write down everything where you think, "Oh I have to tell that to my husband later, that's so sweet.' Or "that's a bit weird; that a four-year-old child should act like that, that would fit a younger child." Or "this little 2.5-year-old can already do that and that, that's quite a thing."

And so, every week another child had to be looked at as if through a magni-fying glass. And the students brought their observations, and Anna Freud was always there. So, you can imagine how much one could learn there. And we always said, she will drop a few pearls. Something that you wouldn't expect, just random. Like, we had a four-year-old child, she had enough of everything at home, she wasn't a disadvantaged child, but she was so greedy, yes, she always wanted to have everything and took it from other children, although she had probably lots more toys than most. And when I was telling her about that child, I said, 'That child irritates me, and I'm not always nice to her.' Well, you could do that, you didn't have to have perfect reports, and that was very nice. 'And because she's so greedy I become angry with her and then I have a bad feeling. I should know better, especially with these things.' And then she said this, 'Imag-ine, if she were a two-year-old, and she'd act like that, you'd find it pretty okay, and you wouldn't be angry.' Which was true, of course. 'If she's like that at that moment, treat her like a two-year-old child in that area, but in the intellectual area, treat her like a four-year-old!' Great. Not always easy to execute what she was saying so easily. She simplified things very often, made it easier than in reality. As a teacher she was outstanding that way.

(Friedmann, interview, 19 March, 2000,
published in English prior to this edition)

Laughing, Manna reports that this girl has become a very good businesswoman. Manna Friedmann remembered the meetings with Anna Freud:

We had a conference with her every week, where one teacher had to present on one child, only on one child. We had 12–13 children in this kindergarten, and these children were observed in the nursery by students as part of their training in the first year. They had to learn what a so-called normal child looks like and learn to distinguish whether it was a passing problem or if the child is really in trouble and maybe needs another sort of help. She was always the one not directly running to a therapist. I had previously worked in a lot of kindergartens, also in Israel and other places, in much bigger ones. It seemed really weird to me at first in such a small kindergarten with 12 children, and then this observing. I thought, good Lord, that's much ado about nothing. But in the 21 years I worked there as a kindergartener, I learnt a lot.

(Friedmann, interview, 19 March, 2000,
published in English prior to this edition)

Anna Freud delivered theoretical explanations, but above all she transmitted her analytical attitude and perspective to those young colleagues and students, most of whom initially understood nothing of psychoanalysis. Manna Friedmann, in turn, learned much from the regular reporting that had to be done on the children. Those reports were then discussed in depth by Anna Freud with the training candidates. Manna Friedmann recalled, 'That was, in fact, my training on the analytical level. There, I have learnt a lot. Furthermore, I participated in a Montessori-course, because in the beginning I did not open that nursery alone' (Friedmann, interview, 19 March, 2000, published in English prior to this edition).

Manna Friedmann also recalled:

In the beginning, it wasn't easy for me, in a clinic, where everybody was psychoanalytically trained, and I was the only one there in educational work. But this thinking, this empathizing deep into the behaviour of the child, I was ... to learn, what it actually means, if a child is aggressive, in order not to say, 'So that, one won't do!' Anyway I did not work like that. I always said I did not work in this nursery in a different way than I had worked in the kindergarten in Israel with 50 children. ... The pedagogical part, that's what I am good at. And naturally, I like to mother people and children, hence this work with these children offered me a lot of satisfaction. But sure, I have learnt why I do something, how I do it [...]

We had a child that was sometimes late, an analyst's child. And then I said to him: 'But why are you so late today?' The mother was very angry and said: 'We had to explain to him why he doesn't go to the toilet.' He was already four years old. Or: 'We had to interpret his fear of the lavatory.' So, I must say that I had no understanding for all that I had learnt. There were also parents who were afraid. They had to be in a different room, know that the children are treated really well. So that's what I went through for ten years.

(Friedmann, interview, 12 July, 1996,
published in English prior to this edition)

Another time, a little boy wanted to bang on a tambourine with a stick and Manna Friedmann took the stick away from him when he did not react despite being asked not to do so. The parents' reaction was: 'We do not want to entrust our child to such a stubborn educator' (Friedmann, interview, 12 March, 2000).

Manna Friedmann remembers an American assistant:

And then I came into the room and there were these children dancing around on the table. On the table. And I heard the teacher say: 'I know you want to know if I still like you [–] I still love you. Yes, I still love you!' And then I said to Anna, 'I can't work with her. This is [–] I can't do that.' And then she was entrusted with the blind children. We also had a kindergarten for blind children, and she was very good at it. Nice person, but she was an American trained teacher.

(Friedmann, interview, 12 July, 1996)

Manna Friedmann related:

She [Anna Freud] came to the Nursery very often. If she had spare time, she came in, sat down, and she left without us knowing, with a collection of observations. A visitor there asked her, 'Miss Freud, what is your favourite pastime? You do so much!' And she said – she had that way where she thinks a bit before answering – and then she said, 'What I'm doing at the moment.'

(Friedmann, interview, 21 November, 1996, published in English prior to this edition)

Anna Freud also believed that education involves a certain degree of discipline. Some felt that Anna Freud had remained more of an educator than a psychoanalyst at heart. Even within the psychoanalytic training she was the 'teacher' for whom it was a matter of course to read the reports of all training candidates regularly and with discipline. There were weekly reports and two monthly reviews. In regular meetings, she decided above all whether a child needed psychoanalysis or not. It was also she who referred the children who needed psychotherapy to the psychoanalysts. With a sure instinct she knew the strengths and weaknesses of the training candidates. Thus, Anneliese Schnurmann received the 'artistic' children, while Alice Goldberger, on the other hand, had a special ability in dealing with children who were not very intellectual.

She was able to find out from each person what they could do well and that's how they ended up. That was also the case with the therapists. I know one therapist who had a deaf child in treatment, and she worked fabulously with that child. What happened? She got all deaf children in treatment. Which maybe she didn't always love, but she learnt because of it. [–] Or Alice Goldberger, for example, who was particularly good with children who were perhaps a bit delayed. She was able to get what was there out of them. Now this group of children Alice got very often, so [–] that Anna Freud always knew that this child goes there, this child is best there, because the students needed cases. [...]

In the opinion of Manna Friedmann Anna Freud was

just such a practical person. That was an art. She also managed to bring something out of people. They didn't even know that they could do that. How could I have known that I was able to give a lecture about a child for an hour with students? But I could. And I did it because it was expected. So, this is [–] of course I could, I did learn to educate.

(Friedmann, interview, 12 July, 1996)

And, as I said, this joy of work and this desire to work that she had, I think that was the driving power in her [–] joy of work, whatever she was doing. She could also cook. When we were at the country house in Wolwerswick, she cooked. Mistress Burlingham cooked too; she did the dishes. [–]

After ten years [from 1966] we changed the whole programme, and we took in children of less well-off people who did not really have difficulties but whose parents had problems with housing and unemployment. The kindergarten was then open from morning, as it is now, until four in the afternoon, so we had much more the type of child [–] I had always worked with. So, of course I liked it much better, although it was hard work, but wonderful. I always preferred to identify with this group of children rather than with those who had everything. So, I thought that was a luxury for me. I once said to Anna Freud: 'This is not really work for me, it's – I'm in luxury here!' And she replied: 'No, that's very important, these children, they need someone who sometimes says no to them.' But they were fabulous children and they all got on very well with their lives.

(Friedmann, interview, 26 November, 1996)

These children, some of them were brought up too liberally, so they were never told no, very few limits were set. And the children found that difficult. And I had to set the boundaries. As she said, a benign super ego had to be built up, so that they would feel that it is much nicer to behave decently than to always have your own will. So, it was really a difficult time to get there.

(Friedmann, interview, 12 July, 1996)

Manna Friedmann always had assistants to support her in her work. One of them was Lottie Kearney, who had turned to Anna Freud for an apprenticeship. When asked by Anna Freud whether she would agree to work with her and whether she didn't want to meet her first, she replied that it wasn't necessary because she usually got along well with people. They got along immediately and later became lifelong friends, along with Anneliese Schnurmann (Friedmann, interview 28 June, 1998). 'And all in all, it was a wonderful job. And I did it for twenty-one years. And I learnt more and more, and more and more could be learnt by the female students who came to watch us' (Friedmann, interview, 19 March, 2000).

When Manna insisted on retiring, Anna Freud brought Nancy Brenner in to continue her work. Nancy Brenner, in her article 'The Third Decade (1978–1988), written about the Hampstead Clinic, reports how she first met Anna Freud in 1973 when she came to London from the USA for an academic year.

I first met Anna Freud in 1973, when I became a visitor at the Clinic for that academic year. I met her again in 1977, when Manna Friedmann was making plans to retire, and I came to be interviewed for the position of Nursery teacher. I knew that Manna, who personified all that the Nursery believed in, would be 'a hard act to follow', but when I was offered the job, I felt privileged and warmed to the opportunity that it presented. However, when Anna Freud told me, 'You realize that you must be another Manna Friedmann,' I had to explain apologetically that I could only be myself!

At Anna Freud's suggestion Manna Friedmann and I spent the spring term of 1978 together in the Nursery. That term taught me how the Nursery was run and provided a period of gradual transition for everyone.

Of course, the most crucial part of the learning for me centred on observations and reports. I remember clearly the first report which I gave, on Sam, under Manna's instruction. Miss Freud sat at one end of the table and I at the other; before I began, she leaned across the table smiling and said, 'I just want you to know that you have my condolences.' That kindly and humorous remark launched my delivery of the first of many Nursery reports under her benevolence.

(Brenner 1988, p. 289)

The importance Anna Freud attached to Manna Friedmann's work in the kindergarten can also be seen from the fact that she wanted to conduct a kind of longitudinal study to investigate the developmental trajectories of some children who showed difficulties when they came to the kindergarten.

In the text by Frances Salo and Manna Friedmann, 'The Runaway Bunny Mother: The Long-Term Influence of the Nursery School Experience' (1988), one learns how a longitudinal study of a baby (Julian) was conducted. He was presented at the Well Baby Clinic at six weeks of age and was further observed and accompanied at home by one of the staff members from his fourth month of life onwards and was later integrated into the nursery school.

In the following, this case report will be discussed in more detail, because it also convincingly illustrates the high degree to which attachment theory was already being applied in the AFC.

The events that negatively influenced Julian's development occurred in the second half of his first year of life, and at his early admission to kindergarten he presented as a highly sensitive child who reacted extremely anxiously in separation situations. This picture was even more striking because everyone who had observed him in his first months of life described him as a well-endowed baby who had a good start in life. During his first 18 months in kindergarten, considerable concern was expressed about his future development, so that some observers felt that psychotherapeutic treatment was necessary to ensure his future mental health. His parents refused psychotherapy, so it remained the task of the kindergarten to help Julian to develop normally. But at first, he experienced his stay at the Nursery School as stressful, and he did not seem to enjoy it very much. Obviously, he was overtaxed in trying to cope with the separation from home.

Anna Freud, who supervised this case, suspected that his entry into kindergarten might be considered premature because of his stressful experiences. She believed that he had lost his capacity for joy due to his experiences in the first year. This is where Manna Friedmann differed from Anna Freud. She saw signs of great developmental potential despite his adjustment difficulties in the kindergarten. Moreover, at the end of the first month, Manna Friedmann felt that she had gained his trust and that she was increasingly able to help him during his panic attacks, whereas at Julian's first visit it seemed that this was only possible for his father:

In most nursery schools children are usually expected to adjust to the environment; in our Nursery School the environment is expected to adjust to the child's needs. Our Nursery School provides the kind of developmental help that most parents of young children provide intuitively: that is, they meet the child at the affective and cognitive levels appropriate to it and thereby increase that child's ability to master difficulties. Most nurseries would say, as Mrs. Friedmann did, that Julian's interference with other children could not go unmodified. But while this might mean that they would restrain the child and attempt to alter his behaviour, what our Nursery School provides is an atmosphere in which the child is supported when faced with regressive pulls, while at the same time knowing what will be expected of him. Within such a framework the teacher says, not 'You're naughty,' but 'You are not ready.' Thus, Mrs. Friedmann provided physical comfort for Julian when he was coping with separation; and she met his bodily needs (feeding, toileting, dressing and other activities integral to the maternal role) within a caring relationship with a new and, above all, consistent object, for as long as it was needed.

The Nursery teachers are also able to discuss the children regularly with their psychoanalytically trained colleagues, and so gain additional support and insight. What good teachers elsewhere do intuitively, from a preconscious awareness, is done here with a conscious awareness of the reasons for doing it. (As Mrs Friedmann said), 'I knew what I was doing before, but when I came here I learned why I was doing it.'

(Salo & Friedmann, 1988, p. 67 f.)

Julian's relationship with the kindergarten teacher continued to be close. Manna Friedmann felt that he trusted her and that she could read him. She delighted in his capacity for joy and his sense of humour. He knew how to secure her attention by doing something she liked. Once when he was looking for her and found her in conversation with someone else, he began to sing 'Happy Birthday' and smiled with satisfaction when he had her attention. Within six weeks, he no longer needed to be constantly by her side, but actively sought the company of the other children. But he needed her proximity so that, by looking in her direction, he could curb his disruptive and provocative behaviour towards the other children.

Julian's favourite book in kindergarten was *The Runaway Rabbit*, the story of a rabbit who wanted to run away and so said to his mother, 'I'm running away.' 'If you run away', his mother replied, 'I will run after you. Because you are my little rabbit.'

When Julian was four years old, the concerns that had been variously expressed over the previous fifteen months grew, and some who had observed Julian in kindergarten felt that he needed analytical psychotherapeutic help to rule out the danger of psychotic development that had already been observed in his grandfather. Manna Friedmann did not share this fear and neither did Anna Freud. In Anna Freud's view, Julian was also not neurotic because he had not become regressive in the face of conflict. So, the care was continued.

Manna Friedmann saw him and his mother much later for separate follow-up interviews when he was 18 years old. He had achieved four A-levels, was in his first semester of mathematics at London University and 'loved it'. He was six feet tall and good-looking. The *Runaway Bunny* was still on his shelf next to the *Encyclopedia Britannica*, and he had told his mother not to take it away. 'Because I'm going to give it to my children' (Salo & Friedmann, 1988, p. 66).

Just how important Manna Friedmann had become for him was demonstrated by the fact that he not only invited her to celebrate his 21st birthday, but that she was given the place of honour on his right (Salo & Friedmann, 1988, p. 73).

After retiring

When Manna Friedmann told Anna Freud that she would like to retire, Anna showed no understanding of her request.

> When I was 60, I told Anna Freud: 'I have to stop now, I have no more patience for these children.' And then she said I should wait until she turns 80, then she would stop, too. By then she was 80 and I was 63, that was 1978, so I asked her: 'What about retirement?' Well, she couldn't, of course, she said she waited too long. [–] She also had too much to offer, while I, as a kindergarten teacher, simply didn't feel like it any more at 63 [–]. And then she said: 'When you retire [–], and I would leave you my two looms, two looms yes [–], would you be willing to teach the students how to weave?' Because she thought it was incredibly important that these people, who only work with their heads, do creative work, just like she did herself. Weaving was absolutely important for her, yes, or to create something. She sewed everything; she sewed her dresses and knitted things for all her friends for Christmas. She was knitting in the analytic hour [–] and she also sewed. Hand sewn like with a sewing machine. And they all had the same dirndl pattern, only she changed the material and it always looked different. Great! And then I said: 'Well, I wouldn't do that.' [–] I politely refused. 'What will you do when you are retired. You are still very creative. [–]' Yes, I have other interests. I started to study music further, as I had studied before, I started to learn the piano. I still can't really play, but I know the theory and all that. [–] And so, she did leave me the looms, although I said I wouldn't do that. Now I already had one that Mistress Burlingham had left me, I have one here, I'm using it here. And now I had two much larger looms, and I didn't know where to put them. So, I took one of them to the museum and they said there was no room for it. And that fits in wonderfully because she has [–] that was so important for her, [that they should be used]. And the other one is with a mother who had two children in our kindergarten who also knows how to weave, she now makes the patterns, the designs and I do the weaving, the carpet bridges and then we sell them for the nursery.
>
> (Friedmann, interview, 12 July, 1996)

Manna Friedmann was never bored after her retirement. She threw herself into refining her knowledge of Hebrew, so that at times she dreamt in Hebrew. Like her brother, she also gave classes in Hebrew at the University of London for 'people of the third age', with whom she worked through passages of the Old Testament she selected and proverbs containing life wisdom, based on which the group learnt Hebrew. She had already learnt basic Hebrew at school in Cologne and was able to deepen her knowledge in Israel (Friedmann, interview, 28 June, 1998).

> I was never interested in political books; instead, I studied Hebrew and music. The book *Hava Nashira* was published again in the year 2001. It is still my favourite book, and it was sent to me by my friend Charlotte Spanier (the eldest child of the K. family, who lives in Jerusalem with her large family).
>
> (Friedmann, 2007, p. 36)

> I have many friends here, so I am very busy. Three times a week I'm usually in the museum weaving, I enjoy that very much; in the afternoons for two to three hours. I must have a structure in the week. Although I'm not pedantic about it. But I must have a structure that I follow. Monday and Tuesday I'm at College and I must do homework for that too.
>
> (Friedmann, interview, 5 June, 1997)

Manna Friedmann often stayed at Walberswick, the country house of Anna Freud and Dorothy Burlingham. On one of these visits, on 11 April, 1971, she wrote down thoughts about her life while sitting on a bench and meditating, that best illustrate her attitude towards life.

> 'Got to look after yourself' could be the title of a pop song and I would understand it in the following way: only when I experience myself as good and at peace within myself can I work and 'live' and make others feel as good. No one who is miserable can have a good effect on others, can be accepted, desired. Maybe it is easier for someone who lives alone to get to know himself and his own potential and to find out what brings joy. [...] For myself it is interesting to note that this feeling of gaining inner peace grows with age, because I am grateful for the gift of life, e.g. being able to experience beautiful things (who gives me this? Foresight? Fate?), just as I am now sitting on this bench in the spring. [...] I often think I have done very well with life, earning my money with things that I like to do well (and at the same time I can do good to others), especially with the children. [...] But these children do not dominate me in the same way as children in residential work, which I loved to the same extent at that time, because it fulfilled my own needs. How right Oscar was when he said that by doing what we do most we meet a need within ourselves. At the time I was arguing with him about it or didn't quite understand what he meant, but he was right, even when he said that this did not diminish the good we do, but that we just shouldn't have this illusion of 'exclusive altruism'. 'We just happen to have this kind of need.'
>
> After the 'abundance' of children over seven to eight hours a day, they go on their way to their families, which means I do not leave them when I return to my

'leisure-pleasure'. There is so much I can do with my leisure. This is what I want to build on, these hours of leisure, and I can do this at my own will and command!

Manna Friedmann loved to read aphorisms and books in German, English and Hebrew. Sitting quietly early in the morning with a cup of coffee and to think was a great pleasure for her.

'Thinking about these things' includes thoughts about Oscar and our relationship in all its aspects. I understand him in so many ways so much better now than I did then. It has been exactly 16 years since we were able to live together and almost 12½ years since he died. Apart from all those years together, I am aware that he has influenced me enormously in my own maturation and in all these thoughts and feelings I am expressing at this moment. I have no desire for another man. I value a relationship with another person in which 'give and take' has room to share interests and views. This 'give and take' can sometimes refer to sharing a joke or having someone to 'wink an eye with'.

As further pleasures of idleness she lists:

To design and weave a pattern, to look at it again, to take it out of the frame and to give it to someone I think should have it for some reason.
    Another pleasure is to make music in harmony (chamber music). The medium is more important than the people with whom I make music. These are often people with whom I have little in common apart from the love of making music. None of my close friends with whom I share my ideas, feelings, views etc. can make music with me. With these friends I love to be together, to talk or not to talk.
    I am very happy to have these friends and my family, also with the fact that they live where they live, e.g., they do not have to be close to me in a geographical sense, as long as I know that they are doing well.
    It gives me pleasure to find a narrow approach to Anneliese's [Schnurmann] chaos that sometimes arises around her, similar to the pleasure I get when I manage to make a child feel comfortable or to create comfort and order for Oscar. I recall Oscar's initial intention, before we were legally married, that comfort and order, as well as sharing thoughts and feelings, could not be created by the same person, especially 'the wife' and slowly changing his mind that he might be wrong, and I might indeed do so. The moments of this realization were perhaps with the happiest in my life. They did not exist all the time and when he returned to his old view, these were the most unhappy moments of my life.

Summarizing the thoughts, she wrote down at the lake in Walberswick, she concludes (original English):

What does it all matter in the end? I am in this world like a soap bubble in the tub of soapy water I gave the children to play with. But as I live in this moment, it is good to become aware of all this joy that I have written down, and there are more of them than I have listed. E.g., the joy of being able to say 'no' to something I don't feel like doing.

I have never really wished to be anywhere but where I am, because I know that wherever you go, you take yourself with you, and being happy with yourself is the best place to be. So instead of wishing to be somewhere, the best thing is to work on knowing yourself and your wishes and if you are able to fulfil them, then it is that you can say 'I am a happy person'.

Accustomed to caring for others throughout her life, this also determined her everyday life after she retired. Until 1995 she also looked after her relatives, with whom she had lived at the beginning of her time in England; all three of them were very old. She visited them daily; one of them still lived in her flat, the other in a nursing home.

So that too was a contact that was important for my weekly schedule or programme. Because I knew I had to go there at that time of day, didn't I? I think [–] if you think, how do I do it best, that later [–], without working, it's not difficult for me, you must make a programme. You must have a fixed programme, because I'm so used to getting up in the morning and going to work [–] that I usually don't go to work now. When I'm done, I go shopping. I must go out and shop or go somewhere. Of course, I go to the theatre a lot, I go to concerts a lot, I read a lot. I'm not bored. I'm not lonely either. I like living alone too, because living alone has enormous advantages.

(Friedmann, interview, 21 November, 1996)

Anneliese Schnurmann is also one of the people she partly cared for. 'Anneliese Schnurmann is a very good friend of mine. I am in constant contact with her. Well, she is my best friend here, so to speak. And we spend every Sunday together' (Friedmann, interview, 28 June, 1996). They already knew each other from their work at Hampstead Clinic and became friends after Anneliese Schnurmann moved into the flat above that of the Friedmann couple in 1959. Oscar Friedmann had asked his wife to keep an eye out to see if an analyst could move into the flat above theirs, as a family with noisy children had previously lived there, which greatly disturbed his psychoanalytical work. After the sudden death of Oscar Friedmann, Manna considered whether she and Anneliese Schnurmann could rent/buy a house together, in which each of them would have their own flat. When they could not accomplish this, they both bought their own flats in 1961.

Claudia Schnurmann, a distant relative of Anneliese Schnurmann's and professor of North American and Atlantic History at the University of Hamburg, carried out historical research in London in the early 1990s and met Manna Friedmann.

Manna has been a real friend to me. In the mornings she would dismiss me into the adventure of the London archives with the saying 'Happy hunting'; in the evenings she would get my frustration or – thank God more often – my glowing reports about great finds. And she really took an interest in these things, asked questions, listened, and thus helped me incredibly. Nothing is worse than being alone at this stage of research. We've been bouncing around the London theatre and restaurant scene together, we've watched films that made Manna's ears go red as a turkey but bravely endured all sorts of frank, true-to-life sequences, and we've chatted, endlessly literally, about God and the world, books, people, dogs (Anna Freud's sneaky chow-chow) and Manna's incredibly exciting life, which she has loved despite all the sadness, all the misery. I have lived with Manna for many, many wonderful months. One highlight was when we sang Cologne carnival songs together – Manna sang Ostermann songs at the top of her lungs, a sight and sound to behold! I often stayed with Anneliese, but the stays were usually shorter – a few times she entrusted me with her flat in Netherhall Gardens, always in fear that the balcony might break off or the façade might collapse.

(C. Schnurmann, interview, 12 June, 2021)

Manna also looked after the son of a Portuguese caretaker family who worked for the Freud family. She taught him and when, in the early 1990s, she visited Cologne together with Claudia Schnurmann, Manna Friedmann insisted on buying a rosary at the 'Black Madonna' in St Mary's Church for the Portuguese caretaker family (C. Schnurmann, interview, 1 June, 2021).

Relationship with Anna Freud in old age

When Anna Freud needed more support, the American Alice Colonna, a former analyst and graduate of the Hampstead Education Programme, took leave from her work at the Yale Child Study Centre

to be a support and help to Anna Freud. This generous and voluntary assignment was carefully camouflaged so that it was presented to Anna Freud as something that was supposedly in the best interests of her guest [...] While Alice Colonna discreetly managed to establish herself as a replacement for the former caring nanny, Manna Friedmann, the retired kindergarten teacher, was also accepted by Anna Freud as a Jewish mother, as the German-speaking nanny with whom they could recite German poems, sing songs from their school days and do all the needlework projects, knitting and weaving, together. In 1981, when Manna Friedmann often came to 20 Maresfield Gardens, 85-year-old Anna Freud announced with joy that it was time for her to take up a new profession, as she was really too old to still care for patients: she and Manna Friedmann would make hand-woven things and sell them under the name 'Mandanna'.

(Young-Bruehl, 1988, p. 338f)

Anna Freud kept people at a distance; they were mainly seen professionally. You didn't come to Anna Freud for a chat, there was no such thing. You had to have a reason [–], you had to have something to talk about or you came to weave.

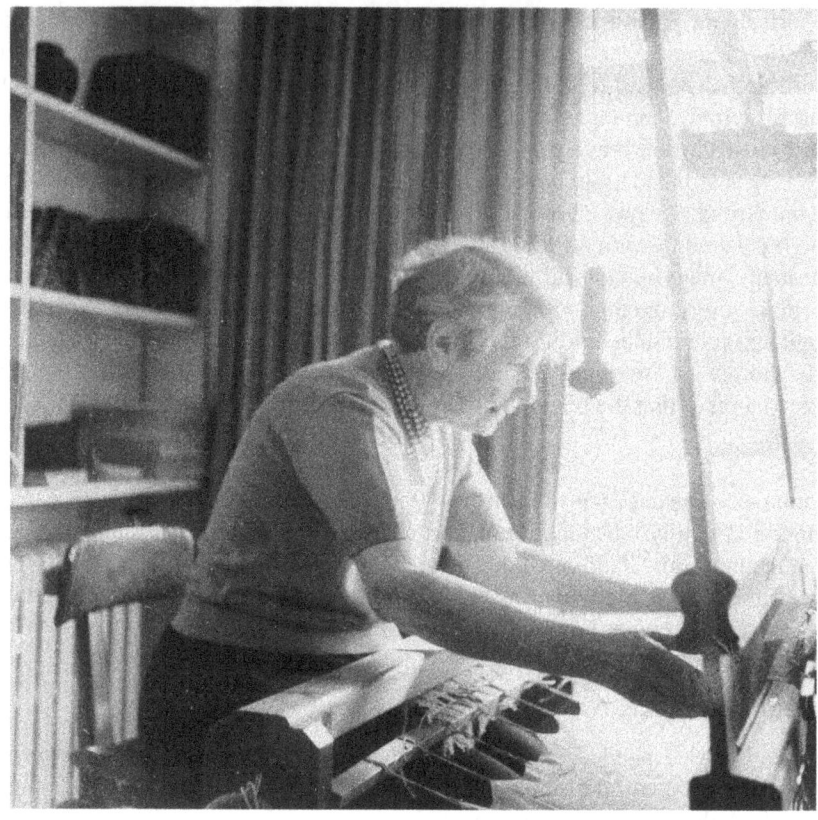

Anna Freud at the loom (credit: Manna Friedmann)

We were also connected by weaving, which she enjoyed enormously. But you always must have help there [-], sometimes. And she had a loom in Wolberswick in the country house and one here. So, we often went there together for the weekend, and that was [-] mainly because of these activities, that we somehow got very close to each other and on a completely different basis.

Personally. I just wanted to say that [-] and then decided against it. That's what Elisabeth Young-Bruehl told me for the first time. Because one felt, as I said, one felt honoured [–] yes, Manna is there with Anna Freud, but that was because I was the kindergarten teacher. And Elisabeth said, quite rightly, I was the nanny for her. The nanny she had in her youth because she was the last of a big family. And when she left, she missed her very much. Anna Freud was a teacher and internally remained a teacher until the end. In 1916, a former student of Anna Freud brought her a poetry album, 'May God keep fresh and long for you these things four: eyes to fathom beauty, soul to sense beauty, mind to remember beauty, hands to make beauty'. Isn't that delightful? Well, she was just such a creative person and when I drew a pattern for her to weave, she said: 'But don't make it too complicated, because don't forget that I write my lectures while I'm weaving.' [–] So not a minute was wasted. I think time was the most precious thing she had. An especially creative person. Today you would call her a workaholic, which I think she was.

(Friedmann, interview, 12 July, 1996)

After Anna Freud had a stroke on 1 March, 1982, she spent three months in hospital. Elisabeth Young-Bruehl (1988, p. 343) writes:

Her motor skills and speech were affected, although her mind remained as clear as it had been when she asked Josephine Stross during the ambulance ride to the hospital: 'Is this the end?' Over the next few months, as she valiantly struggled to make herself understood, to focus her eyes enough to read the headlines in the newspapers and to gain enough control of her trembling hands to do simple knitting, Anna Freud often wished that the end had actually come at that time: 'I never knew you could be so miserable'.

Manna Friedmann told:

She had hoped that I would move in there, as she said that when Manna is here, I don't need a sister. But I refused because I have other obligations. But that was her feeling. And why? Elisabeth Young-Bruehl expressed that very well, and I had never thought about it before. You know, Anna Freud was a person who [–], one had the feeling that it was an honour to help her in any way, to serve, to work and her satisfaction [–] It was somehow a special honour. I can't remember the German words. [–] That was her special art, I think people felt honoured when she asked for something from you. And I think she was disappointed, but I didn't think I could do that. But I was with her almost every day for three hours after she came home from the hospital. And those were good times, but also very sad times, because she lost more and more the use of her voice. Well, that means the voice was very quiet, she couldn't swallow any more, and it got worse and worse. So, I spent a lot of time like that, but before that, when she was in the hospital, I also spent long hours with her. We visited her every day, and she was in a wheelchair. And I took her up to Hampstead Heath and we could sit on a bench, peacefully and there's a little lake and there were birds, and we took some food with us and then we fed the birds. So, she had an almost childlike joy on these little trips and enjoyed it so much.

(Friedmann, interview, 12 July, 1996)

Anna Freud was cared for at home by a new housekeeper since Paula Fichtl, who had worked in Freud's household for over 50 years, had become in need of care herself, and was only reluctantly willing to pass things on to someone else.

Young-Bruehl (1988) describes how Anna Freud was able to live out the last summer quietly with the help of her new housekeeper, paid nurses, her doctors, and the support of Alice Colonna and Manna. Visits usually gave her little pleasure. Only with Manna Friedmann was she comfortable, and this made it very difficult for Anna Freud to let Manna leave in August and September for her annual visit to her brother in Philadelphia. 'I don't agree with your brother claiming you. I am sicker than he is', she said with the vehemence of a small child who does not want to tolerate a rival for the attention of her 'nanny' (Friedmann, interview, 12 July, 1996).

By the time Manna Friedmann returned from America at the beginning of October, Anna Freud could hardly speak and had to support her head with the hand she could control, her right one. 'Sehr schlecht,' she announced 'very bad.' The shaking became so extreme by the seventh of October that a neurologist who had been consulted before came to the house and prescribed an opiate to quell it. Like her father before her, she had been brought to the limit of her tolerance, and she had said in her halting voice, 'I cannot stand it any more.' Early in the morning of October 9, she died in her restless sleep.

(Young-Bruehl, 1988, p. 452)

End of life

After the death of Alice Goldberger, Manna Friedmann became the centre of the meeting of the former children of Lingfield House. She had a special relationship with some of them throughout her life, such as with Judith Sherman, to whom she also gave the letters that the 'Lingfield children' had written to her in Israel.

She came to visit me in Israel [–]. We were of course always in touch. Came to visit me and on that visit, she met the man on the kibbutz whom she married and with whom she has three fabulous children [–] Two doctors and a psychologist. And when I see these children that I see every year, I think to myself [–] I have so many thoughts. First of all, it's a miracle that they are there at all. They were not supposed to be here. But at the same time, I must think how many such fabulous people have been lost to mankind. We don't even know what we have lost. Always humanity – us. Who is 'us'? Humanity. And what they [–] what they had to offer mankind. I mean, there were artists there and writers there and musicians and all kinds of things. And simple people too, of course. But like I said [–] they, uh [–] they made it. But she [Judith] couldn't talk about this all these years [–] of that time. But, as the daughter got married, the daughter asked her and she almost really [–] almost bombarded [her], that she should tell her something. And that's when she started, and it wasn't easy. The daughter, with whom I also got along well [–], she is a doctor, asked me: 'Do you think I pushed my mother too hard?' And then I say: 'No, maybe it's just as well. She never talked about it.' But I [–] She had spoken to me. And then she started. [–] She went back to Ravensbrück.

(Friedmann, interview, 12 July, 1996)

Judith also visited her in Israel, where she met her husband. In her obituary for Manna Friedmann, she describes how, in Israel, Manna not only 'examined' her future husband, an American, but also chose her wedding dress with her (Sherman, 2015). Both later worked as social workers and family therapists and live near New Jersey, about 20 minutes from Princeton. Manna Friedmann found it difficult to understand the couple's decision to move into their own house in a retirement community at the age of 60 (Friedmann, interview 12 July, 1999).

Judith Sherman wrote in her obituary how they, living only an hour away from her retirement home, visited each other.

> When son David visits from Milwaukee or Allen from Arkansas the question always 'When do we see Manna?' And they do. As does Mirjam from Arizona and her son Joshua from California. Zdenka comes from England and Vicky's family from Seattle. Our daughter Ora and her children Ilana, Sara, and Michael are here today and are here frequently. There rooms are decorated with Manna made needle points, their hearts filled with love for Manna – a most treasured person in their life.
>
> (Sherman, 2015, p. 68)

When I arrived at one of the interview appointments a little prematurely, she told me, laughing, that she always comes too early, she knows this 'problem'. In her disciplined way everything was wonderfully tidy with her, as always.

'Manna learned to play the piano in her old age and had a "mute switch" installed so that the neighbourhood was not disturbed by her playing' (C. Schnurmann,

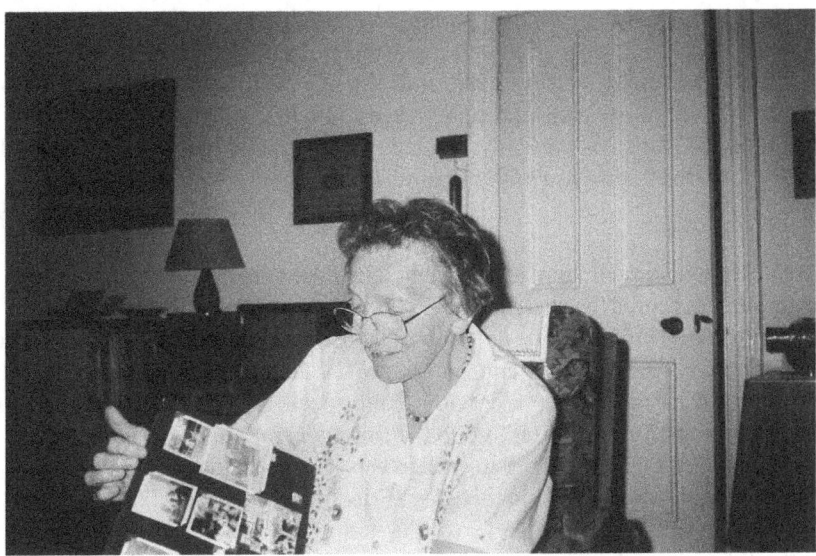

Manna Friedmann showing her photo album to the author, 1996 (credit: Christiane Ludwig-Körner)

interview, 1 June, 2021). She always had to be on the move; too much activity was better than too little. She reported how now, at the age of 82, she was beginning to feel her age. Until recently, she had not considered herself as 'old', but lately she feels more and more how 'only the spirit is still fresh'. She had visited Gertrud Dann a few months previously with Eva, a woman from the Theresienstadt children's group. Her real name was Rahel, but since there was already a girl with that name in the Lingfield group, she was called Eva. That day she enthusiastically talked about the meeting of the Lingfield children that had taken place in the summer of 1997. Manna Friedmann had organized the whole party, assisted by Zdenka Husserl. Laughing, she told how they had cooked far too much and only a third could be eaten. From afternoon to evening, about forty people met in the small flat of an alumnus. There are beautiful photos where she sits relaxed in the circle of alumni and happily looks at 'her big crowd of children'. At that time these 'children' were all over 50 to about 65 years old.

We talk about what has become of these children and whether they coped well with their difficult fate at the beginning of their lives. Manna Friedmann believed that the genetic and original family background was decisive for their later development as well as severe real traumas. Until her old age, she regularly wrote many letters to her large circle of friends and acquaintances and to the many children she had cared for in the past:

People ask me: 'What do you do all day, when you are retired?' I have no time at all. I think it is absolutely essential to prepare for retirement when work stops. And I think that's one of the reasons why psychoanalysts continue to work so long. First of all, it's a given, a psychoanalyst can work for a very long time. Anna Freud saw patients until the end, that is, until she had this stroke. She had always said: 'I waited too long. Now I can't do it any more'. You have to stop before then [–].

When we are all getting older and, and are busy coping with getting older ourselves, all our friends and relatives are much, much worse off than we are. [Laughter.] Well, you can only be glad that you are at least willing and able to help. And that is the case with me now. But I am very well.

(Friedmann, interview, 5 June, 1997)

While Manna Friedmann never wanted children of her own in the past, she sometimes has regrets as she gets older. It was only recently that she realized that one should have children of one's own. 'Those who have children of their own are simply different" (Friedmann, interview, 28 June, 1998). She and Anneliese Schnurmann agreed that they were now, so to speak, the ones who were the mothers of their 'substitute children', up to the third generation. Manna Friedmann was moved by a film that caused her to realize very clearly that genes are immortal and therefore life goes on and on in this way (Friedmann, interview, 28 June, 1998).

I think I can say that at every stage of my existence, I have always thought that it should at least last for a long time as it is now. I have also enjoyed every stage of my work colossally, with the little ones, with the big ones, with the social welfare [work].

(Friedmann, interview, 26 November, 1996)

During our last interview (19 March, 2000) Manna Friedmann was already considering whether she should move to the USA 'sometime' to her brother's daughter (Helen Cohn) or to Tel Aviv to live with her sister's children. Both wanted to have her near them.

At that time, it was suggested (by me) that she should move to Israel (a country she loved and where she had friends and close relatives) and be supported by me and my sister [her Israeli niece and nephew] if necessary. But Helen convinced her that the facilities and availability and care in America were better.

(E. Wolkowski, personal correspondence, 14 June, 2020)

The move was then completed faster than she had imagined. This was after she stumbled in the street in the summer of 2001 and broke her wrist. Her niece Helen, who had moved into a retirement community with her husband in the USA in March 2001, came to London for a month to look after her.

Her arm had required a second surgery while I was there, and it was clear she could not be on her own. I decided to take her back with me to the retirement community, but actually intended to have her live out her life there. Eran was a new father and had 2 little children so could not be expected to come to England at a moment's notice and Chavah had obligations in Israel plus her English would not be good enough to deal with bureaucratic matters should they arise. I was then the only relative who could travel easily but did not want to take on that responsibility: hence, we arranged for her new home in the States. Auntie Matie adjusted very well after some understandable hesitations and the whole community just loved her. She helped with sewing and knitting, and gladly made bags to hang on the walkers of those who needed them and was happy to do any clothing alterations. She started out in the Independent Living section of our Community, eventually needing to transfer to Assisted Living and finally to Skilled Nursing. I was officially in charge of any decisions, including when she had to be transferred to the local hospital for hospice care where she died.

(H. Cohen, personal correspondence, 3 April, 2003)

Manna was perfectly fine when she moved to America, and in good health. After spending some time there, she even complained constantly that she was persuaded to move to America, a culture and environment she did not like. Finally, and with the help of her niece, she got used to it and was very active, swimming every day and attending lectures and social events (E. Wolkowski, personal correspondence, 14 June, 2020).

But still, it was a big change for her, as she was always used to managing everything on her own.

> To make matters worse – speaking of her independence – the unfortunate thing was that her status in America was not 'kosher' (legalized), which made it impossible for her to travel from the USA to London or Tel Aviv. For fear that she would not be allowed to enter the USA on her return journey. So, she got stuck there during her long, good years.
>
> (E. Wolkowski, personal correspondence, 14 June, 2020)

> Until 2011 she was well, and she had no major health problems. In summer 2011 she got a pretty bad cold and pneumonia as a result. Although she recovered, she lost some of her strength and sharpness. At that time, it was decided that she should move to the semi dependent wing of this institution (called 'the manor house'). She continued to swim and attend social events but began to use a walking aid to compensate. In two years, her abilities deteriorated, and she was eventually transferred to the fully supported wing. At that time Manna started to move around the village in a wheelchair.
>
> In November 2013 she got another severe case of pneumonia from which she never recovered. Manna died on 16 November, 2013.
>
> (E. Wolkowski, personal correspondence, 14 June, 2020)

One of her last visitors was Andra Bucci, who visited her shortly before her death. The Italian sisters Andra and Tatiana Bucci stayed in contact with Manna their whole lives and experienced her like a second mother. But they had not seen each other for a long time.

> 'You are real people!' she exclaimed, in a heavy German accent, beaming at the grey-haired women she had loved as children. There were tears. Andra and Tatiana spent nearly seven hours with Manna that Saturday. Judith Sherman, a Weir Courtney survivor who donated the house's archives to the Holocaust Museum, came from New Jersey to see the sisters. They looked at old photos. Manna sang 'Eine kleine Nachtmusik' with every Mozartean flourish. The next day, we had a second, five-hour visit. Andra and Tatiana had brought the doll, the purse and the hat – the going-away gifts that they treasure today as much as they did when they left Weir Courtney 67 years ago. Manna stared at the hat and bag, as if reaching into the depths of her memory in search of their meaning.
>
> 'Oh, wait, yes! Oh, wait a minute. Yes!' she cried. 'Yes!' She held and gazed at the doll that had travelled so far. We talked about Mira and the 'great, great joy' Manna remembered at Weir Courtney when the Buccis found their children. Andra and Tatiana regret that their mother never had a chance to meet her. 'We are lucky,' Manna said. 'No, no,' Andra replied. '*We* are very lucky.' 'We are all lucky,' Manna returned. 'It's good to be alive.' 'Today is a lovely day,'

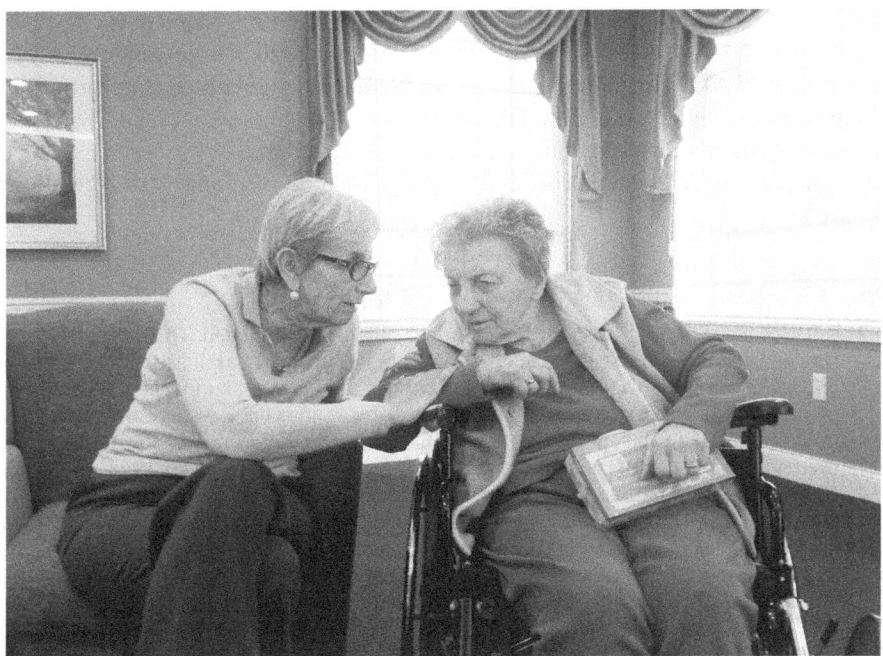

Manna Friedmann in a wheelchair with Andra Bucci, one of the Bucci sisters, in her retirement home, November, 2013 (credit: Getty Images)

said Andra. It was an expression that Manna had often said to herself when she awoke to the English morning.

'I have heard it said,' Manna's niece, Helen, wrote to the sisters and to me later, 'that people often die near or around an important life event.' Helen would always wonder, she said, if the sisters' visit with Manna was one such event, 'as she let go shortly after that'.

(Langer, 2013)

Helen Cohen organized a memorial service for Manna Friedmann, inviting anyone who knew her both in and out of the community. 'It was an amazing time, and Emily Langer (who wrote the Washington Post article) and Rebecca Erbelding of the US Holocaust Museum attended. We spent hours poring over information and the photos from Weir Courtney' (H. Cohen, personal correspondence, 03 April, 2003).

Sources and personal communications

Interviews with Manna Friedmann 12.7.1996, 21.11.1996, 26.11.1996, 23.4.1997, 5.6.1997, 19.9.1997, 15.2.1998, 28.6.1998, 19.3.2000.

E-Mails: Eran Wolkowski: 13 June, 2020; 14 June, 2020; 6 September, 2020; 30 September, 2020; 8 November, 2020; 9 November, 2020; 11 November, 2020; 5 December, 2020; 9 December, 2020 (correspondence originally in English).
Claudia Schnurmann: interview 1 June, 2021.
E-Mails: Cornelia Schnurmann: 2 June, 2021; 6 June, 2021.
E-Mails: Helen Cohen: 3 April, 2003; 28 July, 2023 (correspondence originally in English).

Notes

1 In 1919, the 'Private Jewish reform grammar school' was founded. The head of the new 'Jawne School', as it was then called, was Rabbi Dr Emanuel Carelbach. '"Jawne" is not only a name, but also a programme full of content, which is in significant in the tradition of Judaism. Jawne is the ancient Jewish city which, after the destruction of Jerusalem in 70 AD, became the spiritual centre of the resurgent Judaism. [...] Jawne is located near Ashdod, south of present-day Tel-Aviv and was re-founded in 1948' (Corbach, 1990, p. 21). From 1929 to 1942, Dr Menachem Erich Klibansky was the director of the Jawne School. Thanks to his help, far more than one hundred pupils were able to be rescued as part of the Kindertransport to England. He himself, his wife and three sons were deported to the East and murdered. https://www.yadvashem.org/yv/de/exhibitions/through-the-lens/klibansky.asp (accessed 26 January, 2021).

2 Prof Bruno Zacharias Kisch, MD (1890 Prague - 1966 Bad Nauheim), specialist in heart and circulation, had taken over the chairmanship of the Jawne Board of Trustees as successor to Rabbi Dr Rosenthal. He was co-founder of the German Society for Cardiovascular Research and founded the *Journal for Circulatory Research* in 1927. In 1936 he was dismissed from the University of Cologne (Corbach, 1990, p. 216 f.).

3 Dora Loeb (1905 Bonn–1944 Riga) was a musician (viola and violin). She was the daughter of Walther Löb and Agnes Frank. He was initially a private lecturer in physical chemistry at Bonn University, and later head of the chemical department at the Rudolf Virchow Hospital in Berlin. After his early death, his wife moved with their four daughters to Lessingstrasse 22 in Bonn. All four sisters spent their school years at the 'Städtische Studienanstalt' (now Clara Schumann Secondary School). At the age of 16, Dora left the school to study music, first at the Cologne Conservatory and later at the Leipzig Conservatory. After her studies, she became a music teacher at the Heidelberg Conservatory. She became a member of the Abendroth Chamber Orchestra in Cologne; as a Jew she was dismissed in 1933, then became a member of the Kulturbund Orchestra in Frankfurt/Main. In 1935 she was selected as violist for the Palestine Orchestra in Palestine but returned to Germany due to adverse living conditions. After her return, she worked as a music and drawing teacher at the Cologne Jawne until her deportation to Riga on 7 December, 1941. On 3 or 4 August, 1944, she was shot in the woods near Riga. http://www.familienbuch-euregio.de/genius/?person=468436 (accessed 21 January, 2023)

4 Manna Friedmann seems not to have known that the song originated in the youth movement and was sung more in leftist circles. From Horst Wessel comes 'Die Fahne hoch' (The flag high).

5 Dora Weindling met Norbert-Nathan Wolkowski (1915 Katowice–2002 Jerusalem) in the British prison camp in Atlit (south of Haifa, then Palestine). He became a drawing and art teacher at Jerusalem primary schools and a teacher of fashion drawing and history at a vocational high school for girls. He held these positions after leaving Kibbutz Be'erot Ytzhak (1957). He left his two children (Chava and Eran Wolkowski) on the kibbutz. The painter and cartoonist Eran Wolkowski, born in 1947, was given her flat in London after Manna Friedmann moved to the USA, and Chava became a teacher of children from difficult families.

Publications by Manna Friedmann

Colonna, A. B. & Friedmann, M. (1984). Prediction of development. *Psychoanalytic Study of the Child*, *39*, 509–526. https://doi.org/10.1080/00797308.1984.11823440

Friedmann, M. (1986). Alice Goldberger. *Bulletin of the Anna Freud Centre*, *9*, 313–314.

Friedmann, M. (2007). 1933–1939 Life in Germany. *'45 Society*, *31*, 34–36.

Salo, F., Friedmann, M. (1988). The Runaway Bunny Mother: The long-term influence of the nursery school experience. *Bulletin of the Anna Freud Centre*, *1*, 57–73.

4

Anneliese Schnurmann (31.1.1908–21.9.2006) – Wanderer Between Worlds

When I visited Anneliese Schnurmann for the first time in June 1996, a petite woman opened her door to me, looking at me kindly with her nimble brown eyes. Although she was already 86 years old, she still had a girlish aura about her.

Anneliese Schnurmann was born on 31 January, 1908, in Karlsruhe as the second daughter of a wealthy Jewish family. 'They wanted to call me Anne-Elisabeth and register me as Anne-Elisabeth, but then call me Anneliese, and my father, in his excitement all the way to the registry office, forgot about it and registered me as Anneliese' (Schnurmann, interview, 6 August, 1997).

Her father, Jakob Schnurmann, was born on 3 May, 1861, the eldest of four, in Muggensturm, Rastatt County, Baden-Württemberg. His parents were Samuel

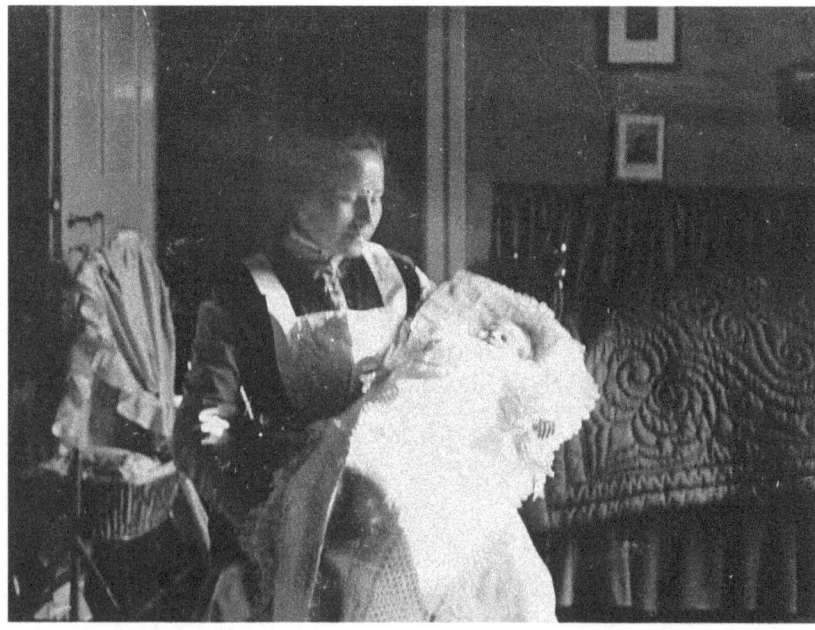

Anneliese Schnurmann with her nanny 'Loline' (Louise Blei) in Karlsruhe, 1908 (credit: Anneliese Schnurmann)

DOI: 10.4324/9781003403906-5

Schnurmann (1835–1915) and Fanny Schnurmann, née Vogel (1839–1912). They continued the old textile company Vogel & Schnurmann, which had been founded in Muggensturm in 1833 by Juda Levi Vogel (1794–1867), the maternal grandfather of Jakob Schnurmann. Samuel Vogel and his brother-in-law Samuel Schnurmann had also bought a bankrupt paper mill (Gramberger & Sack) and other properties in Ettlingen at auction in 1878 and founded the paper company Vogel & Bernheimer, to which a pulp mill was later added, and moved the company headquarters to Karlsruhe in 1878. In 1914, it was one of the most important companies in this industry in the German Empire and had 500 employees. Samuel Vogel, his brother-in-law Samuel Schnurmann, and Simon Bernheimer were the major partners in 1884.

According to Anneliese Schnurmann, her father, Jakob Hirsch Schnurmann, was director of a paper mill – presumably he was involved in the Vogel & Schnurmann company (Schnurmann, interview, 26 April, 1997). Her mother originated from Stuttgart, and as assimilated Jews, her family had already begun celebrating Christmas two generations earlier, while Anneliese Schnurmann's father 'was somewhat more strictly religious'. Even before Anneliese was born, her parents showed great social commitment. At the age of 46, Jakob Hirsch Schnurmann died on 24 April, 1908, the consequence of a riding accident – barely three months after the birth of his daughter Anneliese. It can be assumed that the grief felt by her mother, Alice Schnurmann née Auerbach, overshadowed Anneliese's early childhood. Anneliese Schnurmann said about her father (Schnurmann, interview, 26 April, 1997):

> And he had many women as employees. And the women had children, both legitimate and illegitimate. And then he found that you shouldn't take them away from their mothers. And so, he built a house for children. [...] there were nuns, and they took care of these children. [...] Mother took care of so-called 'fallen girls'. Actually, she was interested in music and painting, but she felt sorry for the girls because they behaved so stupidly [...].

Anneliese Schnurmann remembers how her mother, who owned a gramophone, listened to Wagner operas with her, which Anneliese Schnurmann did not particularly love, but she did treasure the special attention from her mother, especially when she read poems to her. Particularly during the war, these were very nice memories for her to enjoy and which supported her.

Her mother contracted tuberculosis, which led the five-year-old and her sister Leonore (1896–1989) to live with relatives in Marseille for over a year. One year later, while her mother was in a sanatorium in Bonn because of her illness, Anneliese Schnurmann went to live with a maternal aunt in Spain for three months. After her mother's death in 1915, a guardian (a medical officer and staff doctor) was appointed to take the two girls into his family, which they vehemently resisted. They managed to continue living in their parents' house, together with the trusted employees, under the care of the unloved guardian. Upon reaching school age, Anneliese Schnurmann went to school in Karlsruhe for the first few years.

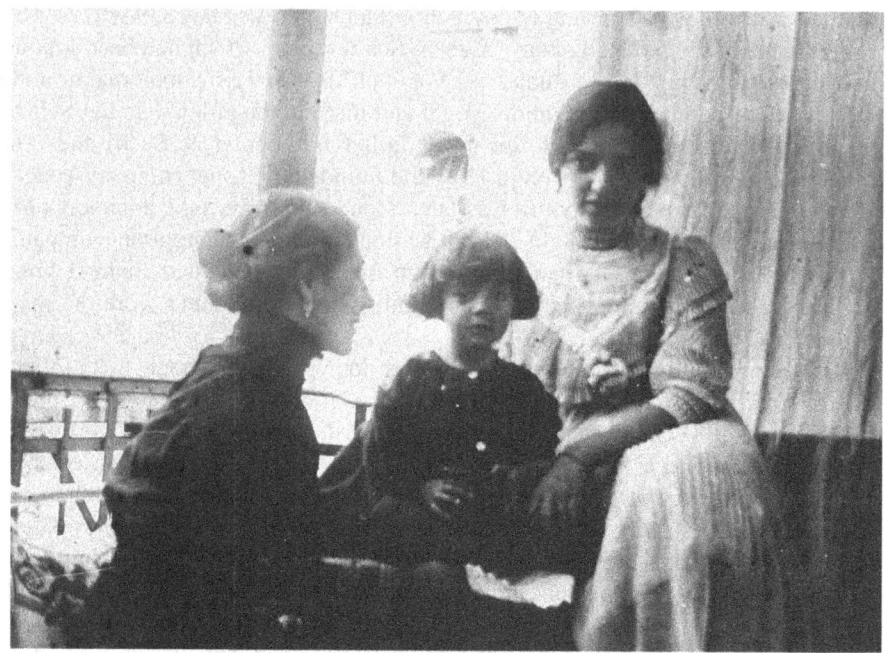

Anneliese Schnurmann with her sister Leonore, probably in 1911/1912 (credit: Anneliese Schnurmann)

When Anneliese Schnurmann was 14, her sister married Moritz Straus (1882–1959),[1] the managing director of Argus-Motoren-Gesellschaft and Horch-Werke (later part of Audi) and moved to Berlin (Humboldt-Strasse 12), and the young couple took in Anneliese Schnurmann. She recalled:

> Humboldtstrasse 12 in Grunewald. When you came over the Halensee Bridge, it was the second crossroads on the left. Exactly, at Humboldtstrasse 12, the Halensee Bridge at the end of Kurfürstendamm. That's where we had animals because food was a bit scarce after the first war. We had a goat and we had chickens, they lived in Humboldtstrasse.
>
> (Schnurmann, interview, 24 November, 1996)

When she later visited her niece Hannah in Berlin, she wanted to see the old house.

> It was completely bombed. I saw it when it was broken. But then it lay fallow for a while and now it's an old people's home, it's there now. And Hannele even went inside, looked around everywhere and talked to people and asked. She was just sorry that all the trees were gone from the garden. I don't know why they were cut down. Such a wonderful chestnut tree in front of the children's room and a walnut tree under which we always ate. That was never again. And there was also a small slope, it went down a bit. And they levelled it, probably for the old people.
>
> (Schnurmann, interview, 24 November, 1996)

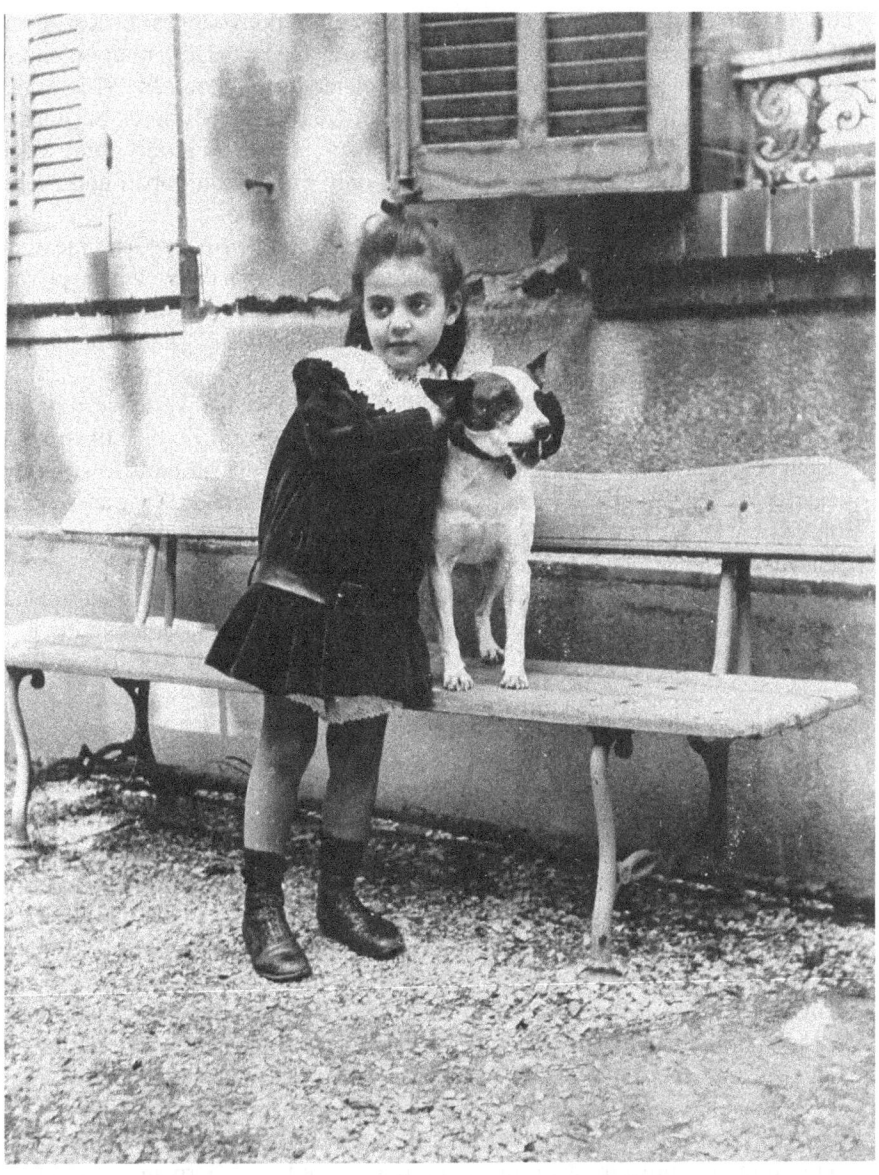

As a six-year-old, one year before the death of her mother (credit: Anneliese Schnurmann)

She saw her two nieces, Hannah and Julia, as younger siblings, and her involvement with them awakened her lifelong interest in child development. She remained in close contact with them and their offspring until the end of her life, but although she got along very well with her nieces, she felt not quite comfortable in her sister's family, 'because my sister just couldn't be my mother' (Schnurmann, interview, 24 November, 1996).

This made her friendship with Susanne Bonhoeffer, the youngest of Karl Bon-hoeffer's (Professor of Neurology and Psychiatry in Berlin) eight children, all the more important for her when she came to her elementary school. In 1921, Anneliese Schnurmann had already started the seventh year at the Bismarck Secondary School in Siemensstrasse in Berlin-Grunewald. "... This was a very long, good friendship with the whole family." They lived only five minutes apart and developed a very close relationship with each other.

More can be learned about the girls' friendship in Susanne Bonhoeffer's memoirs (Koslowski, 2018). When Susanne Bonhoeffer transferred from the Wellmann private school to the Latin branch of the Bismarck Secondary School at the end of the Easter vacations in 1922 with her leaving certificate, she met Anneliese Schnurmann there:

> A black-haired girl, with whom I was walking home together, since we both had to walk along Bismarck-Allee, spoke with such a nice South German dialect that I liked her right away. After a few minutes she told me that she was Jewish. The next day she also asked me what my father was, and in response to my answer she told me that he had made her sister well. Thus began my friendship with Anneliese Schnurmann. Although I did not attend this class for more than half a year (and still missed a lot), I later had the firm awareness that only this school semester had been meaningful for me, because I got to know Anneliese and Bärbel during it.
>
> (Koslowski, 2018, p. 215)

She continues to write about her friendship with Anneliese Schnurmann:

> She thought very internationally – European. How can you say the Lord's Prayer with 'as we forgive those who trespass against us' when you hate the French? she asked me. I fought and argued with her about my national sentiments; I even tried to defend the war, drawing on war poetry and war painting, Red Cross and sacrifice. In the long run, I could not resist her clear logic that a dignified life could only grow in peace and freedom and was based on the will to understand in large and small ways [...].
>
> Anneliese felt distinctly German, even as a citizen of Baden, as a citizen of Karlsruhe, and her dialect was unmistakable. But she had Jewish relatives in Spain, in France, in America. Nevertheless, she was deliberately German and not Spanish like her cousin, because her parents and ancestors had lived in Germany for a long time and she wanted to stay in Germany. She made an effort to teach me the breadth of European thinking. She loved Germany and did not want to hate France, and I began to detach myself from much that had seemed sacrosanct to me until then. Her politics seemed to me much more Christian than mine. She was Christian by nature and disposition, but did not want to give up her Jewish faith (of which, however, she knew no more than I did of the Old Testament) so as not to be unfaithful to the heritage of her forefathers. Only if one was securely rooted in this heritage, if one did not have to be vainly intent on what was not one's due, she thought, could one also allow the other to be valid,

could one honour the heritage of other fathers. We talked a lot about politics. She soon clearly took the lead, I thought.

(Koslowski, 2018, p. 84 f.)

In the Bonhoeffer family, Anneliese Schnurmann found a kind of substitute family, similar to the family-like circle she later found around Anna Freud (Schnurmann, interview, 24 November, 1996). It was a matter of course that she was integrated into the family circle:

At half past four we had vespers; from five o'clock on, people came one after the other, for whom the Sunday afternoon was getting boring at home. Often Anneliese was there, who felt superfluous on Sundays at home, because her brother-in-law came then. Therefore, we arranged it as much as possible so that we were both together at this time, which is why I cancelled other invitations for Sunday simply for 'family reasons'. When there were guests, Anneliese could always join them, because everyone was especially fond of her. She then usually stayed for dinner and enjoyed the sumptuous elaboration with three or four courses. My father loved to eat in the evening, and it suited him well. So dinner was our most upscale meal. But Gert didn't have a lively Sunday at home either, and he joined us first as a friend of Klaus. Dohnanyi's and Delbrück's age-matched children, too, of course. Where there are many children in the house, single children and smaller sibling groups are magnetically attracted. Slowly it became a regular Sunday circle, at least in the winter.

(Koslowski, 2018, p. 283)

But Susanne Bonhoeffer also enjoyed the Christmas atmosphere with other friendly families:

There the trees were mostly of noble fir, with white big candles, very densely hung with tinsel. Against our colourful funny tree, it seemed decidedly distinguished and restrained. One did not exclude oneself but emphasized more the decorative side. Dietrich thought that these were Jewish Christmas trees. It was completely different with Anneliese Schnurmann. There, too, the tree was a wonder, with lots of pretty accessories. We lay on the thick carpet, ate Swabian pastries, put records on the gramophone, read new books or played 'Kasperle' for the little nieces. The most beautiful thing was to light a few candles in the twilight and to tell ourselves made-up stories. Here it was not at all strange for me, but as beautiful as at home.

(Koslowski, 2018, p. 184 f.)

Even long after they had finished school, they attended musical and theatrical events together:

I couldn't do anything with Wagner, although I was very much at home with the German folk and heroic sagas. But there was just too much music for me.

Anneliese and I started laughing so much at a Lohengrin performance about the over-fat Elsa and the blond-haired, very Jewish-looking Lohengrin that we [...] left during the main intermission. We preferred to sit down in a good pastry shop and spent a merry late afternoon. We had both already finished school when Anneliese bought tickets for 'Peterchens Mondfahrt'. We were grown up enough to fully enjoy this nice fairy tale play, which also featured a number of talented children.

(Koslowski, 2018, p. 272)

I came to fully enjoyable, well-rounded theatre evenings through Anneliese, when her Straus siblings took us; that was during the time when we went together to the Pestalozzi-Fröbel-Haus and even later (until my engagement). With them we went to the modern, small plays in the Kammerspiele, in the Komödie and other pretty little theatres, where we siblings otherwise never went, because the seats were much too expensive. We drove up in the car, had wonderful seats, and afterwards often drove to a small but good restaurant to eat and drink something. Then the car took us home again, and I was there on time.

(Koslowski, 2018, p. 273)

[...] When I was taken to the theatre by the Strauses, I finally felt like an only child and, with the knowledge I had acquired, I had something ahead of my brothers, which they sometimes envied. Otherwise, my theatre experiences were always influenced by the impression of the crowd with which we attended. Except with Anneliese, I never went to the theatre with just one other person.

(Koslowski, 2018, p. 274)

Conversely, Anneliese Schnurmann was often taken to the cinema:

However, one of my brothers had to come along to the evening show at nine o'clock, otherwise I was not allowed to go. But since Klaus also watched every good film, I always had him to accompany me. Often we also picked up Anneliese, who didn't like to be alone in the evening. Sometimes Klaus would drag us to the nearby Cafe Engadin, and we would drink juice and beer. Of course, we brought Anneliese home afterwards. 'Include me in your night prayer', Klaus said, when saying goodbye to her. We stayed at the garden door to see that she got inside safely and was not attacked by a robber from the bushes. Only when they had unlocked the front door did we go home.

(Koslowski, 2018, p. 275)

Anneliese Schnurmann celebrated her sixteenth birthday with her entire class at the home of her sister, who had gone out that day to let her celebrate alone and undisturbed. It was a masquerade party, which Susanne Bonhoeffer had decorated with garlands and lanterns. 'Anneliese was enthusiastic about all the preparations – even if she thought the candles in the lanterns under the garlands were harmless only on my assurance that we always had it that way at our house' (Koslowski, 2018, p. 332 f.).

In the middle of the lively celebration,

> [...] flames zig-zagged back and forth through the parlours, the girls screamed and fled, and I had to hurriedly destroy my own work and tear everything down to save the curtains. Helpers came over and praised me for my presence of mind, but I had a very guilty conscience. Luckily no one had come to harm – only the thick Persian carpet had burn marks. To my relief, the insurance company stepped in and it was artfully mended. The Strauses, who soon came home, did not reproach me. [...] Two years later, Anneliese was about to graduate from high school, and I was already engaged. Again, she had invited her class to her birthday, some of whom still knew me from before.

Susanne Bonhoeffer had fun shocking her former classmates, who were astonished that she was engaged to a pastor (Walther Dress). She and Anneliese bought themselves

> [...] in the chemist's lipstick, eyebrow pencil, powder, cream and perfume! Then my cosmetic skills unfolded in front of Anneliese's vanity mirror. Curl on the forehead and in front of the ears rolled into sixes à la Carmen, and the make-up painted on thick like the 'Whore of Babylon'. Young girls in our circles did not behave like that at that time. And now I was a parish bride!
>
> In the best of moods we went to Mrs Straus and involved her in our plan, and she happily joined in. When the chic but solid Grunewald A-level girls came, you could literally hear them swallowing spit when they greeted me. We remained ironclad and serious. But afterwards, to my horror, Anneliese never enlightened the young ladies, and since I never saw any of them again, I probably remained rejected and regarded as vulgar for all of them. [...] Even when an aunt suddenly came to visit, we were not disturbed in the game and in the elevated mood. Mrs Straus, who was sitting at the table with us, did not betray us when this good lady from Baden asked me loudly in a pause in the conversation, pointing: 'Is this also a friend of Anneliese's?' There was now nothing more to make up for, and our inner cheerfulness grew.
>
> In the same outfit, Anneliese and I then went to our house for dinner, since the Strauses were going out and Anneliese was invited to our house. [...] My grandmother was horrified by me and terribly ashamed, especially in front of a distant relative (the so-called Tibet tablet, because he had taken research trips there) – but he of all people found me so 'charming'! My parents just laughed.
>
> (Koslowski, 2018, p. 333 f.)

Anneliese Schnurmann also became the confidante to whom Susanne Bonhoeffer entrusted her poems:

> Finally the time came when I subjected the poems not only to my own criticism, but to Anneliese's judgement. That was not a difficult decision, because she found them all good. Besides, she knew what moved me – why shouldn't she get to read my thoughts formulated?
>
> (Koslowski, 2018, 297)

She could also confide in Anneliese Schnurmann the terrible images and fears that haunted her, the feeling that she was standing on very thin glass and everything was dark underneath – or the feeling of sitting in a sled hurtling downhill. 'The only one who really had understanding for such thoughts and knew them herself was Anneliese Schnurmann. But she was so similar in thinking and feeling that it was no comfort to me (Koslowski, 2018, p. 420).

Eighteen-year-old Anneliese Schnurmann attended dance classes with Susanne Bonhoeffer, who was one year younger:

> Anneliese and I thought: just not as a marriage initiation – don't take anyone who has already passed his exams! [...] Of the fourteen boys between the ages of 19 and 23, eight were anxious to be considered my special knights. This was delightfully non-committal for me – but this reinforced Anneliese's shyness, and I was brutal enough not to care too much, but enjoyed the bevy of my admirers.
>
> (Koslowski, 2018, p. 313 f.)

The dancing lessons were concluded with a masquerade ball with 90 people in the Bonhoeffer family home, on the occasion of which Dietrich Bonhoeffer wore a

> [...] grass-green leotard sewn with reeds and a green creeper wig. Anneliese, who was otherwise decidedly shy, was transformed by her disguise as a cat. She asked me whether Dietrich had probably stuffed his calves. I answered, Yes, of course – pinch it! which she did at the next opportunity under the influence of the champagne and the freedom provided by her costume, to his great astonishment. She was unfamiliar with his unusually powerful musculature and very surprised not to encounter absorbent cotton. When my brothers were present at our parties, Anneliese always had it good; they found her by far the nicest of all my friends.
>
> (Koslowski, 2018, p. 315)

In the winter of 1926, the Straus family also gave a masquerade ball for Anneliese and Susanne's circle of friends, at which Anneliese appeared as a rococo lady with a fan. Anneliese remained a close friend of Susanne Bonhoeffer throughout her life, standing by her in difficult times, not the least of which were in their first years of marriage:

> Anneliese tried to solve my rigidity of soul in other ways. The first time she brought me a record player, 'Electrola' for cranking in suitcase form, the latest

thing! Plus all the records I particularly enjoyed listening to at the Strauses and quite a few others.

(Koslowski, 2018, p. 453 f.)

'Two years later, she had the idea to give me a dog' (Koslowski, 2018, p. 454). Together they picked out Bella at the animal welfare association at Alexanderplatz. In her childhood, a small dog had also helped Anneliese to get over the loss of her mother.

Anneliese Schnurmann often visited Susanne during semester breaks, and later during the Nazi period, when Anneliese was living in Switzerland and did not dare to write to her friend Susanne so as not to endanger her. She heard about how Anneliese was faring through friends of Sabine Bonhoeffer, who also lived in Switzerland:

I dreamed of her all the more for that: 'Uhland 1609', I kept calling, and she didn't answer or had just left again. Or we were sitting in the café, together again at last, and the waiter didn't bring the cake I'd ordered, until I woke up from hunger on a wet pillow. And with every repetition of this dream I hoped: this time it's real, this time it's not a dream, this time she's there – and the whole nightmare is over! And in the daytime I then told my boys about her and taught them to love Aunt Anneliese and the Jews.

(Koslowski, 2018, p. 566)

The relationship between Susanne Bonhoeffer and the Straus family remained close. Not only did she have access to their car at her wedding, but later during the 'winter of starvation' after the end of the war, she not only received care packages from her friend Anneliese, 'which in turn her sister sent her from America to save her from hunger. In addition, parcels from Mrs Straus came directly from the USA to me and also to my parents and siblings' (Koslowski, 2018, 657 f.).

Besides her friend Susanne, Anneliese Schnurmann had much contact with Dietrich Bonhoeffer and his twin sister Sabine and remained close with Sabine until very late in life.[2] She suffered greatly as a result of the murder of Dietrich Bonhoeffer in 1945, whom she held in the highest regard. In 2000, while still in Switzerland, she campaigned for him (1906–1945) to be included in the Yad Vashem Holocaust memorial in Jerusalem. In her letter, she wrote

I presently am in Berne Switzerland. I am 92 years old. Since, at age of 14, I met in School and made friends with Susanne Bonhoeffer, Dietrich's youngest sister, the Bonhoeffer House became my second home, with Dietrich as a friend. With advancing adolescence and adulthood, Dietrich and I had many good talks about religion, politics, and other things. I am Jewish, not baptized and never intended to change my religion, nor did Dietrich try to persuade me to. I know that one of the main reasons why Dietrich opposed the Nazis was their persecution of the Jews. His main preoccupation was the fate of the Jews. As regards his involvement in the conspiracy to assassinate Hitler,

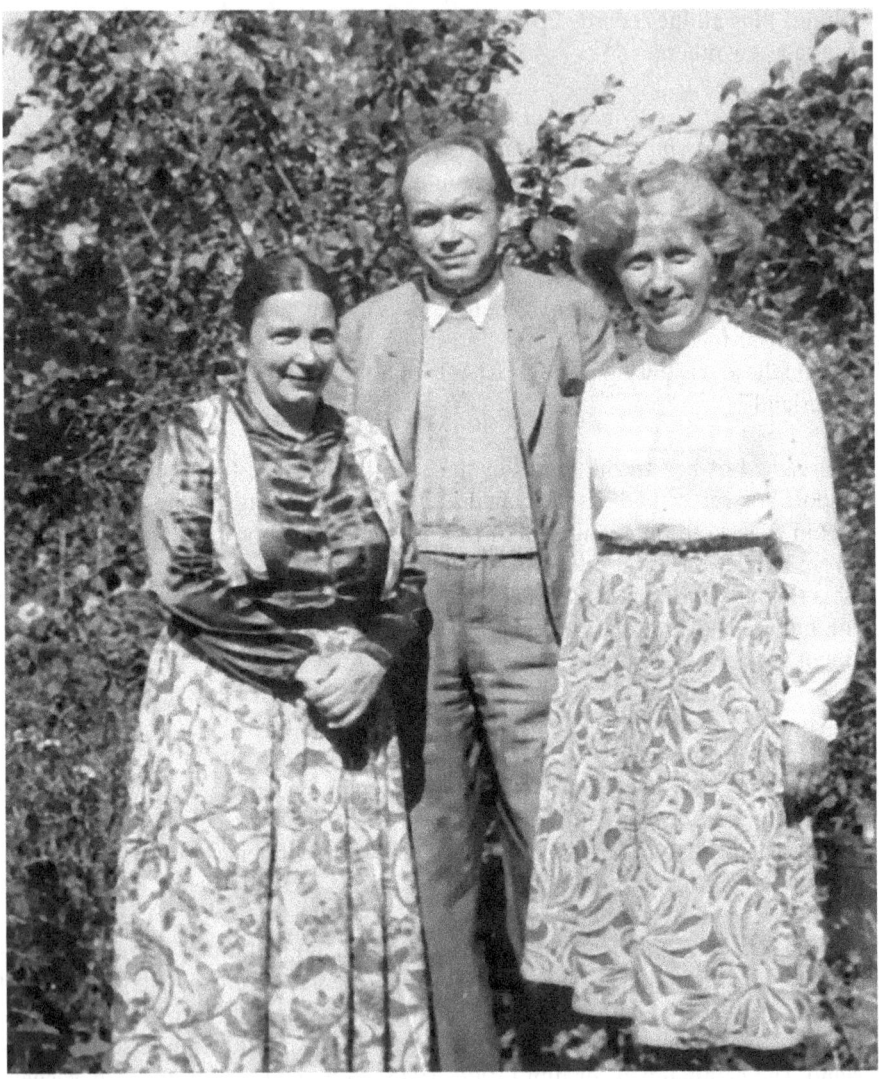

Anneliese Schnurmann (left) with Walther and Susanne Dress (née Bonhoeffer) in Berlin, 1950 (credit: Andreas Dress)

he once said to me: If someone in a car is racing down a hill, running over and killing people (he was thinking mainly of Jews) he has got to be stopped by any means, if necessary by killing him. On numbers of occasions after that he and I discussed related matters, and it was consistently clear that he had totally renounced the antisemitism and anti-Judaism of Martin Luther and all others, most particularly the Nazis. While it is now well over sixty years since I had these conversations with Dietrich, I recall them quite distinctly for two reasons: First, since I am a Jew and heard them as including me during those terrible times, his concern affected me greatly. Second, since I am a psychiatrist and trained to recall statements of importance, they are graven in my mind. Bonhoeffer was a great man and a true friend of Jews in distress, and he should be recognized at Yad Vashem.

(Wise, 2009)

In all our interviews, her eyes lit up when his name was mentioned. Anneliese Schnurmann never married and I [CLK] got the impression that he was her silent love, to whom the following statement referred:

That's such an old story: those you want, you don't get, and those who want you, you don't want! There's nothing you can do [...] Yes, I have always done much with children [...] there is contact. [...] And then, I just felt comfortable here. With the children, I am actually almost more comfortable than at my desk.

(Schnurmann, interview, 24 November, 1996)

She said that she would have liked 'from an early age' to have had children but was denied this, which she regretted very much. In a conversation with Manna Friedmann (28 June, 1998), both agreed that they were now, so to speak, the ones who would be the mothers for their substitute children up to the third generation.

In 1924, When Anneliese Schnurmann went to a neo-linguistic Swiss girls' boarding school in Fetan, Graubünden for a year, she remained in close correspondence with Susanne Bonhoeffer. 'But to Anneliese or Bärbel [...] letters of up to twenty pages were sent off. Sometimes two in three days (and then again nothing for weeks)' (Koslowski, 2018, p. 296). She then lived with her relatives in Spain for three months before applying to a housekeeping school in Germany. However, because of her Jewish religion, the director suggested that she should apply to another school, as he could not guarantee that the girls would leave her alone:

And then I applied to a Swiss housekeeping school on Lake Thun. That was nowhere near as systematic. That was with agriculture and animal husbandry, I think [...]. And that started at six in the morning, where I was supposed to make coffee and had no idea how to do it. And at two o'clock when we were finished, we went swimming and boating, going on excursions and nice things like that for fun. And we had a rotation, always two together, they had to prepare the main course once, dessert once, etc. Whenever it was my turn for the main course, we had lung hash, and whenever I had dessert, we had raspberry tarts.

(Schnurmann, interview, 26 April, 1997)

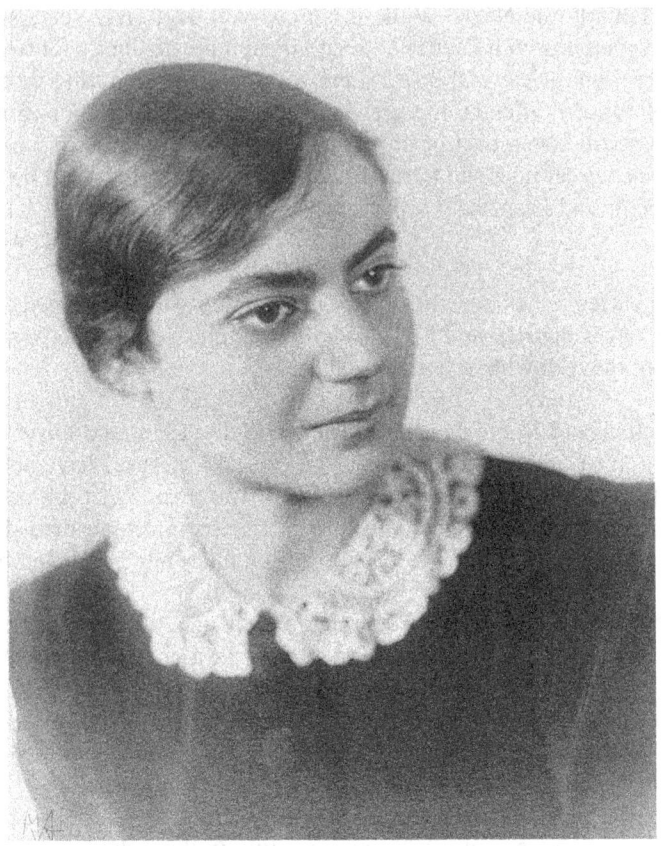

A portrait of Anneliese Schnurmann in a black dress with lace collar (credit: Anneliese Schnurmann)

In 1926, she returned to Berlin and, together with Susanne Bonhoeffer, attended housekeeping courses at the Pestalozzi-Fröbel House, which was run by Anna von Gierke. Susanne Dress remembers:

Starting in the autumn, Anneliese was with me at the Pestalozzi-Fröbel-Haus! She had come from her Swiss boarding school so that we could practise house-keeping together. That was a great joy for me. [...] We were together during the breaks and also during all the practical activities, where one could also have a good conversation. However, her mind was not always on the job, and some things went very slowly. She bore her lack of dexterity with great charm and was popular with everyone because she was always friendly and accommodating.

I still remember some cheerful blunders very clearly. I am stirring our common stock pot, which looks quite cloudy and crunches at the bottom like sand.

Onion skins float on top. But what is that thick lump at the bottom? Oh, the teacher had given Anneliese a tuber of celery and some onions and told her to add them to the soup. She did so unseen, as if in a dream state. Once, in the morning, she didn't show up at Bismarck Square at the appointed time and arrived half a minute later, somewhat dazed. She had dreamed at night that she was supposed to bring a crystal bowl to take a dish home in. And then it was broken. In the dream? In the dream, too – first in the dream and then in reality. Why in reality? Yes, she had gone to the cupboard in the morning, still driven by the idea that she needed a bowl (of which there had been no talk in class) and had packed one carefully so that it would remain safe. That was why she had left late. Then the bowl fell and broke! Did you perhaps also dream that? I ask. At first, I thought so too – but here are the broken pieces. There was no denying it. I went to our class leader and asked that we both be excused from class for the day. Then we went for a nice autumn hike until Anneliese was back to herself and had overcome her overtiredness. In all theoretical subjects she was far superior to me and the whole class; this was recognized by everyone, and on this basis, she could rest a little and afford such little blunders.

(Koslowski, 2018, p. 235)

Koslowski (2018, p. 235f) further states:

At lunchtime, the two of us now often isolated ourselves from the others. We had a right to be together, we thought. Sometimes we went to Nollendorfplatz to the Krokodil restaurant for lunch. We felt insanely grown up about it. Especially when we ordered two cognacs at my insistence after very fatty fresh sausage, which she liked so much. I was sixteen years old and she was seventeen, but she was usually considered the younger one because she was smaller, more delicate and shy. The waiter was probably also thinking hard at first, but I said with the calmest expression I could exhibit: 'The sausage was a little fatty', and so we got our liquor. In any case, we had even more fun together in that half year in housekeeping school than in our half year together in the eighth grade.

(Koslowski, 2018, p. 235 f.)

Anneliese Schnurmann laughingly remembers how she failed the ironing exam there but was good at cooking. 'They all still tease me and say I have an ironing complex. Manna [Friedmann] comes and irons my blouses' (Schnurmann, interview, 24 November, 1996).

Youth Centre Berlin – Charlottenburg

When Anneliese Schnurmann decided to catch up on her secondary school diploma, she turned to the director of the Bismarck Lyceum. He advised her to take private lessons and enter grade thirteen directly, so that she passed her high school exams in 1929 at the age of 21.

She was interested in social issues, and the hardships of the time – especially those of unemployed young people – depressed her, and she wanted to use her assets to help as much as possible. While discussing these problems with the Bonhoeffer family, Paula Bonhoeffer, the mother of the numerous siblings, suggested that something be done for the nutrition and employment of these young people. Thereupon Dietrich Bonhoeffer and Anneliese Schnurmann founded the 'Jugendstube' [transl.: youth centre], a day centre for unemployed young people. Prior to this, Dietrich Bonhoeffer had sought advice from Hans Brandenburg, who was then a mission inspector at the Berlin City Mission. 'Bonhoeffer led Paul Le Seur's "Freie Jugend"', which socialist and communist youth groups attended to engage in discussion. They tried their hand at volunteer work and evening courses for the unemployed' (Bethge, 2000, pp. 229–30).

Bonhoeffer wrote to Hans Brandenburg on 23 October, 1932:

> A woman I know intends sometime next winter to give 430 Reichsmarks per month for the establishment of a youth club for the unemployed. It would mean finding a heated room during the day for useful activities, if possible job preparation. It shouldn't be hard to find leaders or students, probably through the Student Activities or 'academic self-help' […] I'd particularly like to talk over the following questions with you. Is there any possibility that rooms somewhere might be available for free? Does one have to apply to municipal offices for this – and which ones? What kinds of activities would you particularly recommend? Would material for workshops eventually be available from some offices? What could be done with 430 Reichsmarks? It is suggested to this woman that she become part of the 'Emergency group for the establishment of homes and kitchens for the unemployed.' What do you think of this? Since the youth club is to be interconfessional and not affiliated with any party, we could hardly recommend this association. The woman can guarantee the mentioned amount for six months, beyond that she intends to continue it, but cannot yet offer it with certainty.
>
> (*ibid.*)

Anneliese Schnurmann and Dietrich Bonhoeffer then turned to Anna von Gierke, who headed the 'Verein Jugendheim' (Youth Home Association) from 1928 until its dissolution in 1933. Through her, she met Elenore (Nore) Astfalck (1900–1991),[3] a nursery school teacher, horticulturist, youth leader, and lecturer at the Charlottenburg Youth Home, and her friend Johanna Nacken (1896–1963), a handicrafts teacher who also worked at the Berlin-Charlottenburg Youth Home under Anna von Gierke and taught youth leaders (Schnurmann, letter, 8 February, 2000).

Nore Astfalck became a close friend of Anneliese Schnurmann. 'Nore, who was a fabulous, capable person, died at the age of over 90 years, and she was fresh until the end. We celebrated her 90th birthday' (Schnurmann, interview, 24 November, 1996).

Schonig (1996, p. 147) writes about Nore Astfalck:

> She taught schoolgirls in the morning, ran a day care centre in the afternoon, and in the evening, just as intensively, the youth centre for unemployed young

people. From the wealth of her practical experience she pursued her tasks with joy and without looking at the clock.

Anna von Gierke helped to set up the youth centre, with additional contributions from Friedrich Siegmund Schultze and his experience gained through the 'Social Working Group Berlin-East'. In the autumn of 1932, work began in Schlossstrasse in Charlottenburg. In a letter dated 23 November, 1932, Dietrich Bonhoeffer wrote to Anneliese Schnurmann:

> There has been some trouble at the club [...] Z., together with A., seems to have made himself very unpopular with the boys. A few days ago, apparently when he was drunk, he gave himself out to be the club leader. I think we shall have to show him the door as soon as possible. Otherwise there will be a real row. Apart from that, things are still going well. But we are thinking of moving. The premises are getting too small. What do you think about that? Two theology students are working there. There is also a student from the technical college who would be glad to earn 25 marks a month and will spend three evenings a week at the club.
> (Bethge, 2000, p. 230)

Bethge (2000, pp. 230–231) further reports:

> The new premises were ready by the end of November; the boys worked hard to help, and they moved in on 1 December. On 8 December Bonhoeffer invited Anneliese Schnurmann to the opening party:
>   There will be sausages, cakes, cigarettes. The boys worked really splendidly during the last few days, and this is a treat that we must indeed give them. The whole thing will cost 20 marks [...] As for the technical college student, I thought it would be a good idea for him to come three evenings a week, offer shorthand lessons and help in other ways, for which he would receive 15 marks from parish funds and 15 marks from you.

Many types of young people met there. Anneliese Schnurmann remembers one of them 'who was mentally not quite up to scratch. He wasn't exactly feeble-minded, but he had an IQ of maybe 70 to 80 [...]'. Some were sent there by Anna von Gierke, and others learnt about it by word of mouth.

> It was a perfect mixture. One or two were intelligent communists [...] I walked through the city with them, too. We went to Aschinger's once and ate something there. And they were terribly hungry afterwards, and then we got some sandwiches again.
> (Schnurmann, interview, 24 November, 1996)

After Anneliese Schnurmann went to Geneva, this arrangement was continued by Dieter Bonhoeffer, Nora Astfalck and Johanna Nacken. Nora Astfalck came to the realization that it would be dangerous to continue the institution.

And in the meantime, it became Hitlerian and many of them were communists. And then we had to break it up and Nora said it was dangerous. We burned all the index cards and all the written material about this youth centre with every-one before the Nazis could come to investigate. And then nothing happened to them. They went into hiding, disappeared somewhere, thanks to Nora. That was then the end of the youth centre.

(Schnurmann, interview, 24 November, 1996)

According to Bethge et al. (1986, p. 96), after 30 January, 1933, Communist visi-tors encountered difficulties on the street, so Bonhoeffer had them disappear into the Biesenthaler Barracks for some time. Soon the 'Jugendstube' had to be closed. 'Concern for those who were excluded from the work process is now replaced by concern for others, much more radically branded: the Jews. Anneliese Schnur-mann, herself affected by this, had to emigrate.'

University years and emigration to England

In 1929 Anneliese Schnurmann began studying modern languages in Heidelberg, where she first had to learn Old French, which she had not expected at all, and which she did not enjoy. It remains unclear whether she met Karl Mannheim there, who taught sociology as a private lecturer in Heidelberg from 1926, and with whom she later studied at the University of Frankfurt, where he was appointed professor of sociology in 1930.[4]

And I thought, you read interesting books there. But then you started with Old French and English. Well, I found that unbearable. I went swimming in the Neckar. I thought it would be much more interesting to study economics. And then I thought: 'Why don't you take economics in Geneva?' And then I noticed that every professor has his own little theory, and nobody really knows any-thing. So that was not the real thing either. But then I did sociology. That was my thing, at the Institute for Social Sciences.

(Schnurmann, interview, 24 November, 1996)

When the so-called 'Frankfurt School' at the University of Frankfurt, where An-neliese Schnurmann studied sociology under Karl Mannheim, was dissolved in 1933, she continued her studies in Geneva, which she completed with the academic degree 'Licence és Sciences Sociales' in 1935. During her time in Frankfurt, she got to know Teddy Wiesengrund (Theodor Adorno), Max Horkheimer and Paul Tillich.

In 1936 she taught French for three months at the Stoatley Rough board-ing school in Haslemere (Surrey), which had been founded by Hilde Lion and Emmy Wolff with the support of the Quakers after their forced emigration in 1933. Nora Astfalck, who was also on the National Socialists' 'blacklist', and Johanna Nacken, who knew each other from working together on the 'Verein Jugendheim'

Berlin-Charlottenburg, turned to Hilde Lion and helped to build up this school (Anneliese Schnurmann, letter, 2 August, 2000).

Anneliese Schnurmann then returned to Berlin, which she left again in 1937. She herself called this date her official emigration, since she viewed Berlin as her home. Postgraduate studies in psychology and educational science at the University of Geneva and Basel followed. Then, in 1939, during a stay in Basel, she decided to emigrate to England in view of the imminent threat of war and took advantage of the fact that all her friends met up in London and Haslemere, Surrey in the summer. She had two suitcases with her most important possessions and was determined not to return. In Haslemere she taught French to the Jewish children whose parents were still in Germany. She quickly gave up her attempts to teach mathematics as well, realizing that this was not for her.

She then contacted the Women's Voluntary Service, which was looking for a cook for evacuated children in a children's hospital.

> Well, I don't know why I volunteered there – I once cooked at home for eight people for a month in the absence of the cook, but to cook for the whole institute was probably a bit much. And then this matron interviewed me and said: 'I would like to have her, but not as a cook. I want her for the children.' And that was exactly right. And then I was there until 1942, because I didn't like the educational measures of the head nurse. The head of the service, she was good, she had even been a scout leader, but she apparently didn't want to interfere with the head nurse, and she, for her part, was used to sick children, and she treated the healthy children who were only thrown out of their homes because of rashes, bedwetting and similar things as sick children. She wanted to put them to bed at half past five in the evening, did so, and was then surprised when the children were unruly at two in the morning and she left a child of only one and a half years old tied up in the car all day. I said I couldn't watch that. And then Nora, who worked there, said: 'Why don't you go to Anna Freud?' And then I went to London for a meeting. There was a meeting every Wednesday. And there I was thrilled and thought: 'Exactly!' And then after the meeting I went up to her and said: 'Can I work for you? She said, 'Yes'. And that was it. In November '42.
>
> (Schnurmann, interview, 26 April, 1997)

Work in the War Nurseries and as a psychoanalyst

Anneliese Schnurmann turned to Anna Freud to be accepted as a trainee. Together with Ilse Hellmann, who took care of the older children, it was her task to look after the small children whose families from the East End of London had moved to Anna Freud's War Nursery as a result of the bombing.

Anneliese Schnurmann could afford voluntary work in Anna Freud's War Nurseries because she was able to live off an investment of ten per cent of the family assets she had saved. In November 1942 she began working in the Infants and

Toddlers Department at 5 Netherhall Gardens until the War Nurseries closed in 1945 – first for 16 months, during which she cared for ten-day-old newborns and infants up to one year old, and then for ten months with one- to three-year-old toddlers, followed by five months with the two- to three-year-olds. She also worked for six weeks as an assistant in the Montessori children's group.

She sold all the books she brought with her and was able to buy psychoanalytic literature instead (Schnurmann, interview, 24 November, 1996). During the time when the bombings increased and the children were evacuated to the country, Anneliese Schnurmann helped out in the office. She typed, took care of the wages, and said with a smile: 'If I had become nothing [else], I would have been a good secretary.' She told them that at the time when Anna Freud was still alive, they felt 'like a family' (Schnurmann, interview, 24 November, 1996).

She reported how she wandered around London in thick fog and smog.

> It was perhaps 10 minutes, quarter of an hour to walk. And with such a thick pea soup fog together with war lights [laughs], I was always running around in circles. And on some corner, I don't know how he could, a man completely unknown to me, said: 'I'll take you home now', which he did.
>
> (Schnurmann, interview, 24 November, 1996)

Anneliese Schnurmann, who lost her parents early on, suffered from depression and turned to Hedwig Hoffer, whom she knew from seminars. 'I once said: "Can I talk to you privately? My situation is like this and like that. Would you advise me to analyse it?" She said: "Yes, sure!" And then I went to a Dr Friedlander' (Schnurmann, interview, 24 November, 1996). She then switched from the private analysis with Kate Friedlander, which began in 1945, to teaching analysis until shortly before her early death on 20 February, 1949. Kate Friedlander, who later held seminars within the Hampstead Child-Therapy Training Course together with Hedwig Hoffer, Julia Mannheim, and Barbara Lantos, recommended Anneliese Schnurmann to apply for this training in 1947. She was one of the first group to receive analytical training in the Hampstead Child-Therapy Training Course together with Joanna Benkendorf, née Köhler, Alice Goldberger, Ivy Bennett Gwynne-Thomas, Hansi Kennedy, née Engl, Lili Neurath, Lizzy Rolnick, née Wallentin, and Sara Rosenfeld, née Kut (source: *curriculum vitae* A. Schnurmann). Seven of them had worked in the War Nurseries. The training to become a 'Child Expert' lasted four years, full-time (Pretorius, 2012).

Unfortunately, she had just finished her analysis with Kate Friedlander in order to reunite with her family in the USA, whom she had not seen for over ten years.

After the 'Night of Broken Glass' on 10 November, 1938, Moritz Straus was sent to Sachsenhausen concentration camp, but was released. He had to sell his company for far below its value and fled to Switzerland. From there, the family first emigrated to Rio de Janeiro in 1939, as five of his siblings were already living there. Together with his family, he entered the USA in 1941, although the Argus Company foreign patents that he still owned had previously been sold by an acquaintance in the USA without his consent. After the USA entered the Second World War, they were initially classified as 'enemy aliens', but in 1946 they were granted American citizenship (Grieger, 2013).

> While still in US exile, S. filed applications for restitution, which, with regard to the Argus complex, were essentially granted as early as Oct. 1948 through settlement agreements with H. Koppenberg and V. Polak. As a result of this settlement, in Aug. 1949 S. again possessed parts of his former industrial assets and again took over entrepreneurial responsibility in Berlin and Baden but did not move his residence back to Germany.
>
> (Grieger, 2013, p. 49)

When Anneliese Schnurmann came back from this journey, her analyst was already seriously ill. She was able to meet her again but in retrospect she thought: '[...] that was not a good use of time. That the end of the analysis coincided with the reunion of the family' (Schnurmann, interview, 24 November, 1996). Hedwig Hoffer called her to inform her of the death of Kate Friedlander, who died on 20 February, 1949.

It also irritated her that her paper, 'Observation of a phobia', in which she explained the background of an anxiety symptom in a 2.5-year-old girl who had been admitted to the War Nursery at the age of seven weeks, was published in the same year and issue (1947) as the paper 'Neurosis and home background – A preliminary report' by Kate Friedlander (Schnurmann, interview, 24 November, 1996). After her training as a 'psycho-analytical Child Expert' (1947–1950) – as child psychoanalysts trained by Anna Freud were called – she obtained employment as a child therapist at the East London Child Guidance Clinic, where she worked from 1948 to 1951. From 1951 to 1956 she succeeded Hansi Kennedy at the state-run Chichester Child Guidance Clinic, which had been founded by Kate Friedlander (A. Schnurmann, letter, 2 August, 2000). From 1952 to 1973 she also worked at the Hampstead Child Therapy Clinic, participating in research and teaching. She conducted child analyses and helped as a training analyst and supervisor in the training of the Hampstead Clinic Child Experts (A. Schnurmann, letter, 2 August, 2000). From 1961 to 1965 she also trained as an adult analyst at the British Psycho-Analytic Institute (graduated 19 May, 1965). 'I discussed it with Anna Freud. She said: "You are quite right. As a child analyst you should actually be at mother age and not at grandmother age"' (Schnurmann, interview, 24 November, 1996).

She had a conflict of loyalties on this account, because on the one hand she was a 'faithful follower' of Anna Freud, but, on the other hand, the training in child analysis established by Anna Freud was not recognized by the IPA.

She began teaching analysis again with Konrad Gomperts, attended seminars, and throughout her career received supervision from the following psychoanalysts: Margarete Ruben, Joseph Sandler, Paula Heimann, Dorothy Burlingham, Liselotte Frankl, Kate Friedlander, Anna Freud, Ilse Hellmann-Noach, Hedwig Hoffer, Barbara Lantos, Hedwig Schwarz, Julie Mannheim, Ruth Thomas, and Edith

Gyömröi-Ludowyk. She remembers how Edith Gyömröi-Ludowyk conducted the technical–casuistic seminars at her home and where her husband 'always served them excellent Ceylonese tea' (Schnurmann, interview, 23 November, 1997).

She did not get along at all with Paula Heimann in the supervisions and therefore stopped the control analysis with her. While Josef Sandler's 'rather non-aggressive treatment style' was much closer to Anneliese Schnurmann, who describes herself as 'aggressively inhibited', she could not really understand Paula Heimann's attitude, which was influenced by Melanie Klein (Schnurmann, interview, 23 November, 1997), especially since she had internalized Anna Freud's theoretical view through their close work together. She emphasized that she, who had not had any of her cases supervised by Anna Freud, could nevertheless contact her at any time with questions.

> I once had problems with a teaching analyst. And then I went to Anna Freud. I didn't really know what to do, so she gave me some good advice. And to someone else, a student whose case I had supervised. [...] And then I went to Anna Freud and said, 'so and so, that's the case.' And she said, 'This is one of those cases where everything you do is wrong. Calm down, there is nothing you can do.' Yes, well, if Anna Freud said it, I didn't need to reproach myself any further. If even Anna Freud doesn't know what to do, you just can't do anything about it.
>
> (Schnurmann, interview, 24 November, 1996)

Liselotte Frankl, who was pleased with the very good reports from Anneliese Schnurmann, advised her: 'Don't make such nice reports for us in the clinic. You'd rather write your doctoral thesis there'. Anneliese Schnurmann then turned to Karl Mannheim, whom she knew from her time as a student in Frankfurt. Initially, he was a professor at the London School of Economics, but while Anneliese Schnurmann was writing her thesis on psychoanalysis, religion, and behaviourism, which Mannheim had initially suggested, he was offered a professorship at the University of London in the Department of Education. 'And so that's when I started collecting material and spent a lot of time sitting around here in the libraries. In between I was still working at the East London Child Guidance Clinic' (Schnurmann, interview, 24 November, 1996).

Unfortunately, Karl Mannheim died in the meantime and Anneliese Schnurmann turned to another professor in this department. It was also around the time when Kate Friedlander died and, in retrospect, Anneliese Schnurmann understands how unfortunately she had initiated the whole process. Instead of turning to another scholar, who did not get along so well with Karl Mannheim, but who was interested in the subject, she stayed with her dissertation at the Department of Educational Sciences – 'where the stuff did not fit at all' – and the case was rejected. It was of little use to her that her supervisor 'cried out' to Ilse Hellmann when the procedure failed. She had had enough of these 'academic escapades', especially since she had long since realized that clinical work meant much more to her (Schnurmann, interview, 24 November, 1996).

Anneliese Schnurmann worked as a psychoanalyst in her own practice starting in 1965, conducting high frequency adult analysis ('5 times a week'; Curriculum Vitae by Anneliese Schnurmann) and psychoanalytically orientated psychotherapy ('2 and 3 times a week'), which she conducted in her apartment at 11 Netherhall Gardens. She was also a teaching analyst and supervisor at the Hampstead Clinic.

I have been analysing people from the clinic for quite some time. And then some of them came over for the so-called 'One Year Course'. They then found that they also needed psychotherapy, or rather the course participants themselves said so. The courses were often so stirring.

(Schnurmann, interview, 24 November, 1996)

Retirement

In 1983 Anneliese Schnurmann retired but kept in touch with some of the former 'children'. She remained in contact with the Meggy twins, who had been analysed by Ilse Hellmann, and 'Ellen', whose analysis Anneliese Schnurmann took over, about whom Dorothy Burlingham wrote in her book on twins. Another 'former child' is Sandy, whom she had already looked after as a three-week-old baby in the War Nurseries.

I looked after her at night, there was a war going on. And the children slept in the shelter, and she called me when she wanted to go to the toilet. [...] Later she

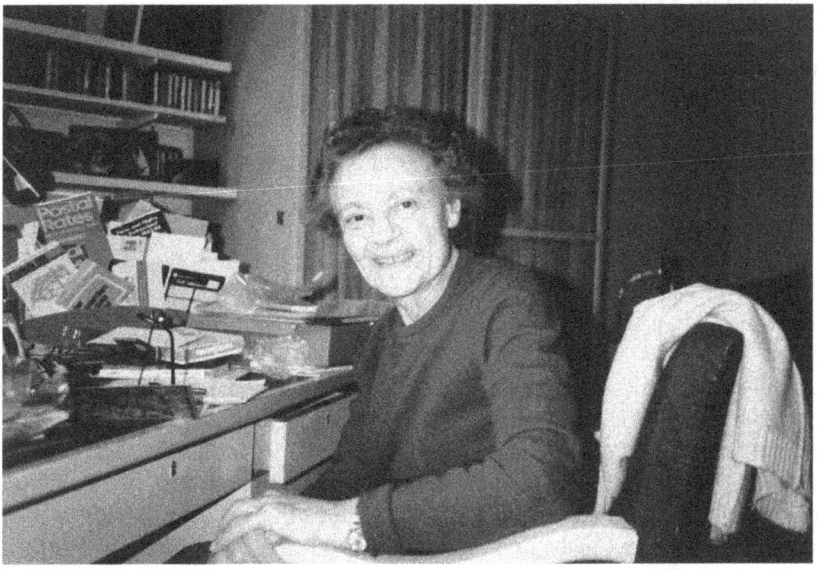

Anneliese Schnurmann at her desk (credit: Anneliese Schnurmann)

was with the 'Junior Toddlers' and there I was. And there was, in a group, there was a Sandy, there was a Lydia – she didn't belong in my group, she belonged in another group – and there was a little boy. And I remember that Lydia, who actually didn't belong in my group at all, sat down on my knees. Then Sandy came and shoved her off and said, 'Mine!' Anna Freud introduced pretty soon that each one had its small group. And it was like families here. And the one child from my family I still see very often, that is Sandy, and I wrote something about her again. I always hope that she doesn't find that [...] Through some kind of influence, Sandy's daughter has taken up a similar profession – with children and in education. I just thought for heaven's sake, what if she ever gets this *Psychoanalytic Study of the Child* article, which I wrote about her mother. But luckily this did not happen.

(Schnurmann, interview, 24 November, 1996)

She also stayed in contact with a then seven-year-old boy whom she treated for speech impediments. In the meantime, he had chosen linguistics for businesspeople as his profession and visited her regularly at intervals with his son.

In a 2001 interview (Anna Freud Centre Newsletter, Spring 2001) she answered the question about her impression of Anna Freud:

I liked Anna Freud from the start. She was always nice and friendly and stayed that way throughout her life. I always knew that I wanted to work with her. She once said that the worst thing about getting old is having to ask your body permission to do things. But she was always available for advice and guidance, up until the time she died.

And to the interview question as to whether psychoanalysis has changed in her eyes in the meantime:

No, not really. I was always interested in child development. But psychoanalysis made working with children very interesting and satisfying. I always loved children, especially the ones between one and three years old. But the older ones always ask the interesting things, like the other day my great-niece asked me: 'Do the flowers know they are here?' It is only the adolescents that I found hard to work with, as they don't follow advice.

Anneliese Schnurmann was a close friend of Manna Friedmann. They knew each other from their work in the War Nurseries. They became friends when an apartment above that of the Friedmann couple became available. Oscar Friedmann had asked his wife to look for a psychoanalyst who could move into the apartment above them. He wished for a quieter tenant, since the noise of the children of the family who had previously lived there had disturbed him greatly in his psycho-analytic work. Thus, Anneliese Schnurmann, who was looking for an apartment at the time, moved into 30 Fitz John Avenue. Until then she had lived in a furnished room. But after her brother-in-law died in 1959, she brought her furniture, which had been temporarily stored in Switzerland, to her home and was happy to be able to give up her hitherto rather provisional life. After she was dismissed by the owner of the house in 1962 and offered a severance package, she was happy to move to 11 Netherhall Gardens, the house right next to her former workplace in the War Nursery (Schnurmann, interview, 24 November, 1996).

Despite their different family backgrounds, Anneliese Schnurmann and Manna Friedmann became close friends. For example, Anneliese Schnurmann learnt everything she now knew about Judaism from Manna (Schnurmann, interview, 28 June, 1998).Since, in Manna Friedmann's eyes, Anneliese Schnurmann had a kind of love–hate relationship with order, whereas Manna Friedmann loved order and was happy to create it for others, she often came to her friend's house to make it 'Klar-Schiff' (transl. 'shipshape'; interview, 28 June, 1998).

In 1985 Anneliese Schnurmann was visited in London by her great-niece, Claudia Schnurmann. In her eyes she was first 'put through her paces' before she was allowed to stay with Julia (Jula) Weiss, a friend of Anneliese and Manna, whom they both knew from their War Nursery time. Julia Weiss (1905–1994) was a secretary for over 21 years at the International Psychoanalytic Publishing House in Vienna, through which she knew the Freud family. She lived in Finchley Road, halfway between the home of Manna Friedmann (Goldhurst Terrace) and that of Anneliese Schnurmann (Netherhall Gardens). So, Claudia Schnurmann also met Manna Friedmann and became friends with her:

> Manna was strict with me for a long time, speaking only English, but then, also thanks to my love for Cologne, we became real friends – age and differences in experience notwithstanding. Manna even visited me in Germany and I accompanied her on a very melancholic 'sentimental journey' through her old Cologne home. I laughed a lot with both of them; we cooked for each other and I encouraged the two ladies to 'alcohol excesses': a can of Pils from Waitrose each; Anneliese first bought the correct equipment for cooking at Liberty before she dared to try a recipe. Her saying at the sight of a slightly failed Coq au Vin is legendary: 'Once upon a time there was a chicken...'; with tears of laughter, we took care of the poor vulture. The two of them were simply terrific. I owe them much, including wonderful meetings with their friends in Bristol and nieces in Switzerland and Israel.
> (C. Schnurmann, personal correspondence, 15 May, 2021)

In an interview (Anna Freud Centre Newsletter, Spring 2001) Annaliese Schnurmann talked about her life in retirement:

> I retired in 1983 when I was 75 years old. I felt I was getting a bit tired and needed rest. Since then I have been busy visiting friends, reading and watching television. I like political programmes like *How to Civilize Capitalism*, *Other People's Children*, etc. I also like classical music, particularly Beethoven. I used to go to the Opera, but I find it too difficult to hear nowadays.

Asked about future plans, she stated: 'I am planning to move to Switzerland to live in a home for the elderly. I am looking forward to this, as I will be closer to my family and will be able to spend more time with my great-nieces'.

She had a very close relationship with her nieces' families and their children until the end of her life. When her friend Manna Friedmann decided to move to the USA in the late summer of 2000, this was certainly one of the reasons why Anneliese Schnurmann gave up her London apartment in March 2001 to move to Switzerland for good. She lived in a retirement apartment in Bern until November 2003, with the option of requesting assistance. After becoming increasingly dependent on nursing care, she was cared for in a retirement home in Wabern, a suburb of Bern. Her great-niece Cornelia Rogger-Müller, a psychiatrist, took care of her during this time (C. Rogger-Müller, personal correspondence, 6 April, 2021).

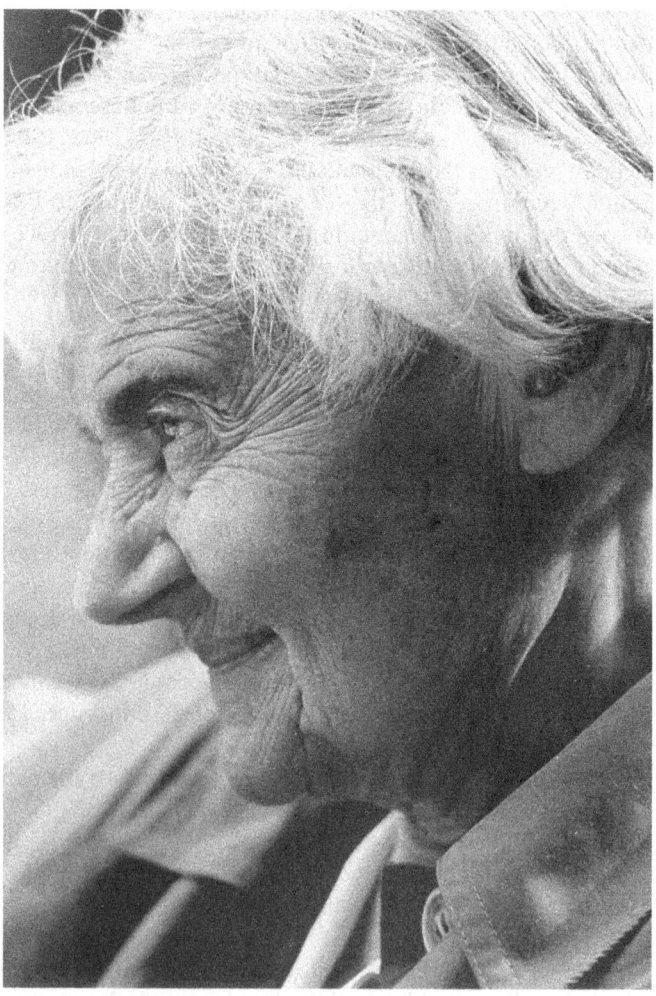

Anneliese Schnurmann, London, 15 September, 1996 (credit: Christiane Ludwig-Körner)

On 21 September, 2006, at well over 98 years of age, Anneliese Schnurmann died.

After her death, the Blum-Zullinger Foundation in Bern received a donation of 200,000 Swiss francs from Anneliese Schnurmann's estate, 'which was used to open a fund for the promotion of Freudian psychoanalysis, in particular for the maintenance of the Sigmund Freud Centre Bern's own premises" (Sigmund-Freud-Zentrum Berlin, n.d.; Wildbolz, 2012). It was natural for her to donate part of her fortune – not only in her young years with Dietrich Bonhoeffer in the 'Jugendstube', but also in her London time – as the author learnt in passing. It was so natural for her that she did not want to talk about it.

When I met Anneliese Schnurmann in the course of my research on Anna Freud's employees, I was impressed not only by her mental and physical vitality (she skied, for example, until a ripe old age), but also by her modesty, her 'personal withdrawal'. Claudia Schnurmann said of her, 'Anneliese had style: completely unexcited, complete understatement, but real class and that certain *"je ne sais quoi"*' (C. Schnurmann, interview, 31 May, 2021). It was far from her to put herself in the foreground in any way. She almost gave the impression to me that, having become rootless herself due to the early death of her parents and forced emigration, she was grateful to be able to give children a substitute home for a while. She is one of those women (and men) whose lives are quickly forgotten, especially since she was a 'wanderer between worlds'. As a representative of many, she should be remembered here.

Notes

1 Straus had already taken over the management of Argus-Motoren-Gesellschaft in 1916 and, after taking over the majority of shares in the Horch automobile factory in 1920, hired Paul Daimler as an engine designer to further develop car and aircraft engines. Under Straus' leadership, the Horch factory became one of the most respected vehicle manufacturers in the world, especially as it became part of Auto-Union (Audi) in 1932.

2 Sabine Bonhoeffer married Gerhard Leibholz, who was friends with the (later) resistance fighter Hans von Dohnanyi. Both studied law in Heidelberg. After his first professorship in Greifswald in 1929, he was appointed to the University of Göttingen in 1931 but had to give it up in 1935. They fled with his family (two daughters) to Oxford in 1938. The family returned to Germany in 1947. Gerhard Leibholz became a federal constitutional judge (1951–1971). Sabine Leibholz-Bonhoeffer, who died in 1999, wrote about her experiences in exile (1983) and about her family (1991) (Schnurmann, interview, 24 November, 1996).

3 Eleonore Astfalck was on the Nazis' blacklist. After the dissolution of the Jugendstube, she worked together with her partner Johanna Nacken in the Stoatley Rough Home School in Haslemere, Surrey, where mainly German and later also Austrian Jewish children aged nine to sixteen lived. In 1946, she returned to Germany and taught at the Odenwald School. Together with Johanna Nacken, she took over the (re)construction and management of the 'Immenhof' (Workers' Welfare Home for children, young people, and mothers) in Hützel (Lüneburg Heath) in 1950 (Schonig, 1996; Berger, 2002).

4 In 1929, Karl Mannheim (1893–1947) was appointed to the Chair of Sociology and National Economy in Frankfurt; his assistant was Norbert Elias. While studying in Berlin in 1914, he heard the philosopher and sociologist Georg Simmel, who was close

to psychoanalysis and whose thinking in turn influenced many psychoanalysts. Karl Mannheim was married to Julia Lange (1893–1955), whom he had met in the 'Sunday Circle' in Budapest. From this time period, the couple also knew Edit Gyömröi (Ludwig-Körner, 1998). Julia Mannheim began her analytical training in Frankfurt, which she continued in London. Later she offered seminars as part of Anna Freud's child analytic training.

Sources and personal communications

Interviews with Anneliese Schnurmann: 26 April, 1996; 24 November, 1996; 8 June, 1997; 23 November, 1997; 28 June, 1998.
Interviews with Claudia Schnurmann: 1 June, 2021; 1 July, 2021.
E-mails: Claudia Schnurmann: 16 May, 2021; 31 May, 2021, 3 June, 2021; 4 June, 2021; 6 June, 2021.
E-mail: Cornelia Rogger-Müller: 4 June, 2021.
Curriculum vitae Anneliese Schnurmann.
Letter from Anneliese Schnurmann: 8 February, 2000.

Publications by Anneliese Schnurmann

Sandler, A.-M., Daunton, E., Schnurmann, A., & Freud, A. (1957). Inconsistency in the mother as a factor in character development: A comparative study of three cases. *Psychoanalytic Study of the Child, 12*(1), 209–225. https://doi.org/10.1080/00797308.1957.11822810

Sandler, J., Kawenoka, M., Neurath, L., Rosenblatt, B., Schnurmann, A., & Sigal, J. (1962). The Classification of Superego material in the Hampstead Index. *Psychoanalytic Study of the Child, 17*(1), 107–127. https://doi.org/10.1080/00797308.1962.11822841

Schnurmann, A. (1946). Observation of a phobia. *Psychoanalytic Study of the Child, 4,* 253–270.

Further reading

Burlingham, D., Schnurmann, A., & Lantos, B. (1958). David and his mother (unpublished).

Hellman, I., Schnurmann, A., & Todes C. (1979). Simultaneous analysis of a mother and her four-year-old daughter (unpublished).

5

Dr Ilse Rosa Hellman-Noach (08.09.1908–03.12.1998) – 'From War Babies to Grandmothers'

When I asked Maggie Williams (née Noach), daughter of Ilse Hellman (after emigrating to England, she changed her surname from 'Hellmann' to 'Hellman' for a more English spelling), if I could interview her mother, who was almost 90 years old at the time, she advised me against it. Her memory was failing, and some things got mixed up. In my first telephone conversation (6 June, 1997) with Ilse Hellman, I was astonished by her young voice, and she was happy to tell me more about herself. During my second telephone call the next day, I unfortunately found it difficult to believe her stories, in which she told me that her parents' families had helped to build up the Salzburg Music Festival and how many artists visited their house on a regular basis. Influenced by her daughter's warning, back then I classified this information as proof of the beginnings of dementia, especially since her daughter did not confirm her mother's statements to me. Not until 2018 – when I was able to turn back to this biography – did I come across the article by Martin Pollner (2014) in the *Alpenpost*, in which he reported on the significance of the Redlich and Hellmann families (the maternal and paternal lines of Ilse Hellman in Altaussee).

Ilse Hellman, born on 28 September, 1908, grew up in a Jewish family of industrialists in Vienna. She was given her second name 'Rosa' after her great-grandmother and maternal grandmother, who came from South Moravia. Irene Redlich (1882–1944), mother of Ilse Hellman, must have been an enchantingly beautiful woman. She was born in Göding, but after her mother Rosa bought a villa in Altaussee she stayed there quite often. She married Paul Hellmann (1876–1938), a Doctor of Law born in Vienna, who had inherited textile factories from his father.

Paul and Irene Redlich were also closely associated with the theatre and film director Max Reinhardt. Their villa in Altaussee and the property, Günthergasse 1 in Vienna, near today's Rooseveltplatz, were cultural meeting places for friends and artists. In addition to the Hellmann and Redlich families, other families based in Ausseerland contributed to this cultural blossoming, such as: Andrian-Werburg, Hofmannsthal, Hohenlohe-Schillingsfürst, Franckenstein, Oppenheimer-Todesco and Wassermann (Pollner, 2014). Paul Hellmann – himself an excellent violinist – owned three Stradivari and was taught by the violin virtuoso Adolf Busch (Taschwer, 2020). He also loved photography.

DOI: 10.4324/9781003403906-6

Ilse Hellman's parents ran a large cultural salon in Vienna and in Altaussee in the 1920s and continued the tradition of the Redlich and Hellmann families, who were already the centre of a dense cultural network in Altaussee and Grundlsee in the 19th century. With the help of their influence and fortune, they succeeded, along with other influential personalities, in establishing the Salzburg Theatre and Festival, of which Paul Hellmann was on the board of directors from 1920 to 1924. Their villa in Altaussee and their flat in Vienna were cultural meeting places for friends and artists. Among her closest friends were Hugo von Hofmannsthal, Richard Strauss, Richard Beer-Hofmann, Egon Wellesz, Jakob Wassermann, Hermann Bahr, composer and violinist Adolf Busch, composer and pianist Ignaz Friedmann, opera singer Friedrich Schorr, the Rosé Quartet and Gustav Mahler. Mahler finished the score of 'Lied von der Erde' when he was staying with Irene's brother Fritz in Göding (Hodonin). The piece was premiered in 1911 at the Hellmann home, but as there was not enough space for a full orchestra, it can only have been performed on a small scale. The Redlich family's close ties to culture are shown, among other things, in the fact that Hans-Ferdinand Redlich (1903–1968), son of Fritz Redlich, i.e., Ilse Hellman's cousin, studied literature and musicology. He had taken piano lessons with Paul Weingarten, was a pupil of Carl Orff, and did his doctorate on Monteverdi. Fritz Wärndorfer, who married Paul Hellmann's sister Lili, was a co-founder and financier of the Wiener Werkstätten, in which Paul Hellmann also invested a large amount of money (Taschwer, 2021). Many other artists, such as Arthur Schnitzler, Nikolas Lenau, Konrad Mautner and Adalbert Stifter, came to Altaussee for summer retreats.

The Hellmann and Redlich families supported young artists. Irene Hellmann-Redlich was friends with Ignanz Friedmann, a pianist, who dedicated the fourth dance of his composed six *Wiener Tänze* to her. She also impressed women such as the English politician Mary Agnes Hamilton, whom she described in her memoirs, 'Remembering my good friends' (1944) as someone capable of gathering artists around her. With her black hair, triangular face, and wide-spaced beautiful grey-blue eyes, she was a Slavic beauty who dressed more elegantly than Parisian women.

Some correspondence is preserved at the German Schiller Society between Hugo von Hofmannsthal and Irene Hellman, whom he appreciated and admired. Of the 29 summers Richard Strauss spent in various accommodation in Altaussee, Grundlsee and Bad Aussee, he lived in the Hellmanns' servant's house in 1917 and 1919. The summit of Loser Mountain is said to have inspired him to write his Alpine Symphony and he also set Heinrich Heine's poem *Bad Weather* to music and dedicated it to Irene. References to the Hellmann family can also be found in the diaries of Alma Mahler-Werfel,[1] née Schindler, in the period from 1898 to 1902 (Mahler-Werfel, 2002).

As a result of the world economic crisis, the Hellmann family fell into financial difficulties, which did not go unnoticed by their friends, as can be seen from an exchange of letters between Hugo von Hoffmannsthal and Irene Hellmann in 1927 (Volke, 1967). During the First World War and the economic depression, the family had to live in Vienna on one floor in the middle of the city centre, but it was still an upper middle-class life with staff and the family villa in Altaussee.

Compared to her graceful, beautiful mother, Ilse Hellman felt rather 'unimpressive'. There is a story of how, as a young girl, she danced at a ball with an older gentleman who raved about her beautiful mother, but also complimented her on being much more amusing (M. Williams, interview, 21 November, 1997). As the only girl with two older brothers (Bernhard[2] was five years older and Ernst just under three years older) she had a special position but tried to 'be in no way inferior to them'. So, for her, it was a given that she would attend the traditional *Schottengymnasium* (transl. secondary school) in Vienna, which only one other girl besides her attended.

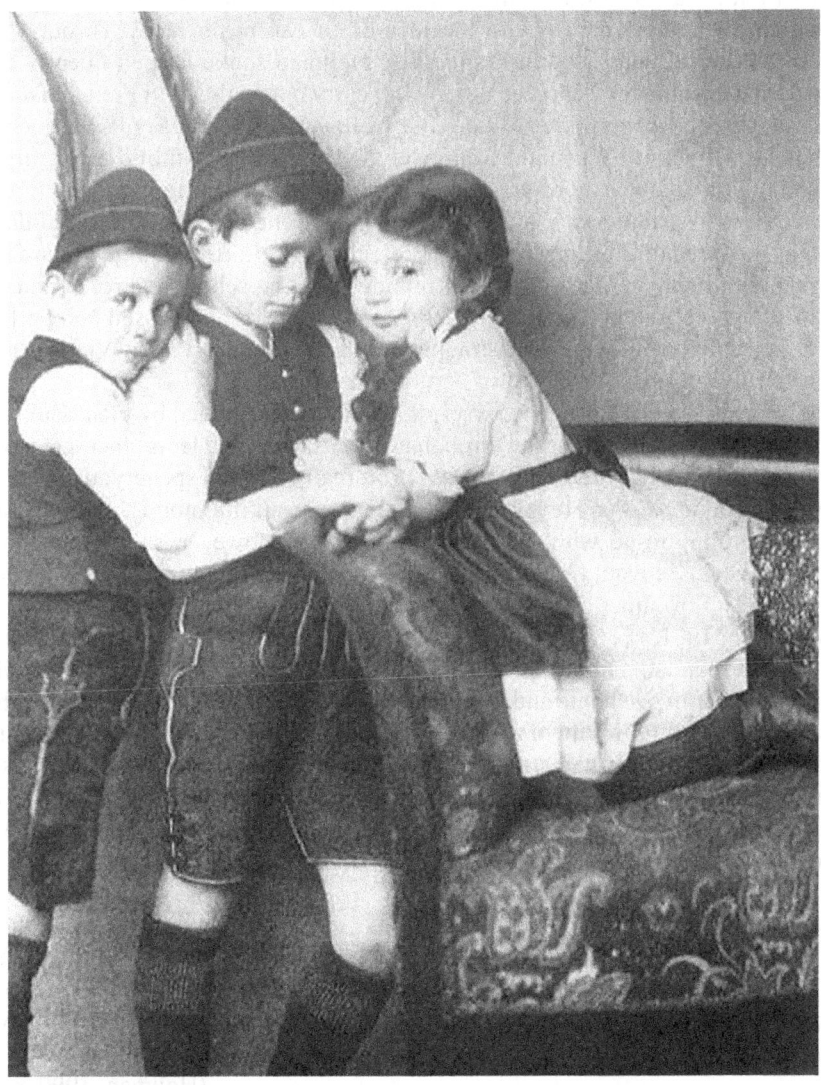

From left to right: Ernst, Bernhard and Ilse Hellmann in traditional clothing, 1912 (credit: Paul Hellmann)

Coeducation had just begun, in which girls were only allowed to attend the school with their brothers. Although it was run by Benedictines, many Jewish children, or children of 'high-ranking' parents attended.

Ilse Hellman's educational background

Ilse Hellman had a French governess who was employed during the First World War and introduced her to the Catholic faith, as Hellman's parents had converted from Judaism to Lutheranism. Occasionally she would take the children to church for a short prayer with the idea of 'It can never hurt'. Through the governess and her later stay in France, Ilse Hellman spoke French fluently and without an accent, which enabled her to later carry out analyses in French. Due to her grandparents' Anglophile attitude, Ilse Hellman also learnt English as a child and spoke it fluently. When she was twelve years old, a Catholic priest urged her and others to take care of poor orphaned children, resulting in her continued involvement in a children's aid campaign. She went out with these children, brought them small presents and later she entered welfare training. She was in training with Ilse von Arlt – who later founded the first school and research centre for social welfare in Austria-Hungary – for two years and passed her welfare exam, specializing in juvenile delinquency. Ilse Hellman lived in Vienna until she was 19 years old.

Her parents did not want her to work at all and were horrified by their daughter, who, however, resolutely pushed through her plans to work. Her mother's reaction to her desire to work with children was: 'You really want to spend your life with dirty little children?' Ilse Hellman felt that her 'so beautiful mother' did not want to have anything to do with the 'dirty sides of life'; however, she herself never anticipated that she would later have to rely on having to go to work (M. Williams, interview, 21 November, 1997).

Starting in 1931, she worked near Paris with juvenile delinquents. Judge Baker had set up a foundation in America which took great care of delinquent youths who could no longer live at home and were too young to go to prison. In France, another institution was set up for them and Ilse Hellman went to France for two years, together with a carer who had also recently graduated. One hour away from Paris, a wealthy French family had made their country house available for children whose fathers were either in prison or whose mothers could not care for them because of psychological problems or being prostitutes.

It was run on family lines, in groups, because it was thought, even in those days, that children who were away from their mothers needed to make firm attachments. So, each staff member always looked after the same small group of children. That was how I started to work in the way that, some years later, was an integral part in the organization of the Anna Freud Wartime Nurseries.

(Hellman, 1990, p. 2)

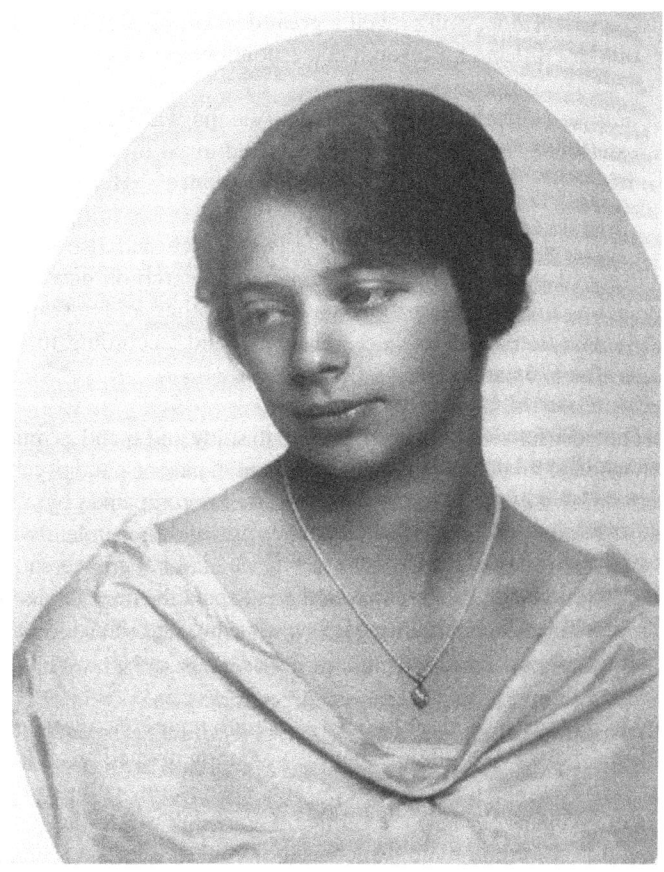

Ilse Hellman in Vienna, 1930 (credit: Paul Hellmann)

She loved this work and between 1933 and 1935 was at the 'Clinique Médico-Pédagogique Paris XIVe', where she worked with children from multi-problem families. In the evenings, she attended courses in psychology at the Sorbonne (1932–1935). After her work permit in France had expired in 1935, she continued her psychology studies in Vienna under Karl and Charlotte Bühler, which she completed in 1937. As Charlotte Bühler valued her work in France, Ilse Hellman was appointed as a research assistant and lecturer. The time Ilse Hellman spent with Charlotte Bühler in Vienna must have been very influential on her. Not only was she involved in Charlotte Bühler's infant research, but she also got to know her assistants, such as Esther Bick née Wander, Liselotte Frankl, Lotte Danzinger, Hildegard Hetzer, all of whom she met later – except for Lotte Danzinger and Hildegard Hetzer – back in London. There she also met René Spitz, who showed great interest in Charlotte Bühler's infant research and visited the institute several times.

According to Robert Emde, Spitz owed a great deal of inspiration for his research to Charlotte Bühler (R. Emde, personal correspondence, 25 September, 1999).

'The first analyst I met and worked with in Vienna was René Spitz. He was so very interested in direct baby observation. I admired him and learned a great deal from him while he studied the "smiling response"' (Hellman, 1990, p. 5).

Jean Piaget was also interested in Bühler's research and Ilse Hellman got to know him during his visits there. Developmental research on newborns was carried out in a Vienna infant home for babies whose mothers did not want their child or neglected it. The home had existed since 1920 and, according to Ilse Hellman (1990, p. 3), is still in existence.

We could choose whatever babies we wanted to study and spend as much time with them as we needed for our observations. We went in pairs: a child psychologist who was already knowledgeable and experienced was accompanied by a student. The psychologist would put into words what she saw, and the student would write it down. We all had to learn shorthand as fast as we could: there weren't any recording machines those days! When I arrived there, I spent the first six months standing next to a research worker and writing down what she said she was observing.

(Hellman, 1990, p. 4)

According to Hellman, Bühler not only wanted to record developmental profiles of children from the very beginning, but also examined whether children develop differently when they are looked after by the same carer, compared to children whose carers often change. Charlotte Bühler extended these studies to the six-year-olds, on whom Ilse Hellman mainly focused her work (Hellman, 1990, p. 4).

Although the university was only ten minutes away from Berggasse 19, Ilse Hellman never met Anna Freud there. Identifying with Charlotte Bühler, who did not have a high opinion of psychoanalysis at the time, she followed her ban on attending Anna Freud's seminars; however, Esther Bick and – then already doctoral research assistants – Liselotte Frankl and Emmy Sylvester opposed this.

Ilse Hellman was fascinated by Charlotte Bühler, a stately woman who made a lasting impression on other people.[3] Bühler had been invited to University College London as a visiting professor in 1935 and to establish a private Child Guidance Clinic (Parents' Institute of Psychology for Subnormal Children in Rowland Gardens, Kensington), accompanied by her principal assistant, Dr Lotte Danzinger.[4]

After graduating in 1937, Ilse Hellman accepted Charlotte Bühler's invitation to conduct a study with her on disabled children at the Parents' Association Institute in London, as she herself could only be in London for a few months at a time. Ilse Hellman replaced a young woman who became pregnant and then another Austrian assistant, a Nazi supporter, who did not want to leave Vienna and said she wanted to be in Austria when the Nazis made the sun rise. Charlotte Bühler is said to have replied: 'I would love to know whether she enjoyed the sunrise over Austria'.

Charlotte Bühler was the director of the institute starting in 1939. Before this, she had learnt of the Annexation of Austria during another stay in London in March 1938 and that her husband had been taken into protective custody on 23 March, 1938. As a result, both had to leave the university in Vienna. After six and a half weeks, Charlotte Bühler succeeded in freeing her husband through connections in Norway, so that the family was reunited in Oslo in October 1938. Her husband then emigrated to the USA in 1938.

When Ilse Hellman emigrated to England, she managed to take some of her family's possessions with her, such as family silverware, paintings and even some

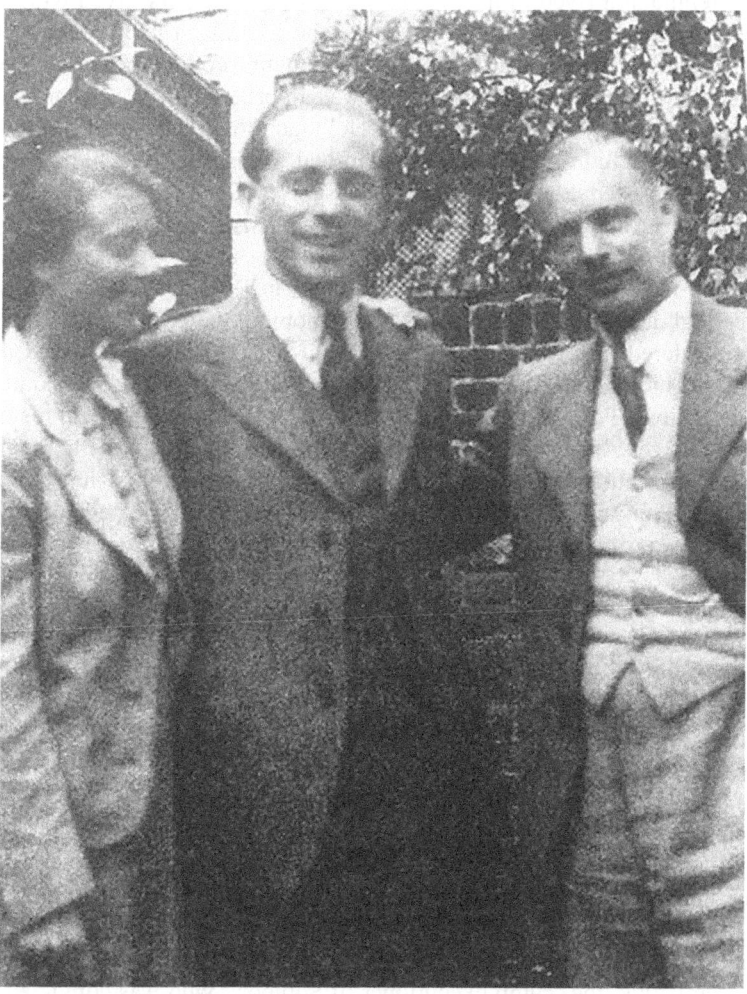

Ilse Hellman with her brothers Ernst and Bernhard in London (credit: Paul Hellmann)

wonderful old pieces of furniture. Her father, Paul Hellmann, had already been imprisoned once, but was released again due to his serious illness. He died of a pulmonary embolism in Vienna on 8 December, 1938.

Her family's fate

After the death of her husband, Irene Hellmann travelled to England, where, unfortunately, she did not stay. Ilse Hellman had a very small apartment in London with very little space for her mother, whereas her brother Bernhard had a house with more room in Rotterdam.

Irene Hellmann arrived in the Netherlands in 1939 and first lived with her son Bernhard, daughter-in-law, and grandson in the Merellaan in Rotterdam, before moving to Bilthoven. Bernhard Wolfgang Hellmann produced wooden jewellery for his family during the first years of the war. In order to have a better chance of survival, the family hid separately. Irene Hellmann then lived on the eighth floor of an Amsterdam high-rise. When she returned to her flat from hiding, she was betrayed and arrested. She was taken by the Nazis to the Westerbrok concentration camp, and on 3 March, 1944, she was deported to Auschwitz, where she was murdered (Sobibor Gedenksteine, n.d.).

Bernhard Wolfgang Hellmann was denounced in 1943 in a shelter not far from Lunteren and deported via Westerbork to the Sobibor extermination camp, where he was murdered. His then seven-year-old son Paul Hellmann survived the war thanks to his hiding place with Helene Kröller-Müller in Ede and Harskamp, near the Hoge Veluwe. For a long time after the war, he lived together with his mother, who had survived Auschwitz and returned to the Netherlands, at the home of Marten Toonder, the author of strip cartoons, which were published in many countries, and his wife Phiny Dik, an author of children's books, until he began his studies. As a child it was difficult for him to understand at first why his mother did not take care of him.

Like many Holocaust survivors, he had long suppressed his terrible experiences, especially as there was generally little talk about them during the war years. Nor did he talk about it with his aunt Ilse, whom he had met occasionally (Hellmann, 2009). He worked as a journalist at NRC Handelsblad until 1995. In the 1980s he had received a cabin-trunk from a Russian friend of Ilse and Arnold Noach with documents and photos of the family, which he first deposited in the attic. When he opened it after his retirement, he received two bags of letters from Irene Hellmann to her daughter. After the death of Ilse Hellman's daughter Maggie, he received all the family documents.

In the meantime, he not only published a book about his grandmother in 2015, but also about his own eventful life as a Jewish child in hiding in Rotterdam. In 2009 and 2010, he was one of the Dutch joint plaintiffs against the Ukrainian Ivan (John) Demjanjuk, the 'camp executioner of Sobibor', who was convicted of war crimes and sentenced in May 2011 for aiding and abetting the murder of approximately 28,000 Jews.

Ilse's other brother, Ernst Richard Hellmann (1905–1980) was able to hide in England. Equipped with a passport from the German Embassy in London, he managed to escape with his Austrian wife Anne Marie, his daughter Christiane, born in 1930, and their son Thomas, born in 1943, and managed to emigrate to Australia in time, where they were able to set up a chicken farm.

Ilse Hellman, concerned about the beginning of the war, also tried, as can be seen from a letter to her American colleague Christine Heinig dated 10 June, 1939, to find a way to emigrate to Australia. The latter had succeeded in obtaining a position as Post Principal of the Melbourne Kindergarten Training College 18 months earlier. When she received the letter, the Australian government was busy deciding how to deal with the stream of refugees. New Zealand did not accept refugees, whereas South Africa and Canada accepted a few. Former Prime Minister Stanley Bruce, then High Commissioner in London, recommended that Australia take in 30,000 refugees. The Australian government halved this number to 15,000 on 1 December, 1939. Ilse Hellman's letter was forwarded several times in Australia and on 6 November, 1939, she received a friendly but not encouraging reply from the Victorian Council for Mental Hygiene: 'There was room and need for the sort of person you are mentioning. Indeed we have another fine Viennese woman here at present, Mrs. Lacerta Finton who has splendid training and experience' (Vickers, 2016).

Ilse Hellman's response is not known. Owing to the influence of Mary Agnes Hamilton, writer and Member of Parliament for the Labour Party and friend of the family, Ilse Hellman was not classified as an 'Enemy Alien' and was therefore not arrested on the Isle of Man, like many other Jewish employees of Anna Freud.

Ilse Hellman's professional life in London

In London, Ilse Hellman met the psychoanalyst Susan Isaacs, who supported her very much and became a close friend of hers (Nölleke, n.d.). Susan Isaacs knew the work of Charlotte Bühler and was in contact with her in London, where she also met Ilse Hellman. Isaacs was replying to readers' letters in the weekly *Nursery World* and was in urgent need of support, as she could no longer cope with the flood of requests from readers.

> So, every week I went to see her. We looked at the letters together; she gave me those she wanted me to answer and replied to herself to the two or three most important ones, which would be printed. My own answers were sent direct to the mothers.
>
> I thoroughly enjoyed my visits to her and learnt from her the way she approached child development and dealt with the difficulties of handling small children. Out of our meetings a friendship developed. It played a great part in my further studies and in my later work in her department at London University's Institute of Education.
>
> (Hellman, 1990, p. 6)

At the beginning of the Second World war, the institute in London, run by Charlotte Bühler, was closed and Ilse Hellman worked as a developmental psychologist
caring for evacuated children who, in the face of the war, had to be quickly assigned to foster families. She was also responsible for the care of women and children evacuated from Gibraltar in early 1941 at the Home for Problem Evacuees, 32
Kimsley Road, Northampton.[5]

At the beginning of 1941, Ilse Hellman received a letter from Anna Freud, who –
through Liselotte Frankl and Susan Issacs – knew about her work.

> Her letter was very amusing: she said she knew I had nothing to do with
> psychoanalysis but knew more about children in homes than most people. Perhaps
> I would like to spend a weekend in Wedderburn Road and see what I thought of it!
>
> (Hellman, 1990, p. 7)

She wrote about this first encounter:

> So I went there, and it seemed very strange to me. Naturally, the whole approach
> to children was based on psychoanalytic principles, and it was quite unlike any-
> thing I had seen before. The children's behaviour, and what was expected of
> them, was very different from other nurseries in terms of discipline and 'do's
> and don'ts'. I'll never forget when I first arrived. It was during the children's
> lunch-time, and all the one-and-a half- to two-years were eating with their
> hands. They sat around a big table, and they could choose what they wanted
> to eat. Usually in a children's home you put food on the plate and tell them to
> eat up! But here there was a little buffet, and they could say what they wanted
> to eat, and if they didn't want it any more no one minded. When I was asked
> what it was like, I said, rather ironically: 'They eat spinach with their hands,
> and it looked rather peculiar, but maybe that makes one emotionally healthier!'
> It didn't make sense to me at that time, but it did when I thought about it later,
> because all the feeding disturbances I had seen in other homes didn't exist with
> children brought up like this.
>
> (Hellman, 1990, p. 8)

Anna Freud hired her immediately after the preliminary interview, especially
since, as Charlotte Bühler's assistant, she naturally brought with her the best
knowledge of developmental psychology and was also a carer. Charlotte Bühler's
former research assistants in turn passed on to Anna Freud a great deal of experience with baby observation and provided suggestions for research. Ilse Hellman
(1990, p. 23) wrote the following on the nature of Anna Freud's observation:

> All members of staff, whether nurses, educators or students, were to refer to all
> aspects of their behaviour, expected or unexpected, whether or not they con-
> firmed or contradicted expectations. New steps forward or regressive moves,
> questions, fantasies and activities were noted.

The war children's home in Wedderburn Road, which offered space for 20 children at the time, was not big enough, and after Anna Freud received financial support from the American Foster Parents' Plan, she was able to take in 50 children at 5 Netherhall Gardens. From March 1941 until the closure of the home in September 1945, Ilse Hellman ran the War Children's Home (Babies Rest Centre). There she was mainly responsible for the older children.

Anna Freud advised her to start psychoanalytic training as soon as possible.

It was my second year at the Nursery, in 1942, that Anna Freud said to me, just once or twice: 'Do you still find analysis strange? Wouldn't you like to become an analyst?' The person who played a big part in my decision to apply for the training was Dr. Josefine Stross, the paediatrician who was responsible for our children's physical care, she had trained as an analyst in Austria. She suggested to me that it would be a good idea if I combined the training with my work at the nursery. It was then that I began to read a lot and came to the conclusion that I really did want to train. But I had no money, because we were paid only two pounds, ten shillings a week, which was only just enough for our needs. Of course we were living and eating in the Nursery, but you couldn't pay an analyst on what was left over.

It was then Susan Issacs inadvertently came to the rescue. She paid for my work in the Nursery World. Anna Freud told me that one of her colleagues had heard that I wanted to start analysis and could take me for ten shillings a session. So I had two pounds ten from the Nursery, and the two pounds ten from Susan Isaacs paid for the analysis.

(Hellman, 1990, p. 10)

The admission interview with Dr Edward Glover MD left her with a bad memory. She did not know at that time that he was against the admission of laypeople. He had studied her documents, knew that she was a Doctor of Psychology from Vienna and asked her the question right at the beginning:

'And what makes you think you'd be good as an analyst?' I found that a very difficult question. I explained that I did feel I could understand people's feelings and I felt I could sense what they needed. 'And you think you can provide that?' he said. I thought I did rather badly because I got cross while I was listening to his questions.

(Hellman, 1990, p. 10)

In a further conversation with Dr Sylvia Payne, she felt accepted and supported from the beginning. In 1942, Ilse Hellman began her training at the British Psycho-Analytical Institute, which she completed in 1945, and became an associate member until 1952, when she became a full member of the British Psychoanalytic Society. She could hardly pay for her teaching analysis with Dorothy Burlingham at first, although Burlingham only charged a small hourly rate. When she had finished her training and started in a permanent position at Hampstead Clinic, she wanted to pay back the money to Dorothy Burlingham, who advised her to donate it to poor children. In this way she supported orphans who lived in municipal children's homes.

Ilse Hellman initially experienced her analytical training as very complicated. It was not only that many of the psychoanalysts were not on site – some were in the war and others had retreated to the countryside – but she also suffered from the tension between Melanie Klein and Anna Freud.

> There were no 'groups' at the time, but different analysts gave very different types of lectures and seminars. My first patient, for example, was supervised by Anna Freud, but I had to present him in clinical seminars to Mrs Klein and Mrs Riviere. I felt I was told things that I was quite unable to understand, and I hadn't read enough yet to help me. So the same material was understood and interpreted quite differently by the different seminar leaders. As a beginner, I found this extremely confusing; but the person who rescued me was Sylvia Payne, who supervised my second case.
>
> (Hellman, 1990, p. 11)

She not only helped her to understand the differences between the theoretical directions, but also trained her in transference interpretation. She also appreciated the courses by Willi Hoffer, who impressed her very much because he could convey Freud's writings very clearly and spread an atmosphere in which everything could be asked, so that different theoretical positions became clearer for her. Her relationship with Melanie Klein, however, was not burdened by this, as she did not let her know that she had done anything wrong:

> She had a very nice way of saying, 'Could one perhaps think that he might have meant something else?' She tried to minimize the feeling that what one was learning or what one was doing was no good. Many of her ideas were of course very interesting to me, since I had done so much work with babies and very small children.
>
> (Hellman, 1990, p. 11)

In addition, Melanie Klein and Paula Heimann, who were very interested in art, knew Ilse Hellman's husband Arnoldus (Arnold) Noach, who was a lecturer of art history, and often invited them both to their homes.

Ilse Hellman was very interested in Winnicott's thoughts, especially as he also showed great interest in her varied experiences with children in institutions. He invited people to meetings once a month, where he sometimes brought in his own cases. At first, she found it very difficult to follow what he was saying, and it was his wife, Claire, who stepped in to clarify. Later, Ilse Hellman conducted seminars together with Winnicott.

Ilse Hellman experienced a big change in the institute when Paula Heimann turned away from the Kleinian view and explained her reasons in 'speech and writing'. It was the time when Ilse Hellman was preparing for her graduation in 1945 and Paula Heimann, as well as Hedwig Hoffer, found it very helpful when she opened her own practice. Hedwig Hoffer knew that her colleagues needed support, especially when they were no longer in supervision after completing their training, and so, in 1946, she offered a weekly seminar at noon in her house for female graduates.

Ilse Hellman was a member of the permanent staff of the Hampstead Child Therapy Course and Clinic around Anna Freud and Dorothy Burlingham. For several years, together with Liselotte Frankl, she was in the youth department of the Hampstead Clinic, where she was responsible for the research projects carried out there, on which she also published (Frankl & Hellman, 1962).

She became a training analyst in 1955 and was a recognized psychoanalyst of the British Psycho-Analytic Society. Together with Dr Rowley, she chaired the British Psycho-Analytical Society's Training Committee for a while. When she started teaching analysis, many Canadians were with her for analytical training, due to the absence of a Canadian training institute.

She was friends with Susan Isaacs, Liselotte Frankl, Sylvia Payne, and Paula Heimann and was a member of the 'Middle Group'. She was very committed to psychoanalysis, although she never completely 'submitted' to it. She was one of the first to oppose high-frequency psychoanalysis in favour of short therapy and counselling work.

In addition to her own practice, she continued to work on research projects at the Hampstead Child Therapy Clinic, such as the simultaneous analysis of mother and child, an idea of Dorothy Burlingham's, which she had already worked on in Austria. Dorothy Burlingham believed that sometimes it is not enough to treat only the child, but that the mother also needs psychotherapy at the same time. The task of an independent coordinator was to decipher the conscious and unconscious interactions of mother and child in the treatment material. The treatment material of the two completely independently working analysts (Oscar Friedmann treated the mother) was evaluated by a third colleague – a 'coordinator'. Ilse Hellman was one of the coordinators (Hellman et al., 1960).

Another study focused on the treatment of young people, and she published on these and other issues. Both Joan Raphael-Leff and Clifford Yorke describe her great ability to teach and introduce training candidates to the world of treatment (Raphael-Leff, personal correspondence, 4 November, 2018).

Gertrud Dann appreciated Ilse Hellman's distinctive sense of humour, which sometimes helped her

to get over the more difficult sides of her. Liselotte Frankl was very friendly with Ilse Hellman. She was a lovely co-worker. With a great sense of humour, but terribly conceited. You had to know what to believe, what is exaggerated. But her humour was wonderful.

(Dann, interview, 14 July, 1996)

Ilse Hellman 'knew how to get into the picture. If she was in conversation with someone, it was quite possible that she suddenly turned to someone else who seemed more important to her' (Dann, interview, 18 September, 1997).

Ilse Hellman is described as a rather extravagant woman with 'mood swings'. In photos taken at the opening of the Freud Museum in London, staff members are welcomed personally by Princess Alexandra. It is easy to imagine that Gertrud Dann, with her rather reserved manner, sometimes felt overwhelmed by the more dominant Ilse Hellman.

Ilse's husband, Arnoldus Noach (1911–1976), a native Dutchman and art historian, survived the Nazi regime in Holland. Ilse Hellman got to know the somewhat younger man through friends, who brought them together after the Second World War. 'I think there is someone you would certainly like to meet. He is the funniest and thinnest man you have ever met' (Douglas, interview, 21 November, 1997). They then met for tea at a friend's house. The couple had known each other for a while before he was offered a position as lecturer in art history at Leeds University through the assistance of Ernst Gombrich, a fellow art historian. Diana Douglas, lecturer at Leeds University and former research assistant to Arnoldus Noach, describes him as 'very English and as someone who attached great importance to being more English than the English'. Arnold Noach is described as a 'language genius' who was fluent in five or six languages. His accent-free English was so good that he could tell from among the English exactly which region someone came from (Douglas, interview, 21 November, 1997). He seems to have held his

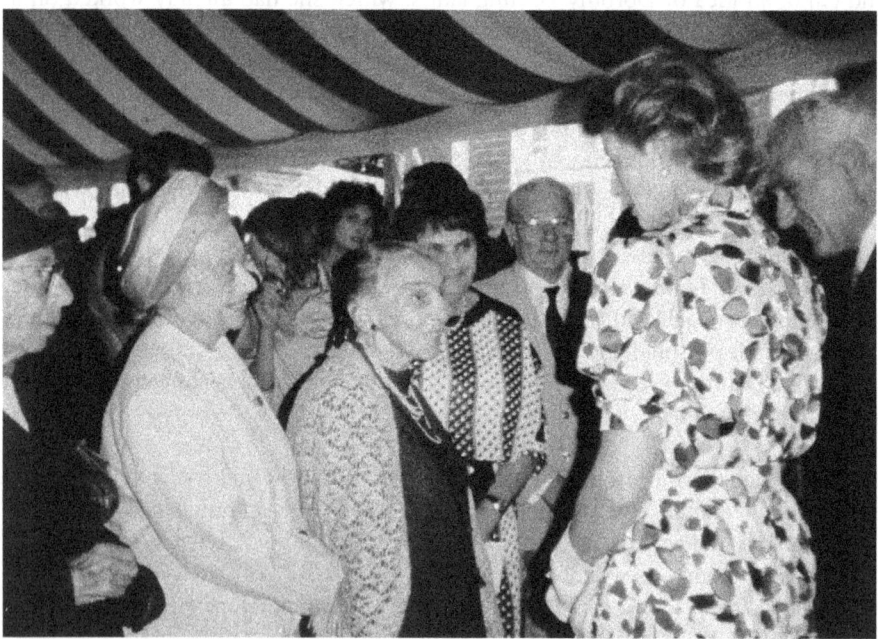

From left: Sophie Dann, Ilse Hellman, Josefine Stross, Hansi Kennedy, in the background Clifford Yorke, with Princess Alexandra of Kent at the opening ceremony of the Freud Museum 1986 (credit: Gertrud Dann)

fellow countrymen in less esteem. There was a Dutch woman in his circle of acquaintances, and he said to his colleague: 'I know she is Dutch, and she knows I am Dutch. And she knows that I know it, and I know that she knows it, but we don't talk about it' (Douglas, interview, 21 November, 1997). Full of curiosity, open to various scientific fields and equipped with a very good knowledge of human nature, Arnold Noach had the ability to stand up to his 'stately woman'. Clifford Yorke describes him as a warm-hearted man. 'His was a fun-loving and warm personality'.

When Ilse Hellman married in 1948, she was in her late thirties and gave birth to her daughter Margaret Irene (Maggie) on 18 August, 1949 at the age of 41. She was highly anxious during her pregnancy due to her advanced age, and she had no more children because of it. The couple must have seemed unusual for outsiders, in terms of their external form alone. He was overly slender and she herself was of small stature, and, according to her daughter's descriptions, 'round as a ball, just like a Viennese woman' and she described the shape of a cone with her hands (M. Williams, interview, 21 November, 1997). The marriage must also have been very complicated, although the couple stayed together for life. Ilse Hellman often amused herself and spoke 'of the rich Hellman and the poor Noach', probably alluding to their different origins.

With her hoarse, seemingly rushed voice, her daughter vividly described to me how the couple communicated with each other and everyday life at home, in which the daughter often lost out. The impression came to mind that Ilse Hellman, in her probably rather extraverted way, was less successful in offering her daughter a calm, clear framework for life. Between psychotherapy sessions, only a short exchange of information was possible. Ilse Hellman had her practice in the house, so she started talking while she was rushing up the stairs until new interruptions came in from outside, often caused by the excited barking of a small round dog or a neighbour or the sick daughter. Meanwhile, her husband stood on a ladder to reach the top books of his huge library. Then the front doorbell rang, and a new patient arrived. Ilse Hellman was still talking and ran down the stairs again. So sometimes the meal was never finished. When the father was at home – the phone was in the hallway – both her father and mother rushed towards the phone from different sides, and usually he was faster. When he had answered the phone, he would call his wife and say, 'Here's that awful analyst for you again', so that the caller had to hear it. With his 'dry humour' he often made fun of his wife's psychoanalytical colleagues. Her mother, she said, often exchanged views on the phone with other colleagues about treatment problems when the patients were out of the house. Maggie Williams recalls how her conversations with her mother were always disturbed by patients. Often her mother only had a short time for her between sessions, so it is understandable that, as a child, she had expressed the wish to become a 'patient'. She hardly ever got to see her mother, because in the evenings she often had to attend meetings or gave seminars or supervised in clinics. Julia Eccleshare writes in her obituary for Maggie Williams (née Noach) that she was mostly looked after by her beloved nanny Gretel, with whom she remained in contact throughout her life (Eccleshare, 2006).

As an adult, Maggie was at least as professionally involved as her mother had been. She was a well-known literary agent, and during the interviews we conducted, I was able to witness how Mrs Williams was repeatedly called to the phone, sometimes with two phones at her ear at the same time – like a broker negotiating – similar to how her mother had been at that age.

Ilse Hellman's husband's job forced him to travel between Leeds, where he lived two to three days a week, and London. It is hard to imagine that Ilse Hellman would have given up her work in London. Since Ilse Hellman kept her maiden name and they had their own social circles, it sometimes occurred at a party that someone would introduce them to each other. 'Professor Noach, you absolutely must meet Dr Hellman'. To which he replied laconically: 'Oh, I know her, she is the mother of my child'. On some weekends Ilse Hellman was also in Leeds, where she supervised a psychiatrist, also a member of the British Psychoanalytical Society. As a result, the couple had their own circles in Leeds so that such strange introductory encounters could happen. When Arnoldus Noach introduced his wife to colleagues, he often commented: 'She is a psychoanalyst, but don't be spooked. She only does it for money' (M. Williams, interview, 21 November, 1997).

Together with the married couple Manna and Oscar Friedmann, Ilse Hellman and her daughter Maggie, who was very fond of Oscar Friedmann, spent holidays together in Bad Gastein (Friedmann, interview, 26 November, 1996). She also attended the inauguration ceremony of the Sigmund Freud Institute in Frankfurt on 10 October, 1963, together with Paula Heimann and Willi Hoffer (then Vice President of the IPA) (Hoyer, 2008).

In 1976, after his retirement and shortly before the age of 66, Arnoldus Noach died suddenly of heart failure. He had had heart problems for 15 years, but continued to smoke, with this attitude to life: 'I could quit smoking, drinking wine, eating good food and would live to be over 90. But neither I nor my friends would then have the joy of life, so what?' (M. Williams, interview, 21 November, 1997).

Ilse Hellman did not accept any new teaching analyses after her 70th birthday; however, many of those she had accompanied during her training came to her later to exchange ideas with her (Hellman, 1990, p. 17). At over 70, she was still working in a cancer hospital (the Royal Marsden). Her job was to help the clinical staff with their hard work. It was a consulting job and not supervision in the usual sense. She regularly went there once a week in the morning, and, together with Martin Israels, a senior lecturer in psychopathology at the University of London, she gave courses on 'Human dying' and 'Dying care'.

The Contemporary Freudian Group of the British Psychoanalytic Society invited her to celebrate her 80th birthday. Until the age of 84, she worked as a psychoanalyst for adults, children, and adolescents, gave lectures and was an honorary member of the British Psychoanalytical Society. She once asked a teenager if he, after reporting enthusiastically about a certain kind of pop music that she could not follow, would not prefer a younger analyst. The boy replied: 'I'd rather have a grandma like you'. Even afterwards, colleagues or patients from earlier times still turned to her for supervision and advice. (M. Williams, interview,

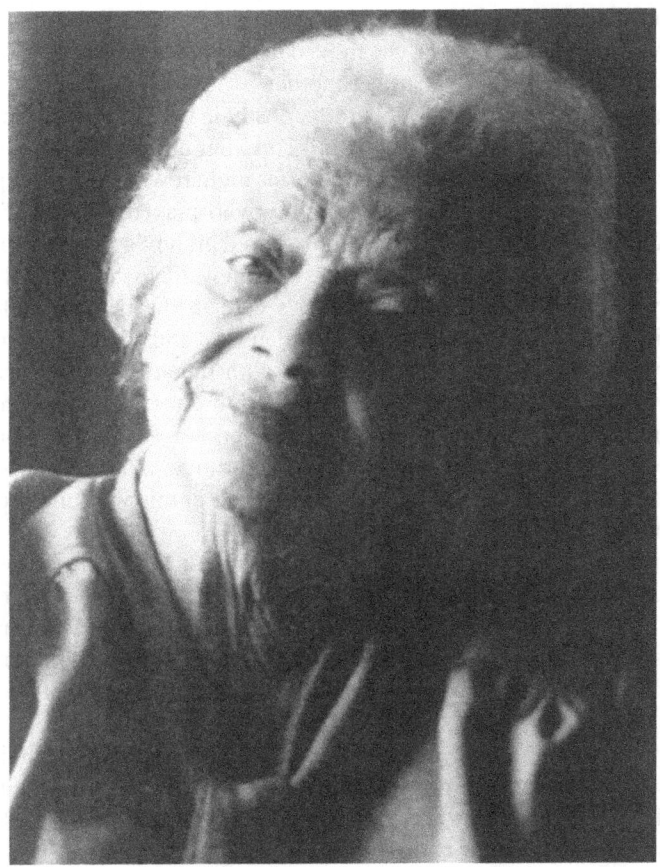

Ilse Hellman as an old woman (credit: Paul Hellmann)

21 November, 1997). In her early eighties she edited a book (*From War Babies to Grandmothers*), published in 1990, in which she and colleagues (Clifford Yorke, Ivy Bennett, Oscar Friedmann, Elisabeth Shepheard, and Liselotte Frankl) reported on various aspects of the work in the War Nurseries.

Until the end of her life Ilse Hellman was still in contact with some of the children she had looked after in the War Nurseries, a pair of twins (especially Meggy, whom she had also analysed) and two other children. Hansi Kennedy (Kennedy, interview, 23 April, 1997) reports how she and many others were invited by Ilse Hellman to celebrate the 50th birthday of one of these children and visit an opera together. The twins visited Ilse Hellman regularly and took her to the opera on her 85th birthday.

As Ilse Hellman's physical weakness grew, her daughter Maggie decided to leave her beloved residential area of Chelsea, where she had grown up, a year after her divorce from her husband (after which she began using the name Noach again).

When a house became available near her mother's home (21 Redan Street, Hammersmith, West London 14 OAW), she moved there with her daughter Sophie, then three years old, to take better care of her mother.

Ilse Hellman spent the last years of her life mostly in bed, heavily disabled by her considerable overweight and high blood pressure, but above all by her blindness. Her zest for life waned and she seemed to prefer nightgown and dressing gown to any other clothing. Her granddaughter Sophie, who played with her frequently, visited her about twice a week. Together they shared granny's 'passion for sweets', especially *mousse au chocolat* (S. Williams, interview, 6 November, 2014).

Maggie Noach had organized her mother's care in the best possible way by always having a woman live with Ilse Hellman day and night for two to three weeks – arranged by a private organization – with the advantage that the carers could cope well with this period of time and be more relaxed and were relieved before becoming burnt out. The motives of the carers were very different: some of them took over the work from a more charitable attitude, others primarily needed the money or did not have their own home but lived in this way, more or less, by changing households.

Diana Douglas, a former employee of Ilse Hellman's husband, seemed to have taken the position of a second daughter in the family. When she was in London, she lived in Ilse Hellman's house (No. 23 Redan Street). Maggie Williams and Diana Douglas reported how she was able to meet Ilse Hellman in an unbiased way, without being caught up by 'shadows from the past', as is sometimes the case with one's own children.

Ilse Hellman spent the last year of her life in the White Horse nursing home. After her death, her remaining professional estate was given to the Freud Archives in London. Her personal papers are with her nephew, Paul Hellmann, in Rotterdam.

Ilse Hellman considered her notes important for a lecture series, *Psycho-Analysis and Contemporary Thought*. This was a series of Freud Centenary Lectures put together by the British Psychoanalytical Society. It included a lecture by Ilse Hellman entitled 'Psycho-analysis and the teacher'.

Other documents demonstrate her enduring interest in early childhood and educational issues, such as the work of Robert and Joyce Robertson, or an article by E. R. Boyce on playing in kindergarten, or *The Educational Value of the Nursery School* by Susan Isaacs. From W. Ernst Freud she had documents on 'The baby profile, Part 2'.

Documents from her colleague Hansi Kennedy on the problems of reconstruction in child analysis are available in the archive, including the manuscript for 'Growing up with a handicapped sibling'. Among the papers that were found in her estate are writings by John Bowlby and Dorothy Burlingham as well as German papers such as a publication by Annemarie Dührssen, '*Zum Problem des Selbstmordes bei jungen Mädchen* [transl.: On the problem of suicide in young women], as well as the essay by Erika Danneberg and Hedda Eppel (1971) *Teamarbeit: Eine Behandlung von Mutter und Sohn* [transl.: Teamwork: The treatment of a mother and son].

Just how much she appreciated her work with Charlotte Bühler is shown by the fact that her estate also contains the paper by Paul Feitscher (1939) on Bühler's and Hetzer's tests for small children, as well as the paper by Lotte Schenk-Danzinger (1963) *Die Grundideen und die theoretischen Fragestellungen in Charlotte Buhlers Lebenswerk* [transl.: The basic ideas and theoretical questions in Charlotte Buhler's life's work], a commemorative publication by her for Charlotte Bühler.

Notes

1 Alma Mahler-Werfel reports a close connection between the family of her stepfather, Carl Moll, and the grandparents of Ilse Hellman – Bernhard (1838–1901) and Lina Hellmann (1850–1930). At the beginning of the diary entries, 19-year-old Alma Schindler was close friends with Gretl (Margarete), one of the couple's five children, as well as with Paul, future father of Ilse Hellman. From the diary entries, one gains an insight into the luxurious life of the Hellmann family. For example, the family had its own box in the Vienna Court Opera Theatre, and Alma Schindler (Mahler-Werfel, 2002) enjoyed attending Wagner performances with Lina, Gretl and Paul Hellmann (Mahler-Werfel, 2002). She seemed to 'go in and out' with the Hellmanns, reports many meals together, concerts and dinners, visits to concerts or the Secession exhibition house, outings, balls and trips to the Hellmanns' property in Altaussee and Grundlsee. For example, she writes how she dressed up for a 'Hellmann ball' (Mahler-Werfel et al., 2002, f.) and danced with the then 23-year-old father of Ilse Hellman. Gretl Hellmann, who was unhappily in love with Max Neumayer, a very good friend of Paul Hellmann, gave Alma a photograph of Klimt, because at that time she was deeply in love with Klimt. 'Gretl can't imagine what infinite joy she has given me. My, my Klimt. Eternally my Klimt' (Mahler-Werfel, 2002). Paul Hellmann later (in 1917) acquired the painting 'Portrait of an Old Man (The Blind Man)' by Gustav Klimt at the Dorotheum, about whose later rightful ownership there was much dispute. The family is also said to have owned another painting by Gustav Klimt, 'Island in the Attersee' (Niederacher, 2018, pp. 12, 25).

In the experience of Alma Mahler (2002) she was – not only through her friendship with Gretl, whom she also gave piano lessons for half a year – a much-appreciated guest in the Hellmann family. The relationship with Paul Hellmann seems 'flirtatious', and the extent to which Lina Hellmann would have liked to see Alma Mahler as her daughter-in-law remains unclear. Thus Alma Mahler (2002, p. 98) writes on 10 March, 1898: 'Nm [afternoon]. I received a card from Paul Hellmann with *hot greetings* from the ice, namely from Svalbard. Only *polar greetings* were intended for Gretl [Hellmann]. Well, of course – a subtle difference had to be made'.

At another place: 'Lunch at the Hellmanns', also N.M. [in the afternoon]. Paul Hellmann is getting a little too cheeky for me, and so is the old man' (Mahler-Werfel, 2002). On 11 April, 1899: 'They all rejoiced mischievously. Paul ran at me and kissed my hand. Gretl literally ate me up. We stayed the whole afternoon. Gretl and Paul took us home on rubber-wheeled bikes' (Mahler-Werfel, 2002).

At the farewell (30 August, 1899) Alma and her sister were given 'charming pendants' by Gretl Hellmann and 'Mrs. Hellmann gave us charming golden brooches – made from veneer – why are we being so spoiled?' (Mahler-Werfel, 2002).

2 The oldest of Ilse Hellman's brothers, Bernhard Wolfgang, was not only born in the same year and on the same day (7 November, 1903), but also at the same hour and in the same district of Vienna (on Alsergrund) as Konrad Lorenz. Both came from wealthy homes and probably met as first years at the Schottengymnasium. They were united by a deep

friendship and common interests. They were close to nature; both hiked frequently, climbed mountains, and observed animals from the time they were children. The Hellmann family in Vienna had plenty of animals to show, such as a large aquarium and a Nile crocodile, which bit both Konrad Lorenz and Bernhard Hellmann several times. The interest in observing behaviour was equally strong among both friends. For example, Bernhard was able to observe an isolated male tilapia in the aquarium and found that when he held a mirror in front of it, it attacked violently. Konrad Lorenz later called this observation 'action-specific energy', which could be 'dammed up' or 'used up'. Another passion of theirs was motorcycling, which was also reflected in later terms such as 'idling action' and 'skipping movement' in Lorenz's behavioural research (Taschwer, 2020a).

When Konrad Lorenz received his Nobel Prize and talked about biographical roots and influences on his career, he mentioned his old friend Bernhard several times. What he did not mention at this point, however, was not only his entry into the NSDAP after the annexation of Austria, but also his resulting betrayal of Bernhard.

3 Charlotte Bühler, née Malachowski, was born in Berlin on 20 December, 1893. In 1916, she married her university instructor, Karl Bühler, who held a professorship in Munich from 1913 to 1918 and in Dresden from 1918 to 1922. She completed a post-doctoral thesis in Dresden in 1920 and went with her husband to Vienna in 1923, where he was appointed professor of philosophy and became director of the Psychological Institute. Although he, too, did research on developmental psychology, his theory of language is better known today. From 1929 to 1938, Charlotte Bühler was professor of child psychology in Vienna.

After fleeing to Oslo, Charlotte Bühler worked from 1938 to 1939 in a child counselling centre, from 1939 to 1940 as a professor of psychology at the teachers' academy in Trondheim, and from 1940 as a professor of psychology at the University of Oslo. She then emigrated via London in 1940 – at her husband's insistence – just in time to flee to the USA. She was given various professorships there, also worked as a senior psychologist and spent the end of her life – even though she had taken on American citizenship in 1945 – in Stuttgart from 1971, where she still had a private practice. She died there on 3 February, 1974 (Charlotte Bühler Institut, n.d.)

4 Charlotte Danzinger, later married Schenk-Danziger, and called herself 'Lotte', since she worked with Charlotte Bühler. She had first studied education, then psychology with Karl and Charlotte Bühler (dissertation 1929 with Karl Bühler: 'Foster Mother and Foster Child', published in 1930). She was paid from the Rockefeller Foundation funds raised by Charlotte Bühler from 1927 to 1935 and was involved in the famous 'Marienthal Study' with Maria Jahoda (as was Josefine Stross). Later, she held a professorship in developmental psychology.

5 Questionnaire for the Personnel of all Colonies, 6 August, 1941 from Ilse Hellman.

Sources and personal communication

Telephone conservation with Ilse Helman on 6 and 7 June, 1997.

Interview with Maggie Williams (Noach) on 21 November, 1997.

Interview with Gertrud Dann on 18 September, 1997.

Interview with Diana Douglas on 21 November, 1997.

Interview with Sophie Williamson on 6 November, 2014.

Interview with Hansi Kennedy on 23 April, 1997.

Publications by Ilse Hellman

Bennett, I. & Hellman, I. (1951). Psychoanalytical material related to observations in early development. *Psychoanalytic Study of the Child, 6*, 307–324.

Hellman, I. (1954). Some observations on mothers of children with intellectual inhibitions. *Psychoanalytic Study of the Child, 9*(1), 259–273. https://doi.org/10.1080/00797308.195 4.11822542

Hellman, I. (1960). Simultaneous analysis of mother and child. *Psychoanalytic Study of the Child, 15*, 359–377.

Hellman, I. (1962). Hampstead Nursery follow-up studies. Sudden separation and its effect followed over twenty years. *Psychoanalytic Study of the Child, 17*(1), 159–174. https://doi.org/10.1080/00797308.1962.11822844

Hellman, I. (1964). Assessment of analysability illustrated by the case of an adolescent patient. *Bulletin of the Hampstead Clinic, 1*, 65–73.

Hellman, I. (1978). Simultaneous analysis of parents and child. In: J. Glenn & M. A. Scharfman (eds), *Child Analysis and Therapy* (pp 473–491). New York: Aronson.

Hellman, I. (1983). Work in the Hampstead War Nurseries. *International Journal of Psychoanalysis, 64*(4), 435–439. https://doi.org/10.1080/00797308.1960.11822582

Hellman, I. (1990). *From War Babies to Grandmothers. Forty-Eight Years in Psychoanalysis*. London: Karnac Books.

Hellman, I. & Frankl, L. (1962). The ego's participation in the therapeutic alliance. *International Journal of Psychoanalysis, 43*, 333–337.

Hellman, I., Dann, S. & Dann, G. (1942). Annual Report of a Residential War Nursery: a thank-you letter. Anna Freud Centre Archives, London (unpublished).

Hellman, I., Friedman, O., Shepheard, E. (1960). Simultaneous analysis of mother and child. *Psychoanalytic Study of the Child, 15*, 359–377.

Hellman, I., de Monchauy, C. & Ludowyk-Gyomroi, E. (1961). Simultaneous analysis of a mother and her eleven-year-old daughter (unpublished).

Hellman, I., Schnurmann, A. & Todes, C. (1970). Simultaneous analysis of a mother and her four-year-old daughter (unpublished).

6

Hansi (Hanna) Kennedy (6.1.1923–30.10.2003) – A Life for the Hampstead Child Therapy Clinic

Hansi (Hanna) Kennedy, née Engl, was born in Colonia, near Vienna, on 6 January, 1923, three and a half years after her sister Susie. Her mother, Gertrud Engl (née Kohn, 1891–1971), was from Žatec/Saaz, Czechoslovakia, with the maternal line then settling in Vienna.[1] Her father, Oskar Engl's (1890–1952), family came from Plzeň (Pilsen) in Bohemia; however, her father was born in Vienna and continued to run the family hat factory. He grew up 'surrounded' by two older and two younger sisters.

When asked about the name Hansi, which she herself had already chosen in Vienna, Hansi Kennedy (interview, 11 July, 1996) told me, laughing:

> Yes, Hanna is my name. But I have always called myself Hansi. At that time, that was also such a modern name. Actually, I think my parents perhaps wanted a boy. But there are many Hansis in my generation. That was a modern name in Vienna.

She attended the local elementary school with Jewish and non-Jewish children from different backgrounds. Early on, she was able to perceive her classmates' fears, which sensitized her to the experience of others (Miller & Neely, 2008).

Her first encounter with psychoanalysis occurred in 1933 when she was ten years old when the Lampl de Groot family moved into her neighbourhood.[2] Hansi Engl wondered about 'the patients', adults and children, who were treated there. 'That's when I used to ask my parents what it was and what the patients there were, and they explained it to me a bit. That was the first contact. That's when I knew something about psychoanalysis" (Kennedy, interview, 11 July, 1996).

She became friends with one of the Lampl daughters, both of whom later joined the resistance in the Netherlands.

> My father told a lot about psychoanalysis through Mr Lampl. He was friends with psychoanalysts in England and was interested in it. Mother was not particularly interested; was a housewife, liked music, settled in England very well.
> (Kennedy, interview, 11 July, 1996)

DOI: 10.4324/9781003403906-7

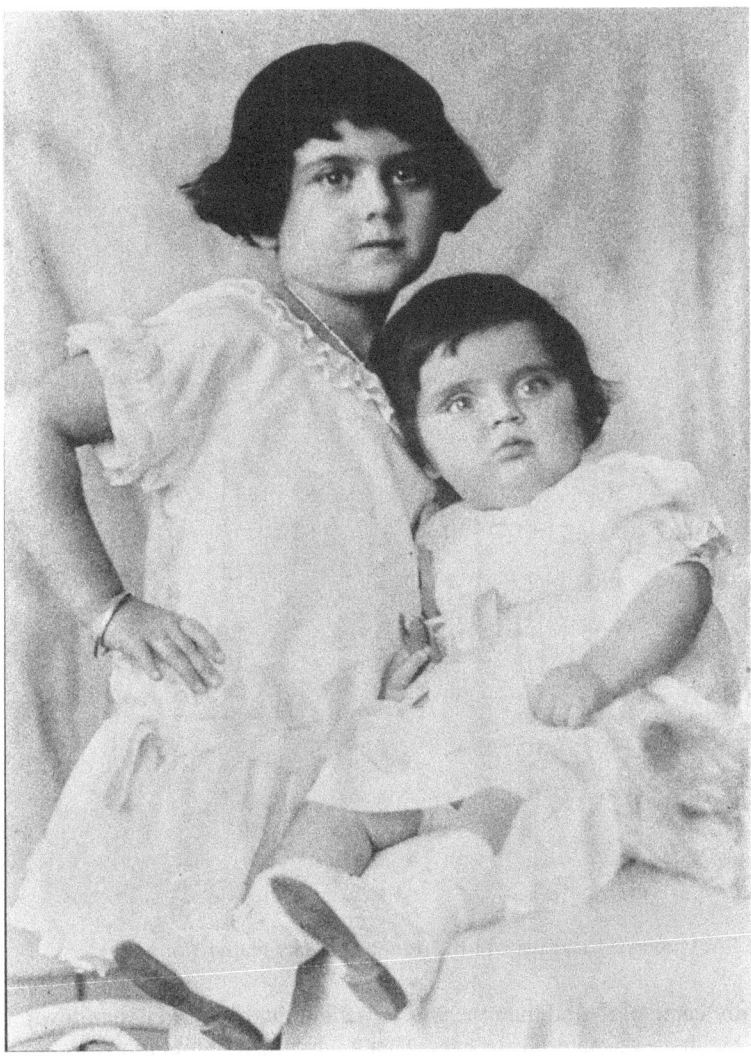

Susie and Hanna Engl, 1924 (credit: Hansi Kennedy)

Her paternal grandparents died while she was still a child in Vienna. When the hat trade faltered in the early 1930s, her father tried to expand his export/import business in London.

He wanted to open a company here. Partly because one of his sisters came from Berlin and said: Hitler would also come to Austria. And so, he went to England in 1935 to establish himself and probably opened the company here, but nothing

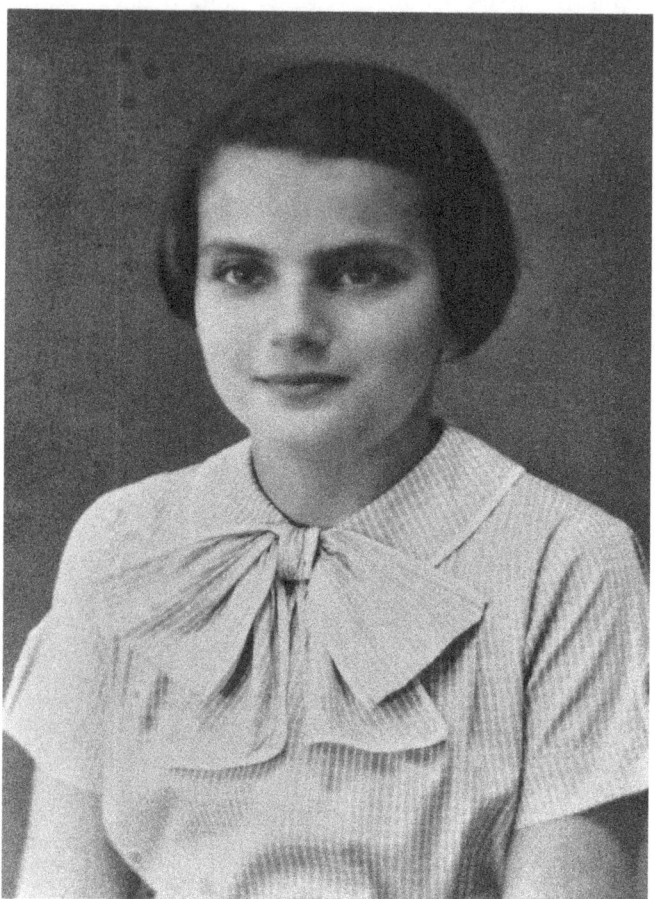

Hansi Engl, about 15 years old in Vienna (credit: Hansi Kennedy)

really came of it, and then the war came and then he closed that down. [–] Then he had hats, or material for hats. That's why the trade relations went better. Father had gone ahead alone, and my mother stayed with us.

(Kennedy, interview, 23 April, 1997)

It was a great time of adjustment for Hansi Kennedy and her family, separated from her beloved father. In addition, her Viennese parents had to abandon their house, the contents were packed, and her mother moved with her daughters to stay temporarily with her parents, who lived in the same street. 'I was just 15 when Hitler came and – was just 16 when I came to England. I already had a British textbook' (Kennedy, interview, 11 July, 1996).

In 1938, when Hansi Engl was in high school, Jewish students had to leave the school; some classmates were already wearing the Nazi uniform. Instead of moving to a new school, Hansi Engl was determined to make her long-cherished dream come true and become a kindergarten teacher. She sought out Hedy (Hedwig) Schwarz, who ran a Montessori kindergarten in Vienna, in order to gain experience in a kindergarten. At the time, Hedy Schwarz was preparing to emigrate to London. She urged Hansi Kennedy not to begin her studies in Vienna, in view of the increasing anti-Semitic conditions, since she would be unlikely to be able to complete them anyway, but to go to London instead. The restrictions imposed on Jews by pre-war circumstances also made Hedy Schwarz doubt the quality of education in Vienna. In any event, Hansi Engl emigrated to London with her family in March 1939. The family, along with her maternal grandparents, lived from August 1939 in the same house in Hampstead where Hansi Kennedy lived until her death. Her sister Susie lived nearby with her family.

> [My grandparents] lived originally upstairs and then rebuilt and wandered around the house. Circumstances caused this. There was little money. My grandparents had some money and a Czech passport; were not Austrians. On 1 April, 1939, they immigrated as tourists, quite simply. Had advantages because of that. Grandfather died after one year; was already ill when he came.
>
> (Kennedy, interview, 5 June, 1997)

Her father had also managed to accommodate niece and nephew in England and to support his sisters in their emigration. Hansi Kennedy felt 'privileged' – compared to many others – that her family was able to escape the Holocaust together with the entire household. In the interview (Kennedy, 5 June, 1997) she reflected that emigration must nevertheless have been difficult for her parents, 'while for the children life was just beginning. It was a bit difficult with settling in and with the language. Then there was the war.' She describes her father as 'very modern' and 'fun loving'.

> My parents had a nice life, had hosted parties. For mother, going to England was already a factor. She then also began to cook. Never whined about what she had lost, on the contrary. She was glad to have her family and built up a social life.
>
> (Kennedy, interview, 5 June, 1997)

Jan Wiener, the daughter of Hansi Kennedy's sister Susie, who decided to pursue a Jungian education and interviewed Hansi Kennedy three weeks before her death, describes her aunt as 'actually a very cultured and knowledgeable woman with a particular love of music' (Wiener, 2003).

Hedy Schwarz was at a London boarding school that a cousin of Hansi Kennedy attended.

> My father was already living in England, he brought my cousin to school, and she immediately connected that, my name with his, and there I had a contact. Hedy Schwarz was the first kindergarten teacher who Anna Freud took into the

War Nursery, in the very early days, before Ilse Hellman [–] And then, Hedy Schwarz, when the War Nursery started [–] she came directly from there into the War Nursery, and she was the first director in Wedderburn Road, before the Baby Home was opened. She was there for a short time, though it was actually for families, a rest centre.[3] My father had some kind of connections with analysts. And he heard that Anna Freud was going to open the War Nurseries. He knew I was interested in that. I'd done so many different little jobs but hadn't really started anything. And so, he said, 'Go there – maybe you want this?' And so, I went and introduced myself, and that's how I got into it. Actually, to have my kindergarten education. That was my main interest. And psychoanalysis was more in the unconscious at that time.

(Kennedy, interview, 11 July, 1996)

Jan Wiener (2003) reveals that Hansi Engl was not immediately accepted at her first job interview. 'Her father, to whom she was very attached, said it was because she was wearing the wrong clothes and was too flighty – too interested in men'.

She was assigned as a student assistant and a workload of ten to twelve hours was a given for all of them. Hansi Kennedy remained in the War Nurseries until its dissolution in 1945.

I was pretty young back then and so I hadn't done anything before, had left school – and then spent four years very closely, I mean long hours, with those children. And then we had a training, and a very interesting one. You learned directly from the observation of the children about psychoanalysis. Then we talked about it, at first without theory. And that was so easy for me, I mean, it was in my bones somehow. […] We held on to that later, that the students had to observe.

(Kennedy, interview, 11 July, 1996)

How much her work was appreciated is shown by the testimonial she received from Anna Freud after the disbandment of the War Nurseries in 1945.

HAMPSTEAD NURSERIES
15 Wedderburn Road, N.W.3.
Tel. Hampstead 6334
28th August, 1945

TO WHOM IT MAY CONCERN
Miss Hansi Engl has been on the staff of the Hampstead Nurseries from August 1941 to August 1945. In her capacity, first as a student worker, then as an assistant, she has passed through all the departments of the Nurseries and has gained experience in the care and upbringing of the various age groups. She has spent 10 months on her baby training with infants from 10 days to 1 year, including milk kitchen duty; she worked for 11 months with the children between 2 and 7 years of age. Periods of varying length were given to nursery

schoolwork. Included were recurring periods of night duty, when Miss Engl was responsible for a shelter dormitory of 50 children, including the night feeding of the young babies.

During her assistantship Miss Engl was employed in all the children's departments in turn.

In addition to this practical work Miss Engl has attended the course and lectures held for the students of the Nursery. The subjects treated were those concerning the bodily and mental development of young children: Anatomy, Hygiene, Nutrition, First Aid; Normal and Abnormal Mental Development, Testing; Emotional and Instinctual Development; Problems of Early Education. Miss Engl also attended some special Seminars on the Theory of Psycho-Analysis and its Application to Education.

Miss Engl proved herself to be an outstandingly good and very intelligent student and worker in every respect. She was from the beginning fully devoted to her work, seriously interested in all the problems involved in it, and spared no efforts in making herself acquainted with the principles underlying the work and their application of the daily handling of the children. She showed excellent capabilities as a baby nurse; was very skilful with the toddlers between 1 and 2 years; and she worked specially well in the department of the older nursery-children. She is well able to occupy groups in a constructive manner. To prepare and use educational toys and material, and to plan a nursery day. She showed equal interest and skill in handling individual children, among them some problem children, over long periods of their upbringing. She is well able to observe, to understand, and to guide children through difficult periods of their development.

As a war-time student Miss Engl has had her full share of hard work and emergency conditions. Miss Engl has made full use of all the possibilities for theoretical study which were offered for the students of the Nursery. She has used her spare time to take a Diploma in Psychology in Birkbeck College.

Her cooperativeness and helpfulness have won her the sympathy and respect of her teachers and fellow workers.

In her speech on the occasion of a celebration in June 1995 commemorating Anna Freud's 100th birthday (published 2009 posthumously by Hansi Kennedy), she describes vividly the conditions under which the children lived during the Blitz and the grounds for their admission to the Hampstead War Nurseries. From her descriptions, it is also clear how much Anna Freud witnessed the children's grief at separations from their mothers.

There was an onrush of mothers who wanted their small children in a place of safety and also accessibility. With some of these children, especially those with bad previous evacuation experiences, the separation from their mothers was extremely distressing, and whenever possible mothers were encouraged to stay, even for a few days, to settle the children in.

Observing the extent of the children's grief made a deep impression on Anna Freud, especially the reaction of a three-year-old boy who turned within a few days from a seemingly healthy child into a grief-stricken one with a compulsive ritual. She often related his story in later years to students to illustrate severe manifestations of separation anxiety.

(Kennedy, 2009, p. 307)

Hansi Kennedy vividly describes Billy's grief, which immediately brings to mind the film about the separation experiences of 'little John' that James and Joyce Robertson later released in the 1960s.

Immediately after her arrival in London, Hansi Engl took correspondence courses to catch up on her A-levels and was able to study psychology starting in 1942, first at Kings College and then on weekends at Birkbeck College, taking her psychology exams at the age of 22.

So I made up A-levels in London in the first year before I was with Anna Freud [–] and then in the war, so about the second year, from the War Nursery, so how we all tried to do that, I did an external university course. It was supposed to be a weekend, it's for working people – part-time [–] and, because it was war and you couldn't do evening classes [–], there's still a college today as an evening class – it was moved to the weekend and Anna Freud gave us that time. So on one day we had our day off and in the second day [–] I think 2½ days it lasted, the training. And namely before anything else, you had to read and study, of course, and we had these terribly long days, we actually had twelve hours on duty with two hours off, sometime during the day. But generally twelve hours on duty and then still coming home and reading books in a hurry. But you didn't have as much social life [laughs] [–].

And there were about five of the many young girls who were working there at that time, so they were doing a university course. Either in psychology, like me, or in social work, social science. [–] I had just got my qualification when the Nursery closed. That was very good.

(Kennedy, interview, 23 April, 1997)

Kate Friedlander employed her as a psychologist at the Child Guidance Clinic she founded in Chichester in West Sussex in 1947, where Hansi Engl worked as a child therapist for four years.

Kate Friedlander, she called me and said, 'I want to hire you, would you like to work as a therapist?' 'I have no training as a therapist.' 'You know more than I can make up, and we need to hire you as a psychologist,' because that's what I had training for, but 'you're going to do treatments, and I'm going to supervise you.' And that's how it went. There I was [for] four years, and in those four years the course started and the training with Anna Freud.

(Kennedy, interview, 23 April, 1997)

When Anna Freud began psychoanalytic child therapy training, partly at the urging of Kate Friedlander, Hansi Kennedy was among the first. After the War Nurseries closed, she went to Dorothy Burlingham for analysis five mornings a week, then went to Chichester for three days to see her patients. Hansi Kennedy was glad to have done her training analysis with Dorothy Burlingham. She wanted a woman analyst who had children of her own (Miller & Neely 2008). 'It was nice because it was a Freud analysand. That's what mainly interested me about it' (Kennedy, interview, 23 April, 1997).

In retrospect, she thinks:

No, so the pioneers in psychoanalysis, they were already quite different from the later analysts, that's something quite different. Although there were so many things going on that you don't do today: 'incestuous relationships' and family histories and so on. [–] In Europe it was still repeated after the war, where there were so few analysts. [–] [Dorothy Burlingham] [was] a quite underestimated analyst, quite underestimated. For me the most important thing in the analysis was [from which line I come from], who I am? A direct descendant of Freud. That she often spoke of Freud in the analysis. That was important to me [–], but [she was] also very human. Yes, she was terribly important for, for Anna Freud. Although professionally, of course, she always stood in the background. But she made everything possible that Anna Freud wanted, yes? [–] She was a supporting hand. She was certainly much better as a practical analyst than as a theoretical, perhaps not so [–], [it] was not important for her, yes? But the human part was always different.

(Kennedy, interview, 23 April, 1997)

The people who were in the War Nursery could do the training course in two years instead of three. And then the clinic [Hampstead Child Therapy Clinic] was opened, after those four years, that developed so very nicely, and from the first day the clinic opened, I worked there.

(Kennedy, interview, 11 July, 1996)

And we were then the first generation, after our training and most in my group had already finished in '49. Two years, later the course was three years; only much later it was four. But most of us did it in two years.

(Kennedy, interview, 23 August, 1997)

There was Sara Rosenfeld [Sarah Kut].[4] She had already trained as a kindergarten teacher in Germany; a bit older than me. She was a very good friend of mine. We worked in the War Nursery for four years and then in the clinic for many years. Yes, and Hanni (Benkendorf née Köhler) started at the War Nursery on the same day as I did, and was there all the time, and was also on the course, and they didn't do their traineeship in West Sussex, but with Dr Bonnard and Dr Frankl in East End London Hospital [sic]. There was another group who were employed there and after the war did their child analysis there. Augusta Bonnard. She was also trained by Anna Freud. A psychiatrist – English.[5]

(Kennedy, interview, 23 April, 1997)

In 1949, Hansi Engl married Gerhard Helmut Kahn. He was working in his father's paper importing business, and, as a soldier, had taken on the English name Gerald Kennedy. When she met him while playing tennis, he was already using this name. During this time, she was working strenuously in West Sussex but quit in 1951 after becoming pregnant.

In '51 I left West Sussex … my gynaecologist didn't want me to be making this long trip. I was having problems. Yes, I had already lost a child in the first pregnancy. And when I was pregnant the second time, he said, 'I want this to stop; this long journey.' And then I left West Sussex. Dr Friedlander died before that, too. She died very young. [–] And – so Anna Freud then had opened the clinic in 1952. But in '51, when the money actually came and the house was bought and all the preparations were made, so while I was pregnant, I was actually already [–] I mean I wasn't employed, but I participated. But in the months when my child was born, the clinic was opened, eh, that was '52. So, February '52 we saw the first patients. [–] I didn't stop. I lived very close to the clinic, of course, as I still do today, and I was there for two hours or so. Then I worked there for 40 years. First a few days and later, when my children were older, full time.

(Kennedy, interview, 23 April, 1997)

I never stopped working. I was very proud, I only stopped for two weeks [laughs] when I had my kids. But I really only [went to work] by the hour. I used to get these really crazy kids in treatment that couldn't go to school anyway. So, I could divide it up like that, you know? I could see them in the mornings, or as it suited me.

(Kennedy, interview, 11 July, 1996)

She was supported by her mother, who also took care of her children. In 1955, three and a half years later, her second son was born. 'One can reconcile it. It's nice to have a profession that you can combine. Especially if you don't practise at home. I didn't practise at home until my children were older' (Kennedy, interview, 11 July, 1996).

I was the first one to get married of that group of people who did the training. And when I told Anna Freud that I was getting married, she said, not very enthusiastically somehow, 'You are lost for the course.' You lose somebody you've trained. And also, [she] didn't always call me by my married name, it took at least two years before she actually called me by my married name. [–] And then many years later she once [–] my children sometimes came to parties then back then [–] and that's when she met them, and we were invited to Walberswick.

Then Sara Rosenfeld and some others also [got married]. And we all went on working, yes. And then at one point she said, 'Well, now I can see that you all are actually bringing something to it with your families.' [–] I had been working for many years before I had children. Once you have children of your own, your attitude toward the patients' parents changes. You see the difficulties. You see that it's not so easy. And that the role of parents, sometimes [–] I wouldn't even say [–] you make mistakes, but you just can't always strive for the ideal. And that maybe it is actually not good to always strive for the ideal.

(Kennedy, interview, 11 July, 1996)

[...] No, [Anna Freud] was always terribly nice, and to my children, and at Christmas she would come with presents. In later years, sometimes I was [–] of course, sometimes I was invited there [–] and she would say stay for lunch, and [she] even came here to my house once. I really enjoyed that, but it was [laughs] exhausting. It was exhausting, because through all of this it was formal [laughs] yeah, yeah [pause]. And she had different relationships with everybody. [She had a] very different relationship with Dr Yorke. That was a medical relationship. He was allowed to discuss certain things, like health-related things, with her. And she had a different relationship with me, through this long-term collaboration, so the War Nursery was always the common thing, there were few people who were there that long. [Pause.] And with the Danns it was quite different again.

(Kennedy, interview, 11 July, 1996)

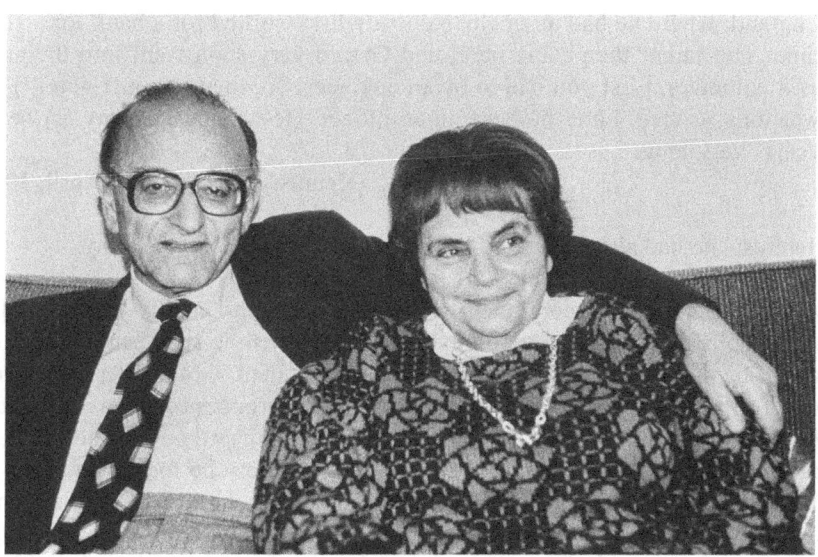

The Kennedy couple, 1988 (credit: Hansi Kennedy)

I married a German who grew up in Mannheim. My husband. [Pause.] Well, that was a complicated story. But you could go into the English army. At first only [–] without arms, and so later [–] my husband then became an officer but was not yet my husband. And was sent to Germany. And so, before they were sent to Germany, they could change their name [–], so that if they were captured, they would be treated as English prisoners of war, not emigrants. And then so my husband [–] they all changed their names, looking in the phone book and then kept that. [...] And he called himself Gerald. Gerald is the English version. And he took the H of Helmut as a middle name. Gerald H. Kennedy. [–] And we had a cousin who was in the American army parachute regiment, and he had then also changed his name to Kennedy [laughs]. My children now have cousins in America named Kennedy [laughs]. It's quite funny; life is funny.

(Kennedy, interview, 23 April, 1997)

His mother was ill, and her husband did not want to abandon her, especially since they had a factory. So, Gerhard Helmut Kahn was sent to school in Neuchâtel in 1934, where he took his baccalaureate in French. I mean, he certainly could have had a very academic education and had a great advantage because of that, after he knew languages. So, his French was absolutely [–], English, German and French were fluent, and, in the war, he was mainly in Italy, and there he was also able to speak very fluently in Italian. And of course, that helped him later commercially very much [–] he was in the import/export business. [–] His brother was in Italy and after the death of his mother in Mannheim on 6th September, 1937, Gerald Kennedy emigrated to England, where he had an uncle. Kennedy first worked for a bank for a short time. The father then came here, and Gerald very soon went into the army as a volunteer. First you had to be an engineer. So, then you just dug [–] not weapons service. Later he became an officer. He was in the army for seven years. Very long!

(Kennedy, interview, 23 April, 1997)

Her husband had already started studying during his time in the army.

And then, he always continued to study. So, he was mainly interested [in] philosophy and later anthropology. And then, when he took early retirement at 63, he did a university degree as a mature student. Got his degree. He did that full time. And when he [d...] [doesn't fully pronounce the word 'died'], he was just going to do a PhD. Yes. He didn't finish that. But he travelled all over the world in running the stationery business he took over from his father and built up. He was particularly interested in the Mayan civilization in South America, where he often went. So, I travelled with him a lot. [–] But he was very happy with the opportunity to do what he always wanted to do and couldn't do before.

(Kennedy, interview, 23 April, 1997)

Her husband died in 1988 at the age of 68.

> It's interesting how it works with emigration. It takes at least a generation, [so] that most of one's real friends, except for my professional colleagues, are actually all originally from Germany. They all live in this area, too. It's different with our children. My son married an English woman who came from Manchester, who is interested in it, but has no relationship at all with the emigrants, they came from Manchester. My other son married someone who was semi-continental. The mother was from Germany, the father was English, so there it's a little bit slower, but actually with the next generation it's different, they feel really English. I don't feel English. You also have problems with the language. Already when I open my mouth. You can tell right away where I'm coming from, and I can tell right away. [...] We didn't speak German for various reasons. First of all, we didn't speak German during the war. We had just married after the war, relatively shortly after [–] in 1949. Then we had this problem: between Austrian and German. [laughs] So my children somehow have an ear for German.
>
> (Kennedy, interview, 5 July, 1997)

Hansi Kennedy also spoke to her mother in English except when they wanted to discuss something unsuitable for the ears of her sons. She became a grandmother late in life.

> Yes, I have two children (Steven and Tony) and now also, terribly late, two grandchildren. And when I said to my son Tony, 'I had already given up all hope,' he said, 'We waited until you retired so you would have time.'
>
> (Kennedy, interview, 11 July, 1996)

After the time in which the interviews were conducted, another grandson was born.

Hansi Kennedy became a mainstay at Hampstead Clinic. At the age of 29, she was already one of the first to work in continuing education.

Anna Freud acknowledged the suggestions and achievements of her female employees. On the occasion of the death of Sara Rosenfeld in 1973, a close friend of Hansi Kennedy during her time in the War Nurseries, Anna Freud said:

> It is a fact that our Training Course might never have been started if there had not been, among others, two girls, Sara and Hansi, who had proved their worth in the Hampstead Nurseries to an extent to make it quite impossible for us not to offer them further training and a further career. Our first efforts at training were built up around them and, I suppose, we learned as much from teaching them as they learned from being taught by us.
>
> (A. Freud, 1973b, p. 1, as cited in Miller & Neely, 2008, p. xxviii)

And Hansi Kennedy mentioned in a lecture she gave in Mexico City in 1993: 'Some of the first graduates of the Training Course were now offered staff positions as child analysts, though Anna Freud continued to refer to them for some years and with some pride as "our former students"' (Miller & Neely, 2008, p. xxvi).

Analytic treatment of the children

Starting in 1952, Hansi Kennedy worked as a psychoanalytic child therapist at the Hampstead Child Therapy Clinic and in her own practice. From the interviews with her, it became clear how she later repeatedly met children from her earlier work in the War Nurseries and the Child Therapy Clinic:

> I gave a little lecture there on the War Nursery for the Freud Museum as part of Anna Freud's centenary (1995). And that's interesting for a lot of people who don't know about it. Our students, even today, know relatively little. There were two kids sitting in that room who were formerly there and two other people who were on the staff who I could hardly [–] I could hardly remember them. People kept showing up. One of the kids, for example, became a very famous actor. And he brought his kids to our Nursery. And there's kind of, there's certain connections there. When Anna Freud died, it was in the news and in the paper. I happened to be in the house and the phone rang and a former War Nursery child called and had read that. [–]
>
> I'm still getting letters today, too. So, it goes there [to] Anna Freud or to the museum and it's then sent to me, from children who want to know about their parents. And I can't help all of them [most of them], we don't have full stories. I at least have no way now, maybe somewhere in America there are still documents, but they were not full stories and sometimes we had false stories. We didn't take it very seriously, the protocol. Who the parents were, where the father was. We sometimes [–] I have a whole lot of photographs of the children, and I still know most of the children. So sometimes, instead of a big answer, I send them photographs of their childhood and that's also some piece of childhood, an important one. But these are the kids who somehow lost their parents, or somehow were in homes, or never heard about their father. Of course, many didn't know what happened to their father [...]
>
> And then we had these families, one was looking after two or three children in particular. So, I was looking after a little girl from about eight months to five years. [That] was my child, my first child. And we continued to visit them, of course, you know? They had a relationship with us and [–] I even did some writing, quite early on [–] I then brought her back after [–] first I went to visit her in the East End and then I took her to Hampstead once and then [pause], so not special, not a special paper, but interesting.
>
> (Kennedy, interview, 11 July, 1996)

This is the girl she described in 1950 in 'Cover memories in formation', reprinted in the book by Miller and Neely in 2008. Hansi Kennedy was 27 years old at the time and had not quite finished her education.

> And so, we have, many years I had [a] relationship with this child. There's quite a number of children, former children, who somehow reappeared in the clinic as

patients or brought their own children to the clinic later. Or continued to have a relationship with Dr Stross at the Well Baby Clinic.

(Kennedy, interview, 11 July, 1996)

Yes, but of these young children described by Sophie Dann in this essay, most were adopted. I think the only one who was not adopted, he was then sent to Lingfield House, to Alice Goldberger's home and when he came to me, he was [–] I think nine years old, or ten. [...]

The little ones were not sent to treatment, because Anna Freud thought that they should first see how they could develop and how they could adapt. From this group then, in later years, because they were also relatively young, the children who came to Alice Goldberger, those were the ones under five, the others were over five. There we had some children in treatment. Some were with Mrs Ludowyk and some were with Sara Rosenfeld, a colleague in the clinic. And Mirjam, who has now emigrated to America, but she also died in the meantime. Some analysts had [–] had German speaking analysts, but the children then also spoke English very well, actually they forgot German. Alice Goldberger treated a boy, that is also published; no, it's not published. [...]

The twins, that was actually a different relationship, we also talked about the fact that some of the children who were in the War Nursery, yes, who had kept contact with us, through Anna Freud or through Jimmy Robertson. Because he actually did the follow up. And if they needed help, you know, they were sent to the clinic and could have that. And some through Ilse Hellman. [–] So, my interest was actually, I always wanted to work with children, I like children. I have this, today I do prefer the company of children [laughs]. At least with my grandchildren [–] I enjoy talking to children. I find it interesting. And I find it also, in terms of analysis, that of course you can sort out very much still, maybe more easily. So, it's an important intervention [-] although if the family is very disturbed, it's not so.

(Kennedy, interview, 11 July, 1996)

From Alice Colonna's speech (2003) at Hansi Kennedy's funeral:

Whether in delight with her grandchildren or children at the nursery school or patients, it was clear how much Hansi loved children. She was able to 'put herself in the skin of the child' as Anna Freud advised and yet equally able to retain her outside stance as a helping, supportive adult.

At her funeral, her son Steven (2003) gratefully recalled that his mother did not resort to any therapeutic techniques in dealing with her sons.

Certainly, as children we were grateful that therapeutic techniques were left behind at the front door. For Hansi, therapy was a way to address life's problems, rather than a way of life – and no substitute for the give and take of normal family discourse, and even the occasional raised voice.

Her collaboration with the Sigmund Freud Institute
Frankfurt

Anna Freud was meant to go to Frankfurt and [give] seminars, we were still to start a children's analysis training, with the Mitscherlichs. And Anna Freud was supposed to go [there] and at the last moment she couldn't go, and she kind of sent me. That is, she asked me if I would go, and then she wrote that she couldn't come, but I would come. And I wasn't very well known or anything at that time, young and inexperienced. And she said, 'Under the same conditions as me, you have to go.' Of course, I don't think the Mitscherlichs were very happy [laughs] about that. But they invited me. And when I went to Frankfurt for the first time, with certain feelings [–], and at that time [–] my husband was already working with Germany on business [–] just before that he was in Frankfurt and had rented a room for me [–] so, not the institute, but he. And I was picked up. They wrote that someone would pick me up from the airport and that was Lore Schacht. Lore Schacht, who of course I didn't know before, she was still [a] very young student, [a] candidate. She was very excited, as Lore Schacht can be, and said: 'Imagine what just happened, I wanted to find out where the hotel was, and when I was there at the traffic light, I asked a driver next to me where this hotel was, and he said: "Oh, the hotel where the Führer stayed!"' And that's when she said, 'Ten years after Hitler [pause], or twelve [–] it was more than ten years, somebody in the car tells me where the Führer lived, so that's terrible,' and so on. And that made it so easy for me to make that first visit to Germany, really very [easy], I never forgot that. We still tell each other these stories.

I went a few times, that was like five or six times over two years. And it actually went quite interestingly. I met people that I still [pause] know today, and so they're in Stuttgart and now in [pause] but they never continued a children's analysis training. [–] They wanted to at that time, but somehow that didn't work out. They did this child therapy training in Frankfurt. That's about the same as the Hampstead Clinic. There is also a relationship with the institute, that's where the analysts [–] we've only ever had analytically trained, training analysis in our course. And that's what they did in Frankfurt. Although the child therapists [–] it's not all child therapists in Germany [who] are in real analysis, but in Frankfurt they [are]. Yes. [–] Yes. That was in the early 60s.

(Kennedy, interview, 23 April, 1997)

She complained to Alexander Mitscherlich:

I then just, I mean I saw one side of it too [refers to Mitscherlich], I was then invited, then they received me very nicely, then [–], with champagne in the apartment and so, terrible [–]. I mean, Anna Freud never did that.

(Kennedy, interview, 23 April, 1997)

Director of the Child Therapy Course and Clinic and the Anna Freud Centre

During Anna Freud's last years, Hansi Kennedy shared the management of the centre with her. After Anna Freud's death, Hansi Kennedy continued to run the centre together with the psychiatrist Dr Clifford Yorke. It was renamed the Anna Freud Centre in 1982. Clifford Yorke was the medical director and was responsible for the diagnoses, she for the child therapy department and the administration. Hansi Kennedy emphasized that as long as Anna Freud was alive, nothing was done that she did not know about.

> She was always kept informed, until her last day of life, so to speak. But the correspondence, etc., she gave me letters and I answered and then she signed it, for years actually. And after she died, we were still directors for five years.
>
> (Kennedy, interview, 23 April, 1997)

> So [–] I [–] five years before Anna Freud died, Clifford Yorke and I then became directors, with her. And at that time, she told me, 'It's much better to have a little distance like this' [laughs]. I was, of course, very friendly with most of the staff that grew up with me. And then also of course [with] very young students who [–], even those who were in supervision with me. We were usually also friends, yes. That's always [–] I say that's much easier when you have a little distance. [–] I mean, that was very interesting, because of course she did [keep the distance]. You could always go to her and discuss anything, in person or not in person, but it was a one-sided discussion. I always tell the story when she was already very sick and very alone, and that's when I often went to her house with Dr Yorke, so we had meetings at her place and she always wanted to know everything and [–] mentally she was always quite alert, until her last day. There was one day where I had this feeling, this is at the weekend, on Friday or something, and she said, 'What's happening for the weekend, is anybody coming?' 'No, nobody's coming.' 'Would you like me to visit you? I'm here.' 'Only if we have something to discuss'. [laughs; pause] So, then I always found something like that to 'discuss'. Then I didn't ask that any more, like that. [laughs] But that was very typical, all these years.
>
> (Kennedy, interview, 11 July, 1996)

In 1987 she was replaced in the management by George Moran, who came from America.

> Then there was a young man, he was good, and he was very friendly with Peter Fonagy, and they worked very well together. And he then became director and he wanted to continue working with us and then he made Clifford medical director, I became principal child analyst, child therapist. He had little clinical experience, but he was good. [pause] And the first thing he did, he found

money in America to renovate all the houses. Yes, he took over the financial side completely. And other things he started slowly, especially the link to University College, that was almost finished when Anne-Marie [Sandler] came.[6] He was doing a PhD with Peter Fonagy. And that was finished at that time, and I guess he was very friendly with him and so he wanted to make a connection there, a link through education and so on and get that research done. He became very ill, suffered from muscular atrophy. It's horrible [–]. He was a very young man, was married young, had an eight-year-old daughter, and he was really [–] worked there with us almost until the end. But it was horrible to see. He couldn't drink, he couldn't eat, he couldn't [pause] he could walk for quite a long time, but he couldn't use his arms [–]. Duncan McLayne then became the medical director. He was already a psychiatrist in our time. First, he did the training with us, child training and then he became [–]. I was going to [–] when George became director [–] I was actually going to retire. That was the idea. To then make this change. [–] Anna Freud was also very good there in these things, when somebody [–], she would, when somebody worked seriously, she would acknowledge that. She always told me such beautiful things, that I myself would then take over the leadership. And she always said that, but she also always did it. For example, there was a guest who gave a lecture that was actually terrible, and we were all sitting there impatiently and so Anna Freud would stand up and she would pick out a good point and talk about it. She left most of it. So that's nice, isn't it? That was always an example for me. I had to do that sometimes in later years, too. But it's a very good way. It's good. [–] Yes.

(Kennedy, interview, 23 April, 1997)

Scholarly work

Even though she always considered German her language, she published only in English.

I once had to give a lecture in German; in Vienna and sitting in the front row was Rudi [Ekstein] [–] uh, what was his name, oh it's terrible with names, a child analyst from Los Angeles, from Vienna.[7] It will come back to me. Well, anyway. He was sitting there in the front row and as I saw it, it bothered me terribly to speak German. He still spoke Austrian. He did his training in Austria. And at the end, he came and spoke to me, and I said, 'So sorry that you had to listen to me and my German.' 'German is very good, you don't know Austrian.' [Laughs for a long time.] But it's not very good. Professionally, German is very hard for me and so when I really had to give lectures in German, I wrote them in English and had them translated and then I put them in my own language. You know, I already had a feeling [of] what I wanted to say and how I wanted to say it. [Pause.] Sometimes I had to sit down with the dictionary and do the translating and I found that terribly difficult, even though I always tried to read German the week before and kind of readjust. I did my training in English. You think in

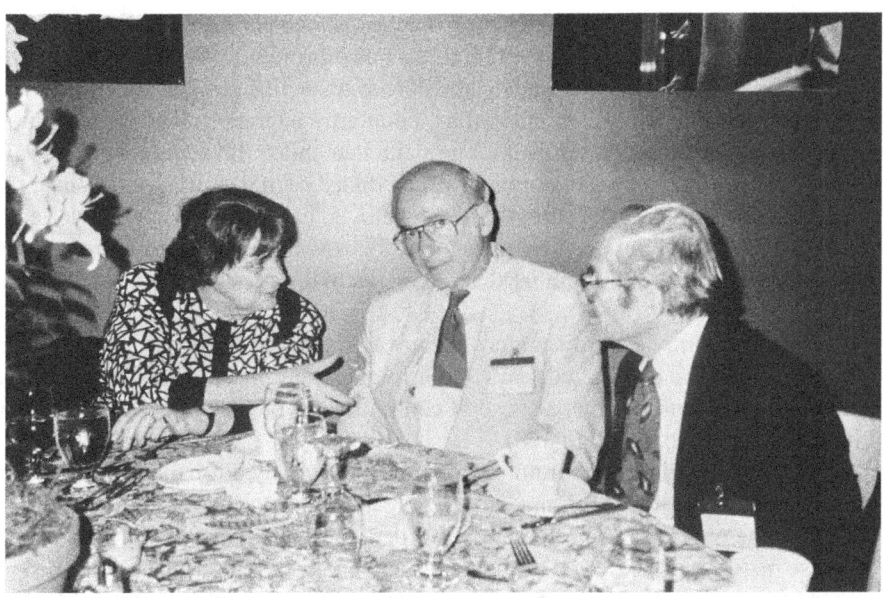

Hansi Kennedy next to Theodor Cohen, child psychoanalyst, in Philadelphia, 1992 (credit: Hansi Kennedy)

English, and you don't have the words and so you can't find the exact words. When I read it in German, I know that's not what I want to say. But Anna Freud had a secretary who came from Switzerland, and she was very good at translating. And she translated it and then I put it into my own language. And that was relatively easy. Anna Freud didn't have anything translated, you know, so what she wrote [was] in English [–]. And then all her later papers came out in German. And she translated everything herself.

(Kennedy, interview, 23 April, 1997)

In addition to child analysis, Hansi Kennedy was involved in research and engaged in psychoanalytic training. Ehud Koch (2012, p. 378) describes his supervision with Hansi Kennedy:

Mrs Kennedy had been recommended by fellow students as being especially helpful in work with younger children. I had earlier been impressed by her astute observations in the context of diagnostic discussions and those of the Profile Research Group. Her language reflected her involvement with *Joe Sandler* and the Index Research Group. Her focus was often on attitudes towards the self and self-esteem and affect regulation. Her amusement at the incongruous was appealing. An attractive, forty-ish mother of two late latency boys, she welcomed me into her consulting room on the first floor of her north-west London home. [...] My recollection of Mrs Kennedy was that of a 'participant observer and commentator' rather than a directing teacher. She made the occasional suggestion of an intervention or interpretation, but more often she would reflect on what my patient was experiencing and defending against. [...] Mrs Kennedy was sympathetic and non-judgmental of my countertransference reactions, even noting Miss Freud's query, 'How does he stand that child?' She was very attuned to object loss, which was a major reconstructed feature of the girl's experience, she having suddenly lost the care of a much beloved nanny at two and a half years. As I think back, I believe Mrs Kennedy's focus was much more on the ego and affective life of the child rather than on instinctual forces.

When he later came back to London, she always received him very kindly: 'Over tea and biscuits, we exchanged news of our lives and families. I believe there was a mutual affection and, for me, a sense of continuity with the Hampstead Clinic that I had valued' (Koch, 2012, p. 378).

She was among the collaborators who published widely. Probably influenced by Anna Freud's way of writing, she wins over readers through precise descriptions of the cases she presents. She often eschews (dry) theoretical discussion and instead lets case histories speak for themselves. Miller and Neely (2008) have compiled all of her 54 publications, most of which she wrote alone, but also with well-known colleagues such as Anne-Marie Sandler, Mary Target, Peter Fonagy, Rose Marjorie Edgcumbe, Clifford Yorke, Robert Tyson, etc., and 61 lectures.

I have, actually [–] my heart has always been in the clinical work. And the other was interesting; and you develop when you write something. You learn a lot more from that than if you just work in the clinical sense. I mean, though [–] when it comes to thinking! Most of what I've written is clinical [–] actually all of it.
(Kennedy, interview, 23 April, 1997)

Mary Target (2010, p. 313) recalls how she was appreciatively accepted by Hansi Kennedy when she began research at the Anna Freud Centre. She worked for over six years with her, along with Peter Fonagy, Rose Edgcumbe, and George Moran, benefiting from her vast clinical experience, the many cases she had either treated herself over her long professional life or the cases of younger colleagues who were in supervision with her, resulting in numerous publications. A book Target had planned on the theory and technique of child analysis at the Anna Freud Centre sadly did not come into being.

This was partly because Hansi felt it was not really her or our work, or the Centre's collective work; we represented the Centre's tradition and approach using many examples from colleagues seen and understood through the eyes of our group; it was best left as a resource for scholars and clinicians, and that is what we have let it be. It was typical of Hansi in my experience, to devote many hundreds of hours of work but be genuinely uninterested in taking credit, or even particularly in seeing the work presented, the point was to think and learn something, and work it through in the group. Others might be interested

and could take what they wished, but she would not push it at them. I always felt
that she was solid and secure in her experience and clear in her own interests,
but that she felt no need to try to persuade others to be like her.

(Target, 2010, p. 313)

I remember how she mentioned at our last meeting (Kennedy, interview, 5 June,
1997) how uncomfortable she was when the clinical experiences of so many female colleagues were then incorporated by so few into their publications in a way
that made it possible to identify where these findings originated. She experienced it
as an appropriation or 'an adornment with borrowed plumes'.

Kennedy's thinking was clear, disciplined and sophisticated, with a depth that
demonstrated her understanding of development and of the mind of the child.
Unburdened by concerns of what was and what was not analysis, and whether
child analysis was equivalent to adult analysis, she followed the children, first in
the War Nurseries, then in the Hampstead Nursery School and the children she
and others analyzed in the Hampstead Clinic, later Anna Freud Centre.

(Miller & Neely, 2008, p. xv)

Mary Target (2010, p. 314) writes:

She developed early into a very astute clinician with a wry, penetrating sense of
humour and an even-tempered awareness of both the dangers and opportunities
within life's adversities. In Anna Freud's last years Hansi shared the Centre's
directorship with her, then following Miss Freud's death, Hansi continued to direct it jointly with Dr Clifford Yorke. Hansi took on Miss Freud's role of knowing the details of work with all the cases of staff and trainees. It was absolutely
clear, when in my Ph.D. research I read the diagnostic discussions and weekly
reports of all 800 past child analytic cases, someone had been there before me!
Hansi, like Anna Freud in her lifetime, had contributed to every meeting, supervised many of the cases, and treated a large number.

In reviewing Miller and Neely's book, which includes reprinted articles by Kennedy, Mary Target (2010, pp. 314–315) writes:

Hansi was an inspiring and towering figure in the Anna Freudian tradition of
child analysis. When she spoke one could be sure that she had something sub-
stantial, often surprising, to contribute based on unsentimental thinking about
a large number of cases, which she would be able to explain and link to theory
in a convincing and clear way. When she wrote, as we see in this selection, her
papers are similarly vivid, theoretically clear, clinically concise but drawing on
a wealth of observation. Most of Hansi's ideas were about fundamental aspects
of psychoanalysis (adult as well as child), for example, the nature of memories, and the roles of reconstruction and insight in therapeutic action. She was
ahead of her time, and her quietly radical approach has stood the test of time

well. For instance, her completely clinically rooted approach to memory and insight is consistent with extensive later research (and psychoanalytic writing, for example, by Joseph Sandler) on recovery of memories in treatment, and its therapeutic impact and meaning. Similarly, she cogently argued that acquiring particular insights was much less important than developing the process of self-understanding, within an analytic relationship. Her developmental line of insight together with the description of its function closely prefigures later work at the Anna Freud Centre on the development and therapeutic role of 'mentalization'.

Mary Target (2010, p. 315) is not the only one to regret that Hansi Kennedy did not write more.

But then, she would not have been Hansi, keener to listen than to speak, to read than to publish. She was always ready to recognize ability and new ideas even in inexperienced colleagues and was straightforwardly receptive to men in an institution sometimes known locally as 'the nunnery'. (However, her willingness to listen and appreciate was not endless; on one occasion after listening to opinionated men expound their thoughts at length to senior women colleagues, she was heard to remark, 'Next time, I come back as a man.') She willingly moved aside to enable Dr. George Moran, then in his mid-30s, to direct the Centre only a few years after Anna Freud's death in 1982. Hansi supported George in a wise, enthusiastic and effective way as he shouldered this daunting responsibility. During that time, they wrote an important paper integrating much of Hansi's earlier thinking together with George's developing approach, on the aims of child analysis (Kennedy and Moran, 1991). Hansi then supported George and the Centre through his shocking progressive disability and death after five years as Director, only nine years after the death of Anna Freud. Hansi's appreciation of institutional continuity and stability, emphasised by Miller and Neely, was surely much called upon in those dark years.

Hansi Kennedy served on the editorial board of *The Bulletin of the Hampstead Clinic* from its inception in 1978 until her retirement in 1993, and on the editorial board of *Psychoanalytic Study of the Child* from 1984 to 2002. Along with Joseph Sandler and Robert Tyson, she edited the book *The Technique of Child Psychoanalysis. Discussions with Anna Freud* (Sandler et al., 1980).

Her time in retirement and the end of her life

She was very successful in the transition from active working life to retirement. When Mary Target tried to get her to teach about the tradition of the Anna Freud Centre, she emphasized how much she was enjoying retirement.

Hansi once said to me, declining my request to emerge from contented retirement to teach about the Centre's tradition, that one of her new pleasures was that she was no longer asked about everything, 'What would Miss Freud have thought?' I think current colleagues and students reading this book might surprise Hansi beyond the grave by asking a different, very good question – 'What would Hansi Kennedy have thought?' We read here what she did think about memory, sado-masochism, the superego, trauma, play, insight and interpretation... and much more.

(Target, 2010, p. 316)

From the interview with Hansi Kennedy on 11 July, 1996:

I don't see children now. I do some supervisions for the clinic. And sometimes I see parents in between. Actually, I don't want to – they didn't do it then either, but I promised myself; when I saw all these old ladies always in the clinic in the front row on Wednesday afternoons, and they fell asleep or said the same thing every week [laughs] [–] I promised myself that I would leave before [laughs] I reach that stage. Yes, and this one gives me pleasure. I can now [pause]; I've had so little time in my life [pause] through this, you see, through this actually heavy work very early on, to do things that I really wanted to do. And I lost my university, yes, so where you have time to pursue your interests. And that's what I promised myself I would do today. So. Now I can go to art classes and listen to music whenever I want. Yes! So, I'm enjoying that. And as a grandmother I have time [–].

She now found time to attend courses in art, philosophy, and architecture at the University of the Third Age, expanded her circle of friends or was able to revive old friendships and follow her love of music – especially opera – undisturbed.
  From the eulogy given by her niece Jan Wiener (2003):

Music was a central pleasure for her and strongly linked the generations. Family outings to The Wigmore Hall or Covent Garden maintained strong links between the generations. Her tastes were broad, ranging from the pieces we have chosen today to more modern composers such as Britten, Stravinsky, Bartok, and Shostakovich. Hansi and Gerald loved visiting Aldeburgh in the days when Benjamin Britten and Peter Pears were at their best and they were also patrons of the English Chamber Orchestra. But Hansi's greatest love was opera – a love shared with me and with my mother – and in her last weeks, she took great pleasure reliving performances she had attended over the years with the help of a comprehensive card index and boxes of programmes.
  Last but far from least her house was always the hub of family life both for her own family and for Gerald's – and beyond. She enjoyed and appreciated her extended family and took pride in all our achievements. Scarcely a day passed in recent years that she did not see or talk to her sister Susie who lived just down the road. Her greatest pleasure, however, in her last decade came from her grandchildren.

Hansi retired from life as from her work with dignity and acceptance and her lively interest in others remained intact to the end. She was clear that her personal analysis, all those years ago, had given her the capacity to undertake the necessary internal work to face her imminent death. Hansi was easy to love and I know that I am not the only one here to feel that my life will be much the poorer for her absence.

From the spring of 2003, Hansi Kennedy felt tired, groggy, and had no appetite, which she dismissed with a shrug of the shoulders, which she referred to her age, since she had just turned 80. Although she felt increasingly unwell, she took a long walk to celebrate her granddaughter Catherine's birthday in early July and then travelled to Europe with her friends, where the severity of her illness became clear.

From the speech by her eldest son, Steven Kennedy (2003):

She sensed before the doctors that she had an incurable cancer and told everyone that she did not want her life prolonged by useless treatments. Her worst nightmare was of a slow and painful decline, of dependency and loss of her faculties – and all that she was spared. She spent a couple of weeks in the St John's Hospice when she was no longer able to live independently at home. They did a great job alleviating her symptoms and she made many new friends among the wonderful nursing staff and volunteers. She was able to return home last week and joked about the beauty of the plants and flowers in her living room as enhanced by the

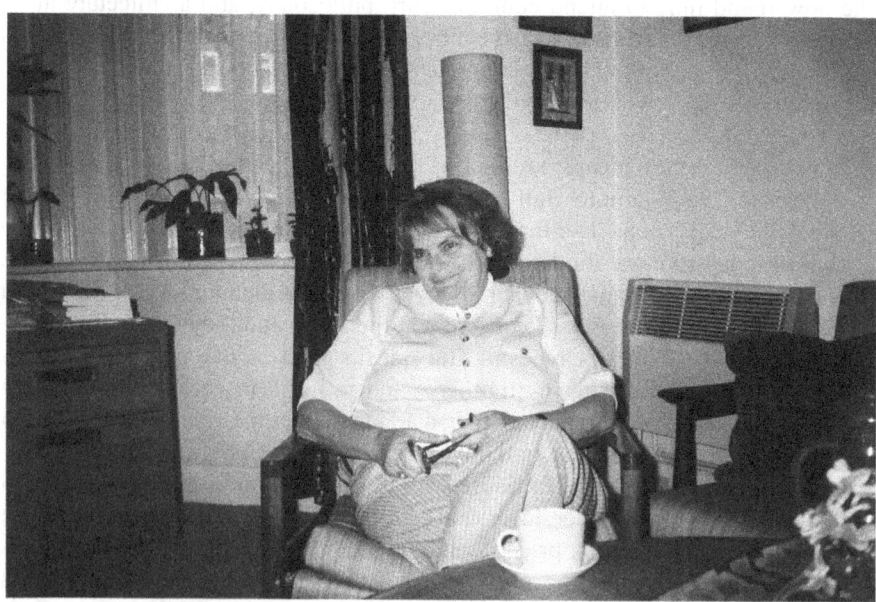

Hansi Kennedy on 28 April, 1997 (credit: Christiane Ludwig-Körner)

morphine in her medication. She enjoyed and participated fully in a lively family evening last Wednesday and a Chinese take-away meal. She was still chatting, joking and helping Catherine make a stuffed animal out of old socks and ribbons 10 minutes before she fell peacefully into a final sleep in her chair.

She did not want a religious funeral, but one 'without much fuss'. Accompanied by music she loved and a few personal speeches – as she had led her life – she found her final resting place next to her husband's grave in Willesden Cemetery.

Notes

1 Gertrud Engl, née Kohn had three sisters. Frieda died at a very early age, Helene, married to Otto Heinrich Grünfelder, died in 1919, aged about 28, leaving behind her daughter Hannah Ellen. Her sister Nellie Rosenfeld emigrated with her second husband Emil Rosenfeld and daughter to England, too. Her first husband, Emil Schermer, died in the First World War (S. Kennedy, personal correspondence, 8 November, 2021).
2 Jeanne de Groot, who was Dutch, went into analysis with Freud and married the psychoanalyst Hans Lampl in 1925. Their two daughters were born in 1926 and 1928. They emigrated to the Netherlands in 1938, where they established the Dutch Psychoanalytic Institute in Amsterdam. Hans Lampl died in a serious traffic accident in 1958. Jeanne survived but was seriously injured. Together with Anna Freud, Dorothy Burlingham and Marianne Kris, she became one of the 'four old ladies' of psychoanalysis (Mühlleitner & Reichmayr, 1992) and https://www.psychoanalytikerinnen.de/niederlande_biografien.html#Lampl (accessed 3 January, 2019).
3 She was accepted as a member of the British Psychoanalytical Society in 1943 and as a teaching analyst in 1951.
4 Sara Kut, married Rosenfeld (1920–1973), born in Russia, lived in Berlin, Tomasiusstrasse, before her escape to Great Britain. In the Questionnaire Foster Parents Plan she wrote: 'girls' high school, kindergarten teacher seminar, worked in a private kindergarten before the war', hired on 8 July, 1941, to work in the War Nurseries. She worked as child therapist in East London, at the Child Guidance Clinic, and Hampstead Therapy Clinic.
5 Augusta Bonnard (1903–1974) had already come from Russia to England as a child, studied medicine, was briefly in Vienna to receive psychoanalytic knowledge and completed psychoanalytic training with Anna Freud, a member of the British Psychoanalytical Society. She was part of Anna Freud's staff in child therapy training starting in 1952. Augusta Bonnard was director of the East London Child Guidance Clinic after the war, which she reopened in 1945 at the London Jewish Hospital and where she worked as a consultant psychiatrist until her retirement in 1968. She also had her own psychoanalytic practice and worked at Great Ormond Street Hospital, UCH, the Tavistock Clinic, and the Lasker Clinic in Jerusalem (Noelleke, Women Psychoanalysts. Biographical Dictionary. https://www.psychoanalytikerinnen.de/england_biografien.html#Bonnard, accessed 15 March, 2019).
6 Anne-Marie Sandler had first (1951–1954) undergone child therapy training with Anna Freud (training analysis with Augusta Bonnard), which was followed from 1965 by psychoanalytic training at the British Institute (training analyst Edith Ludowyk-Gyömröi). She was the director of the Anna Freud Centre from 1993–1997.
7 Rudi Ekstein (1912 Vienna–2005 Los Angeles), psychoanalyst, studied psychology, philosophy and history at the University of Vienna and received his doctorate there in 1937. His teachers there included Anna Freud, Willi Hoffer and August Aichhorn. In 1938 he

fled to London and from there to the USA. In Boston, he was trained as a psychoanalyst at the Social Works School (training analysis with Eduard Hitschmann). He also earned his second doctorate in the philosophy of psychoanalysis there. He then worked at the Menninger Foundation in Topeka, Kansas, from 1947 to 1957 and at the Reiss Davis Child Study Center in Los Angeles from 1957 to 1976. The application of psychoanalysis in education and teaching was a focus of his work and his work with psychotic, autistic children. https://de.wikipedia.org/wiki/Rudolf_Ekstein (accessed 12 September, 2022).

Sources and personal correspondence

E-mails: Steven Kennedy: 16 October, 2020; 24 October, 2021; 26 10, 2020; 19 December, 2020; 13 January, 2021; 15 January, 2021; 5 April, 2021; 8 November, 2021; 9 November, 2021 (original correspondence in English)
E-mails: Jan Wiener: 26 October, 2020; 28 October, 2020; 29 October, 2020: 12 January, 2021; 13 January, 2021; 16 January, 2021; 5 April, 2021; 8 November, 2021 (original correspondence in English).
Hansi Kennedy, *curriculum vitae*, unpublished.

Publications by Hansi Kennedy

Berger, M., & Kennedy, H. (1975). Pseudobackwardness in children. Maternal attitudes as an etiological factor. *Psychoanalytic Study of the Child, 30*, 279–306.
Burgner, M. & Kennedy, H. (1980). Different types of sado-masochistic behavior in children. *Dialogue: Journal of Psychoanalytic Perspectives, 4*, 49–59.
Edgcumbe, R., Kennedy, H., Sandler, J. & Yorke, C. (1978). Some reflections on infantile neurosis. *Bulletin of the Hampstead Clinic, 1*, 101–109.
Fabricius, J. & Green, V. in collaboration with T. Baradon, J. Davids and H. Kennedy (1995). Termination in child analysis: A child-led process? *Psychoanalytic Study of the Child, 50*, 205–226.
Fonagy, P. Moran, G. S., Edgcumbe, R., Kennedy, H. & Target, M. (1993). The roles of mental representations and mental processes in therapeutic action. *Psychoanalytic Study of the Child, 48*, 9–48. https://doi.org/10.1080/00797308.1993.11822377
Frankl, L. in collaboration with I. Harris, H. Kennedy and V. Thompson (1961). Some observations on the development and disturbances of integration in childhood. *Psychoanalytic Study of the Child*, 16, 146–163.
Kennedy, H.E. (1950). Cover memories in formation. *Psychoanalytic Study of the Child, 5*, 275–284.
Kennedy, H. (1969). Film review: Young children in brief separation. *British Journal of Medical Psychology, 42*, 191–193.
Kennedy, H. (1971). Problems in reconstruction in child analysis. *Psychoanalytic Study of the Child, 26*, 386–402. https://doi.org/10.1080/00797308.1971.11822278
Kennedy, H. (1977). The Hampstead Centre for the Psychoanalytic Study and Treatment of Children. In: B. Wolman (ed.), *International Encyclopedia of Neurology, Psychiatry and Psychology*. Aesculapius.
Kennedy, H. (1976). Film review: Young children in brief separation: A critical of five films by James Robertson and Joyce Robertson. *International Journal of Psychoanalysis, 57*, 483–486.

Kennedy, H. (1978a). The analytic treatment of two siblings, A foreword. *Bulletin of the Hampstead Clinic*, *1*, 119–120.

Kennedy, H. (1978b). The Hampstead Centre for the Psychoanalytić Study and Treatment of Children. *Bulletin of the Anna Freud Centre*, *1*(1), 7–10.

Kennedy, H. (1979). The role of insight in child analysis: A developmental viewpoint. *Journal of the American Psychoanalytic Association*, *27* (Suppl), 9–28.

Kennedy, H. (1980a). Dorothy Burlingham, 1891–1979. *Psychoanalytic Quarterly*, 49, 508–511.

Kennedy, H. (1980b). Dorothy Burlingham. Funeral tributes. Bulletin of the Hampstead Clinic, 3, 71.

Kennedy, H. (1980c). Dorothy Burlingham: Hampstead Clinic memorial contributions. *Bulletin of the Hampstead Clinic*(3), 78–79.

Kennedy, H. (1981a). Die Bedeutung der Einsicht in der Kinderanalyse. In: G. Biermann (ed.), *Handbuch der Kinderpsychotherapie*. Reinhardt Verlag.

Kennedy, H. (1981b). Reports by chairmen on the work of study groups at the Hampstead Clinic: Study Group on developmental disturbances. *Bulletin of the Hampstead Clinic*, *4*, 295.

Kennedy, H. (1981c). Vergangenheit und Gegenwart in der Sicht des Kindes: Folgerungen für die Kinderanalyse (Vol. 1). Österreichischen Studiengesellschaft für Kinderpsychoanalyse.

Kennedy, H. (1982a). Die Hampstead Clinic: Ein historischer Überblick. *Studien zur Kinderpsychologie*, *2*.

Kennedy, H. (1982b). El papel del insight. *Psicoanalisis*, *1*, 51.

Kennedy, H. (1982c). Questions soulevées par la reconstruction en analyse d'enfant. *La Psychiatrie de l'enfant*, *25*(2), 369–386.

Kennedy, H. (1982d). The Hampstead Clinic: A historical perspective. Sigmund Freud Gesellschaft Bulletin, Anna Freud Memorial Issue. Vienna.

Kennedy, H. (1983a). Anna Freud. 1895–1982. *Psychoanalytic Quarterly*, *52*(4), 501–506.

Kennedy, H. (1983b). Anna Freud: Funeral tributes. *Bulletin of the Hampstead Clinic*, *6*, 11–12.

Kennedy, H. (1984). The 'baby at the breast' experience: Memory or fantasy? Some further thoughts on reconstruction. *Bulletin of the Hampstead Clinic*, *7*, 15–24.

Kennedy, H. (1985a). For or against child placement: A clinical illustration. *Bulletin of the Hampstead Clinic*, *8*, 245–252.

Kennedy, H. (1985b). Growing up with a handicapped sibling. *Psychoanalytic Study of the Child*, *40*(1), 255–274. https://doi.org/10.1080/00797308.1985.11823032

Kennedy, H. (1986a). Memories of Anna Freud. *American Imago*, 53, 205–209.

Kennedy, H. (1986b). Trauma in childhood. Signs and sequelae as seen in the analysis of an adolescent. *Psychoanalytic Study of the Child*, *41*, 209–219.

Kennedy, H. (1988a). The pre-history of the Nursery School. *Bulletin of the Hampstead Clinic*, *11*, 271–275.

Kennedy, H. (1988b). Trauma in childhood: Signs and sequelae as seen in the analysis of an adolescent. *Psychoanalytic Study of the Child*, 41, 209–219.

Kennedy, H. (1989a). Sadomasochistische Perversion in der Adoleszenz. Eine entwicklungsgeschichtliche Betrachtung. *Zeitschrift für psychoanalytische Theorie und Praxis*, *46*, 181–198.

Kennedy, H. (1989b). die Erfahrung als "Baby an der Brust": Erinnerungen oder Phantasie? *Studien zur Kinderanalyse*, Jahrbuch 9.

Kennedy, H. (1993). Developing resilience in high-risk Nursery School children. In: M. H. Etecady and B. Pacella (eds), *The Vulnerable Child* (Vol. 1). International Universities Press.

Kennedy, H. (1994a). Book review: Robert Coles, "Anna Freud: The dream of psychoanalysis". *Psychoanalytic Quarterly*, *63*, 587–590.

Kennedy, H. (1994b). Doris Wills, 1908–1993: Memorial tributes. *Bulletin of the Hampstead Clinic*, *17*, 57–62.

Kennedy, H. (1996). Memories of Anna Freud. *American Imago*, *53*(3), 205–209. http://www.jstor.org/stable/26304490

Kennedy, H. (1996). Memories of Anna Freud. *American Imago*, *53*(3), 205–209. http://www.jstor.org/stable/26304490

Kennedy, H. (2001). The technique of psychoanalysis with the prelatency child. In: R. Tyson (ed.), *Analysis of the Under-Five Child* (pp. 262–281). Yale University Press.

Kennedy, H. & Moran, G. S. (1984). The developmental roots of self-injury and response to pain in a 4-year-old boy. *Psychoanalytic Study of the Child*, *39*, 195–212. https://doi.org/10.1080/00797308.1984.11823426

Kennedy, H. & Moran, G. (1991). Reflections on the aim of child analysis. *Psychoanalytic Study of the Child*, 46, 181–198.

Kennedy, H. & Yorke, C. (1980). Childhood neurosis vs. developmental deviations. *Dialogue: Journal of Psychoanalytic Perspectives*, *4*, 21–33.

Kennedy, H., Moran, G., Wiseberg, S. & Yorke, C. (1985). Both sides of the barrier. *Psychoanalytic Study of the Child*, *40*(1), 275–283. https://doi.org/10.1080/00797308.1985.11823033

Sandler, J., Kennedy, H. & Tyson, R. L. (1975). Discussions on transference. The treatment situation and technique in child psychoanalysis. *Psychoanalytic Study of the Child*, *30*, 409–441.

Sandler, J., Kennedy, H. & Tyson, R. L. (1983). *La tecnica della psicoanalisi infantile: seminari con Anna Freud*. Italy, Bollati Boringhieri. https://books.google.de/books?id=RauZoAEACAAJ

Sandler, J., Kennedy, H., Tyson, R. L. & Freud, A. (1980). *The Technique of Child Psychoanalysis: Discussions with Anna Freud*. Hogarth Press and the Institute of Psycho-analysis. https://books.google.de/books?id=gGl-AAAAMAAJ

Target, M. & Kennedy, H. (1991). Psychoanalytic work with under-fives: Forty years' experience. *Bulletin of the Anna Freud Centre* (14), 5–29.

Yorke, C., Kennedy, H. & Wiseberg, S. (1980). Clinical and theoretical aspects of two developmental lines. In: S.I. Greenspan and G.H. Pollock (Eds.). *The Course of Life, 1: 619–637. Washington: U.S. Department of Health and Human Services.* Revised and reprinted as *The Course of Life*: *Middle and Late Childhood.* pp. 135–160. Madison, CT: Int. Univ. Press, 1991.

Yorke, C., Kennedy, H. & Stanley, W. (1983). Algunos aspectos clinicos y teoricos de dos lines de desarrolo. *Revista de la Asociación Psicoanalítica de Buenos Aires*, *5*(2), 221–248.

Yorke, C. in collaboration with Kennedy, H. (1987). On the concepts of fixation and regression: Their clinical relevance. *Bulletin of the Anna Freud Centre*, 10, 119–135.

Yorke, C., Kennedy, H. & Wiseberg, S. (1991). Clinical and theoretical aspects of two developmental lines. In: *The Course of Life, Vol. 3: Middle and Late Childhood.* (pp. 135–160). International Universities Press.

7

Anna Freud – Interweaving Life, Work and Research

Anna Freud, herself an emigrant, became homeless and created not only a network for children who either had to live in underground tunnels or survived the Nazi terror, but also offered a home for mostly young women who often did not know the fates of their families during the Nazi regime. In addition to giving many of these women in the war nurseries work and support, she also gave them a task that helped them to make sense of their lives again. Anna Freud not only offered them theoretical explanations for the developmental processes of children, but also conveyed her analytical approach to the young staff members and students (trainees), most of whom, when they started at the Hampstead War Nurseries knew nothing about psychoanalysis. Thus, Hannah Fischer, who was the youngest pupil to enter the Hampstead at the age of 16, remembers Anna Freud talking about 'pedagogical love':

> She was referring to a special kind of love that we as educators must be prepared to give to children, so that the children feel accepted and secure with us; a kind of love that does not demand love in return – as is natural for parents – that belongs to children and sees in the children of one's own group representatives of the totality of children. In contrast to parental love, which belongs to a measured number, i.e., to one's own children, pedagogical love for the child entrusted to one's care is inexhaustible, transferable from one child to another, from one group to another.
>
> (Laible, 1982, p. 17)

In my interviews with the staff, when they talked about Anna Freud, not once did they question her personal integrity and performance. They all had a great appreciation of her work; they spoke of her with affection and respect, even though they emphasized that there was always a certain distance to her:

> Through my work in the archives, I have come to appreciate how humble and unpretentious Anna Freud was and that she always gave priority to what was in the best interests of the child. There is, for example correspondence from 1941 between Anna Freud and a US fundraising organization. They suggested that

DOI: 10.4324/9781003403906-8

she send photos of the children sitting desperately in ruins with torn clothes and bandages in order to increase the donations. Anna Freud replied politely but firmly with a no because she wanted to protect the dignity of the children.

(Inge Pretorius with Alexander Frohn, interview, 2018, transl. I. Pretorius, amended for this edition)

From Manna Friedmann's point of view (Friedmann, interview, 12 July, 1996) Anna Freud

[...] had also been a practical person. It was an art. She also managed to create something out of people. They didn't even know what they could do. How did I know that I could give a lecture about a child for an hour with students. But I could. And I did it because it was expected. So that's [–], of course. I could, I did learn how to educate, you know? [...] And, as I said, this eagerness, this desire to work that she had, I think that was the urgent force in her, the joy of work, whatever she did. She also had a tremendous charisma, I think you call it, you can't teach that; a person has it, maybe you can learn something. But she had it, right? She had a great deal of intellect [–] and talent. And at the same time, she had something tremendously youthful and almost childlike. She had a childlike way of expressing joy and feeling joy. When she saw or experienced something beautiful, she could get so excited. If she liked something less, she would just shake her head or something. In fact, she quite liked it when someone didn't agree with her completely. She wanted to have opposition to discuss it. So, maybe you could call it controlling, staying in control somehow. [...] And indeed, many [–], more often people have said: 'She runs the clinic like a family'. But that was also how the father worked. The way people worked in the household. And the clinic was like a family, and she ran it like a big family. And yet she was not a maternal figure. She was not maternal. She was much more like an abbess. [...] With this tremendous mind, and a teacher, she was a born teacher.

Anna Freud was full of ideas, but she also took suggestions from her co-workers. It was the staff who wanted more psychoanalytic knowledge and encouraged Anna Freud to train them in courses. This led to the development of child analytic training.

She trained and gathered about her a body of people who were able to utilize and extend her findings as these emerged, and who, through comprehensive methods of data collection and recording, provide a wealth of material on which she continued to build. She gave every help and encouragement to her staff to work independently and follow their own interests. In her appraisal of the work they produced she could be generous in her approval but on occasion quite forceful in her criticisms. At the time these could be quite shattering for her recipient but, in retrospect, they were usually felt to be just. Anna Freud's conscientiousness and tireless commitment to work made her also expect of others what she expected of herself. However, no one knew better how to bring out the best in others, and she often saw capabilities which were unknown to their possessor. She offered freely of her time to discuss early drafts of papers and had an unerring ability instantly to point to significant, original thoughts or unusual clinical features in any report or presentation. Her rigorous intellect, clinical acumen, and phenomenal memory impressed one afresh in every meeting or group discussion she attended.

(Kennedy, 1983a, p. 505)

At that time, when I was interviewing Anna Freud's staff (which included Joyce Robertson), I was quite familiar with her writings. But it was the accounts of her collaborators that made me understand the special way in which Anna Freud gained her insights: not at her desk or in the application of theoretical knowledge to methodological problems, but inductively, in the practical experience of dealing with the fates of often severely traumatized children. She sought appropriate solutions to the everyday problems that came her way. Today, her methods would perhaps be called 'applied field research'. This was already her way during her time in Vienna when she and Dorothy Burlingham had succeeded in building a creative force-field with the people working with them. When, in 1927, Eva Rosenfeld and Anna Freud founded the Burlingham–Rosenfeld School in Hietzingen, they attempted to implement reform approaches as developed by John Dewey – e.g., with the implementation of project teaching. The teachers at the private school were Peter Blos, then a biology student, who brought in his friend Erik Erikson (art student) to join him – both of whom later became well-known psychoanalysts. August Aichhorn joined in 1931 and was the headmaster until the school closed in 1932.

Anna Freud was a follower of Montessori education and was already putting these ideas into practice in the Jackson Nursery. When Lili Esther Roubiczek wanted to link Montessori education in Vienna with psychoanalytical thoughts and suggested a meeting between Maria Montessori and Anna Freud, Maria Montessori refused. She forbade any fusion of her theory with psychoanalysis and Lili Roubiczek, who had established the famous 'Haus der Kinder" (transl. 'Children's House') in Vienna, increasingly turned to psychoanalysis (Eichelberger, 2001).

In the Children's House, the children were also ascribed psychological competences. The kindergarten teachers created a psychoanalytic therapeutic environment oriented towards supporting the ego, which offered the children the opportunity to work through conflicts on their own.

(Zwiauer, 2001, p. 152)

With the same attitude, after the War Nurseries were closed, she built a kindergarten from the realization that mothers who came for counselling at the Well Baby Clinic needed further support in dealing with their young children.

And Anna Freud recognized how important it was for candidates in training to observe normal developmental processes. In the first ten years, the kindergarten offered 'a half-day programme for children of the largely middle-class catchment area' (Kennedy, 1982a, p. 133).

> The fact that many of the children had attended the Well-Baby Clinic and play group for mothers and toddlers prior to entrance into the Nursery School, further facilitated longitudinal developmental observations. [...] Since 1966 the Nursery School has concentrated on children from under-privileged and disadvantaged families. Most live in overcrowded conditions or poor economic circumstances. Some children are from immigrant families quite often with limited ability to speak English, others come from one-parent families; some of the mothers have to go out to work. Nursery school education is of special importance for such children and must aim to provide for whatever developmental needs are left unfulfilled by the parents.
>
> (Kennedy, 1978b, p. 8)

The pedagogical spirit that already prevailed at the time in the Hietzing School and in the Jackson Nursery was to enable fun, independent learning. The children had a joy for learning and were eager – as we would put it today – for self-efficacy and the desire to be able to develop. It can be seen, for example, in the case description of 'Julian' (Salo & Friedmann, 1988), where the focus was on developmental potential. The development-orientated therapeutic approach, as represented by Fonagy et al. (2018), Fonagy et al. (2019) and Robert Emde (2011), among others, has its precursor in the spirit of Anna Freud.

Anna Freud (1962) emphasized the importance of the early mother–child relationship, and her co-workers practised this approach, which today has earned the name 'attachment theory'. Hansi Kennedy spoke about this in a posthumously (2009) published speech from June 1995 at a ceremony commemorating Anna Freud's 100th birthday. Very vividly she describes the conditions under which the children lived in the Blitz and the reasons for admitting them to the Hampstead War Nurseries. It is also clear from her descriptions how much Anna Freud was able to empathize with the children and understand their grief at being separated from their mothers.

> With some of these children, especially those with bad previous evacuation experiences, the separation from their mothers was extremely distressing, and whenever possible mothers were encouraged to stay, even for a few days, to settle the children in. Observing the extent of the children's grief made a deep impression on Anna Freud, especially the reaction of a three-year-old boy who turned within a few days from a seemingly healthy child into a grief-stricken one with a compulsive ritual. She often related his story in later years to students to illustrate severe manifestations of separation anxiety. Here was an onrush of mothers who wanted their small children in a place of safety and also accessibility.
>
> (Kennedy, 2009, p. 307)

Her portrayal of 'Billy's' grief is immediately reminiscent of the film about the separation experiences of 'Little John', released by James and Joyce Robertson in 1969.

Anne-Marie Sandler writes (2012, p. 49), 'Anna Freud was convinced that children developed best in stable relations within an intact family and that the role of the mother was crucial in establishing healthy bonding' and elsewhere (2012, p. 51), quoting Anna Freud: '"the attachment of the small child to his mother seems to be to a large degree independent of her personal qualities and certainly of her educational ability"' and '"the figure of the mother is for a certain time the sole important representative of the whole outer world."'

This attitude is also reflected in the fact that all the female staff members from the War Nurseries described here had 'adopted their children'. They were in close

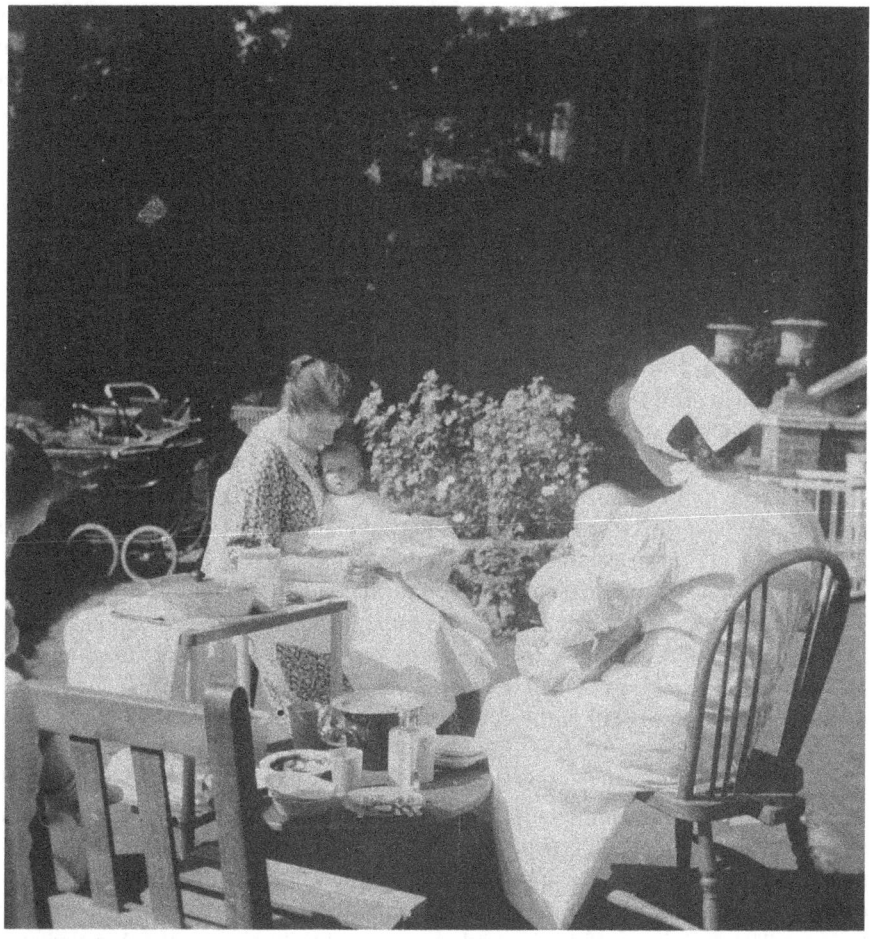

Anna Freud (left) and Sophie Dann feeding babies (credit: Gertrud Dann and AFC)

contact with many of them for the rest of their lives. They also represented a substitute family for some of them who had lost their family. Edit Ludewyk-Gyömröi, for example, took on the role of a mother of the bride for 'her therapy child', since she had lost her mother in the concentration camp (Ludwig-Körner, 1998). Ilse Hellman went with 'her' therapy children to the opera as adults on their birthdays. Anne-Marie Sandler looked after her teaching analyst Edit Ludewyk-Gyömröi at the end of her life in an apartment in her own house (Ludwig-Körner, 1998). Many psychoanalysts today would judge and condemn this behaviour as a serious violation of abstinence.

Surely no one today would withhold from a child as Alice Goldberger did in misunderstood loyalty to Jackie Young's adoptive mother. Dealing with the aftermath of the Holocaust would also warrant a different approach today. It is abundantly clear from the stories – especially those of Manna Friedmann – how difficult it was for her to talk to her brother about the loss of her family in the Holocaust and how the children in her care (e.g., Judith Sherman) could not talk to their children about the Holocaust at first either. Judith S. Kestenberg is an exception, who, together with Vivienne Koorland (1993), wrote the children's book *Als Eure Grosseltern jung waren* [transl. 'Talking to Children about the Holocaust']. Unfortunately, Holocaust denial has long been practised in the psychoanalytic community, apart from a few exceptions (e.g., Brecht & Friedrichs, 1985; Ermann, 2004; Kamm, 2010; Schlesinger-Kipp, 2012; Wachtler & Ulrich, 2013).

Her research efforts

Anna Freud and Dorothy Burlingham (1943, pp. 12–13) list the four main objectives of their work in the book *War and Children*, which she continued to pursue throughout her life and work at the Hampstead Child Therapy Courses and Clinic:

1. Emphasizing the importance of prevention by paying attention to children who had to be separated from their parents to enable them to have as much contact as possible in order to establish or maintain a bond.
2. The treatment of physical and psychological damage in children.
3. Conducting research: Whether it is to understand war and separation traumas and coping with them, or the effects of outside care, in order to gain more knowledge about normal and deviant developmental trajectories.
4. Further training of staff in the competent handling of children.

The experiences from the war children's homes flow into the concepts of child analysis: the concept of the importance of attachment, the effect of separation, the influence of substitute mothers, group education, the consequences of traumatization and their treatment, etc. In the Hampstead Child Therapy Clinic, children and adolescents could continue to be cared for who had need of therapeutic treatment due to (war) traumas. The experience of dealing with traumatized children from the War Nurseries continues to inform work with war refugees today, as Wiese (2019) pointed out.

Anna Freud accompanied all her projects with scientific interest. The close observation of children of different ages, which had already been practised in the Jackson Kindergarten and War Nurseries, has been maintained to this day (Krivanek, 2014). As early as 1951 she wrote the lecture 'Observations on child development' (Freud, A., 1951). She was often invited to America for lectures and training at Radcliffe College. The candidates for training went through the various departments of the War Nurseries, and from the notes recorded on the cards, which formed the basis for discussions, Anna Freud and her staff later created development charts for each child. Willi Hoffer added photographs and films of children from the Jackson Creche.

Anna Freud writes:

Besides being guided to observe and understand the growth of the child's body and his intelligence, students were instructed in the principles of psychoanalytic child psychology, which led to an understanding of the function of the instinctual drives in early childhood and their role in character development. The habits of the child and the most common behavior problems were the subject of systematic lectures and discussions. All theoretical teaching was given in close connection with the practical work of the students in the various departments, and constantly illustrated by the living examples which the rich case material of the Nurseries provided. Advanced students were put in individual charge of problem children and received guidance in the handling of their difficulties.

(Freud, A., 1945/1987, p. 538)

In her modest way, Anna Freud writes about her method of observation: 'no more than the by-product of intensive, charitable war work', and, as all attempts to raise funds specifically for this research were unsuccessful, the observing, recording and classifying of material 'had to be relegated to the spare off-time of the workers and was undertaken as their voluntary effort' (Freud, A., 1951, p. 145).

But she also recognized, as Midgley (2007, pp. 942–943) writes:

Anna Freud recognized that the War Nurseries were 'ideal for the purposes of observation':

The variation in the case material made it possible to see children, almost from birth, in contact with their mothers or deprived of mother care, breast fed or bottle fed, in the throes of separation or reunited with their lost objects, in contact with their mother substitutes and teachers, and developing relations with their contemporaries. The stages of libidinal and aggressive development, the process and the effects of weaning and toilet training, the acquisition of speech and of the various ego functions could be followed closely.

(Freud, A., 1951, p. 146, as cited in Midgley, 2007)

As is apparent in her speech for René Spitz's 79th birthday, Anna Freud was one of the first to do action research, reflecting on the pros and cons of different research approaches; she did not follow a preconceived plan of observation. She highlighted the differences of her way of observing children to Spitz's practice: Spitz tried to observe the children in a more experimental laboratory situation by specifically trained personnel at defined times. She said, 'Where he sets up experiments, I engage in so-called action research, i.e., activities which are geared to educational, or humanitarian, or therapeutic aims, the observations coming in as a by-product' (Freud, A., 1971. p. 25). Anna Freud gained support for her research from those whose work involved caring for children, such as children's hospital nurses, nursery school teachers, and so forth. Anna Freud continued, 'While his researchers follow a preconceived plan, I use as the basis of my investigation, apart from the analytic finding, also the accidental and fortuitous happenings as they occur in everyday life' (Freud, A., 1971, p. 25; Ludwig-Körner, 2017).

Anna Freud was one of the early analysts who conducted direct observations of children and research. She supported Ernst Kris in conducting longitudinal studies in the early 1950s when he set up a longitudinal study of child development at the Yale Child Studies Center. She also prompted her co-workers to collect accurate data (Midgley, 2007). For example, Sophie Dann not only kept an 'Air Raid Chart Hampstead Nurseries', where she recorded exactly how the children reacted to the bombings, but also a 'Sleeping Chart Hampstead Nurseries':

> The helpers in the Baby Department had learned to note down special babies' time of falling asleep and waking up in the day. The night-nurse did the same while on duty. I then drew a chart to show the sleeping times. A date surrounded by a red square meant a day the mother had come to visit the child. Red vertical lines show when a child had to be woken up to be fed. Horizontal green lines show the times the baby was outside on the terrace. At that time, I did not insert the air raids.
>
> (S. Dann, n.d., original English)

Based on Dorothy Burlingham's desire to conduct research into the development of twin children, Sophie Dann made detailed notes of how the children developed physically, their relationship to each other, to their mother and how the mother in turn behaved towards her children. These depictions were included in three colours in Dorothy Burlingham's book of twins (Römer, 1998, p. 121). Of all the children in Bulldog's Bank, the Dann sisters – as Anna Freud wanted them to do – regularly wrote 'observation charts'.

> When the Bulldogs Bank was closed, we asked Anna Freud: 'What should we do with [the charts]?' She said, 'It would be quite good if we had them at the Anna Freud Centre.' And they wrote one day, they couldn't do anything with the stuff and gave it back to me. That was when I was still working in the library. We then asked the asked the Vienna Library and they said, 'Yes, they'll keep it.' A lot of people come there for research. Our CVs are there too – all four of them.
>
> (Dann, interview, 15 July, 1996)

Ernest Freud, grandson of Sigmund Freud, headed the Development Profile Research Group. Humberto Nagera, who joined the staff of the Hampstead Clinic shortly before the Cuban revolution, was engaged in expanding its development profile. The many experiences and data thus gained from the Hampstead Nurseries, the child analyses, and their supervisions, as well as the work in the Hampstead Child Therapy Course and Clinic, led to the creation of a profiling scheme in the 1960s for the diagnostic assessment of disturbed children, the so-called Hampstead Index (Midgley, 2013; Pretorius & Malberg, 2017; Sandler et al., 1962; Rosenblum, 1967).

It was Dorothy Burlingham's idea to create such a psychoanalytic index in order to obtain an overview of the many reports of the various collaborators. This index was then scientifically edited under the direction of Joseph Sandler and co-workers at the Hampstead Clinic (Bolland & Sandler, 1965). It included brief records of the structures, character traits, defence mechanisms, symptoms, transmissions, etc., of the children who were in treatment in the children's ward. In 1955, 60 children were already in analysis and an index was drawn up of all of them (diagnostic interviews with children and families) to systematize the material (later known as the 'Diagnostic Scheme' or 'Profile'). It was used to study mental illness in the child, paying special attention to whether the developmental trajectories were harmonious or unbalanced, or where, how, and why the developmental process lingered too long (Laible, 1978, p. 56). The focus was on developmental factors and included the entire spectrum of mental illness. In 1964, an adult profile was also created. The work in the Well Baby Clinic with pregnant women and infants led to the creation of the 'Baby Profile' by Ernest Freud (1971). Pretorius and Malberg (2017) provide up-to-date information on the revised diagnostic profile, its historical background and current integration.

Her own research at the Hampstead Child-Therapy Clinic included many such observational studies, including that of blind children and longitudinal research on the children of the Hampstead War Nurseries and child survivors of the Holocaust (A. Freud and Dann, 1951). In this respect Anna Freud's work could be seen as a precursor of the infant observation research of the 'baby-watchers' such as Stern (1985), Murray (1988) and Brazelton and Tronick (1980).

(Midgley, 2007, p. 955)

Pedagogy or developmental child analysis?

The Anna Freud–Melanie Klein controversy

Although it is not possible to give an overall appraisal of Anna Freud's work here, a few groundbreaking aspects of her work should be highlighted.

When Anna Freud published her book, *Introduction to the Technique of Child Analysis* (original title: *Einführung in die Technik der Kinderanalyse*) in 1927, the British group around Melanie Klein reacted with open criticism, and there followed a decades-long disagreement about child analysis. This controversy between Anna Freud and Melanie Klein also concerned the relationship between psychoanalysis and pedagogy. Besides analytical work, there must always be a piece of educational work as well – according to Anna Freud, while Melanie Klein vehemently rejected this point of view. A major point of criticism by Melanie Klein was that psychoanalysis had to tolerate expressions of drive necessarily condemned by educators.

Anna Freud never denied her basic pedagogical profession even though this attitude contributed to the intensification of the controversial discussion with Melanie Klein (Edgcumbe, 2000). In the speech she gave at the International Psychoanalytic Congress in Innsbruck in 1927 on the theory of child analysis, she stated:

> But now a word on the pedagogical mindset of the child analyst. If we have recognized that the powers we must fight while healing the child neurosis are not only internal, but also partially external, then we also have a right to insist that the child analyst learns to correctly assess the external situation, in which the child exists, just as we require that he is able to appreciate the child's internal situation. For this part of his task, however, the child analyst needs a theoretical and practical pedagogic knowledge set. This allows him to figure out the educational influences, under which the child sits, to criticize them, and – when necessary – to take this work out of the educator's hands for the duration of the analysis in order to set them right himself.
>
> (A. Freud, 1928b, p. 162)

While Anna Freud's interest in psychoanalytic pedagogy and in researching the normal development of the child is obvious and became clear in her projects, Melanie Klein rejected the idea of psychoanalytic education (Spillius *et al.*, 2011). In her opinion, the infant has an inner world from the very beginning. It consists of primitive images, which are not an expression of the real parent–child relationship, as they are distorted by introjection and projection processes. They unfold in the transference, which, in the Kleinian view, young children are also capable of, analogous to adults. The main task of the child analyst, in the Kleinian view, is to contact the child's unconscious. Therefore, interpretations, especially the interpretation of the negative transference, play an important role in child analysis.

Anna Freud, on the other hand, believed a child could not yet develop a transference neurosis. Her main arguments were:

> The child, unlike the adult, is not prepared to undertake remaking his love relationship, because – one could say – the old version is not yet exhausted. His original objects, the parents, are still available as love objects in reality, unlike neurotic adults in their fantasies.
>
> (Freud, A., 1987b, p. 51)

Melanie Klein and Anna Freud also differed in terms of timing the beginning of child analyses. According to Melanie Klein, the psychotic parts should be analysed as early as possible to ensure normal development, while Anna Freud saw child analysis as indicated only in severe cases of infantile neurosis. Everything else, in her opinion, called for good pedagogy. Melanie Klein, on the other hand, pleaded for a 'prophylactic analysis'. Melanie Klein and Anna Freud did, however, agree on one thing: a five-hour-a-week setting. Marianne Horney Eckardt (personal correspondence, 6 June, 2004) recalled how she and her sister Renate had to go to Melanie Klein's analysis as small children and spent most of their time lying under the couch instead of on top of it, as they were meant to.

It is, therefore, understandable that one finds psychoanalytic concepts based on Anna Freud in the counselling and preventative measures used in current infant care and psychotherapy (e.g., the development of a positive relationship).

The time after Anna Freud: What happened next?

In my conversations with Hansi Kennedy in the 1990s, it became clear that shortly after Anna Freud's death in 1982, the institution she had built up began to change:

> Yes, there are still people in Vienna who have worked with me. But it's slowly changing. There are a lot of people now. Because of the loyalty to Anna Freud, people stayed at the clinic for [such] a long time that the staff generation was actually old. And even secretaries, it's quite unusual to be a secretary for 25 or 20 years. But that was the same, it was all very familiar. [–] But that has changed now. They haven't stayed.
>
> (Kennedy, interview, 23 April, 1997)

According to Hansi Kennedy (Kennedy, interview, 11 July, 1996), Anna Freud had a great talent for attracting people to her work. In Hansi Kennedy's opinion, the War Nurseries were

> [...] the largest and also the most expensive, i.e., the best-funded home. But for our families, for our children that we looked after, we had to send a personal letter to the donors once a month, very briefly, to say what the money was doing. And then they also received clothes or personal gifts. And the donor for my children was Anna Mänchen,[1] who came to visit for the first time after the war and she wanted [–], and there were many analysts [–], she wanted to meet their children. And I took a photograph of [them] in the East End and presented it to her in a garden here and that's where she met them. So that was so very nice personally, somehow a sign of special recognition. It all went through Anna Freud, of course. And through that she had a lot of people in America who didn't give money themselves or found it themselves through rich patients and that was a lot and that was much easier when Anna Freud was alive than it is today.

After the death of Anna Freud and the passing of the generation of psychoanalysts who still knew Sigmund Freud or his daughter personally, the income from donations to the Anna Freud Centre decreased. More serious than the material restrictions, however, was the fact that Anna Freud's theoretical concepts and therapeutic methods were increasingly disregarded. This may have been because her 'Child Expert' training was never considered fully valid by the International Psychoanalytic Association. Graduates of her training were only admitted to the British Psycho-Analytic Society if they had undergone additional training there.

On the other hand, there was growing international pressure for intensive research into psychotherapeutic work, also to prove the effectiveness of these methods. In comparison to Melanie Klein and others, Anna Freud made efforts in research such as the creation of the Diagnostic Profiles. But the methods Anna Freud used to research her own actions and those of her collaborators were less and less in line with the standards applied at the universities, which were increasingly under the influence of the natural sciences.

The extent of the impact of these changes was already apparent with the sale of the two Anna Freud Centre houses in Maresfield Gardens (numbers 21 and 12) in 2019 and the establishment of the Kantor Centre of Excellence, and with it the dissolution of the traditional psychoanalytic kindergarten. With the dismissal of longtime staff, who still represent the tradition of the Anna Freud Centre at the end of 2020 (such as Tessa Baradon, Carol Broughton, Jessica James, Inge Pretorius, and Duncan McLean), the direct line to the Well Baby Clinic and the psychoanalytic Parent–Infant Psychotherapy and the corresponding psychoanalytic training seems to have been cut off.

Thus, this book becomes – unintentionally – not only a retrospective of the valuable work of Anna Freud's 'family-like network', but of an entire epoch. It is striking how little her work is taught in psychoanalytic training institutes today. It seems her successful work – compared to that of Melanie Klein, for example – is almost underestimated at present.

I would like to close this book with a quote from Veronica Mächtlinger, who was able to experience Anna Freud during her psychoanalytic training. I would wish that her approachable and encouraging attitude would inspire psychoanalytic training today and in the future.

> The sharpness and discipline of her thinking, the seemingly classic clarity and simplicity of her formulations and spontaneous remarks are all well known. Whereas it seems to be less well known to what extent her thinking remained flexible and tolerated insecurities and doubts. Working with her was like a lesson in the ability – also essential for experienced analysts – to endure insecurities and doubts, to remain sceptical in the face of an apparently seamless understanding of a clinical phenomenon. In the early phases of training, this unerring insistence that something was not yet fully understood could have an unsettling effect – especially when, as a beginner in handling the complexity of analytic material, after lengthy discussion, one finally discovered some line of understanding and therefore believed to have the answer to the riddle in hand. Unsettling – not discouraging. I never experienced Anna Freud

as discouraging, not once intimidating, which wouldn't have been out of the question – considering her immense abilities, her mastery of psychoanalytic theory deepened by decades of work, practical experience, and not least the fact that she, to a certain extent, embodied the history of psychoanalysis. That she, despite all this, didn't come across as intimidating may have something to do with the fact that she consciously resisted this temptation – one that many an analytic instructor succumbs to. In technical seminars, she let the participants develop their thoughts freely, at most giving only small nudges to get the discussion going. Most of the time, she tended to share only towards the end how she would have acted in the situation in question, what she would have said. In her work in child analysis, her suggested interpretations were surprisingly simple; her formulations were never long or convoluted, even if a complex theoretical idea lay hidden behind them.

(Mächtlinger, 1984, pp. 12–13)

Note

1 Anna Mänchen-Helfen, née Anna Aronsohn (1902–1991), was in Vienna with Anna Freud in analysis. She later became one of the most influential child analysts of the San Francisco Psychoanalytic Society of Anna Freud's school. https://www.psychoanalytik-erinnen.de/oesterreich_biografien.html#Maenchen (accessed 12 October, 2019).

References and Bibliography

Bateson, J. (2004). *The Holocaust Survivors at Weir Courtney, Lingfield*. The RH7 History Group. Retrieved 14.04.2020 from https://www.rh7.org/factshts/holocst.pdf.

Bateson, P., Barker, D., Clutton-Brock, T., Deb, D., D'Udine, B., Foley, R. A. *et al.* (2004). Developmental plasticity and human health. *Nature*, *430*(6998), 419–421. https://doi.org/10.1038/nature02725

Berger, M. (2002). Wer war Eleonore Astfalk? [Who was Eleonore Astfalk?]. *Sozialmagazin, 6*, 6–9.

Berger, M. & Kennedy, H. (1975). Pseudobackwardness in children. Maternal attitudes as an etiological factor. *Psychoanalytic Study of the Child, 30*, 279–306.

Bethge, E. (2000). *Dietrich Bonhoeffer: Theologian, Christian, Man for his Times; A Biography*. Fortress Press.

Bethge, R., Gremmels, C. & McNeil, B. (1987). *Dietrich Bonhoeffer: A Life in Pictures*. Fortress Press. https://books.google.it/books?id=D4mk0YSmvk4C

Bildungswerk Stanisław Hantz e.V. (n.d.) Bernhard Wolfgang Hellmann. https://sobibor.de/de/bernhard-wolfgang-hellmann/

Bolland, J. & Sandler, J. (1965). *Hampstead Psychoanalytic Index: A Study of the Psychoanalytic Case Material of a Two-Year-Old Child*. International Universities Press.

Brazelton, T. B. & Tronick, E. (1980). Preverbal communication between mothers and infants. In: D. R. Olson (ed.), *The Social Foundations of Language and Thought* (pp. 299–315). Norton.

Brecht, K. & Friedrich, V. (1985). *Hier geht das Leben auf eine sehr merkwürdige Weise weiter. Zur Geschichte der Psychoanalyse in Deutschland* [Life Continues in a Very Strange Way. On the History of Psychoanalysis in Germany]. Psychosozial. https://books.google.it/books?id=TALbAAAAMAAJ

Brenner, N. (1988). The Third Decade (1978–1988). *Bulletin of the Anna Freud Centre, 11*, 289–294.

Budritzski, E. v. (1929). Fürsorgetätigkeit im Obdach [Care in homelessness]. *Berliner Wohlfahrtsblatt, Beilage zum Amtsblatt der Stadt Berlin, 8*, 70–72.

Burgner, M. & Kennedy, H. (1980). Different types of sado-masochistic behavior in children. *Dialogue: Journal of Psychoanalytic Perspectives, 4*, 49–59.

Burlingham, D., Schnurmann, A. & Lantos B. (1958). David and his mother (unpublished).

Burlingham, D. T. & Freud, A. (1942). *Young Children in War-time: A Year's Work in a Residential War Nursery*. G. Allen & Unwin for the New Era. https://books.google.it/books?id=qeQpnQEACAAJ

Burlingham, D. T. & Freud, A. (1943). *Infants Without Families: The Case for and Against Residential Nurseries.* International Universities Press. https://books.google.it/books?id=mBtFAAAAYAAJ

Caldwell, L. & Taylor Robinson, H. (eds) (2017). *The Collected Works of D. W. Winnicott, Volume 5 1955–1959).* Oxford: Oxford University Press.

Charlotte Bühler Institut (n.d.) Charlotte Bühler. Available at: https://www.charlotte-buehler- institut.at/charlotte-buehler-info/

Collona, A. & Wiener, J. (2003). Speech at the funeral of Hansi Kennedy (unpublished).

Colonna, A. B. & Friedmann, M. (1984). Prediction of development. *Psychoanalytic Study of the Child, 39,* 509–526. https://doi.org/10.1080/00797308.1984.11823440

Corbach, D. (1990). *Die Jawne zu Köln. Zur Geschichte des ersten jüdischen Gymnasiums im Rheinland und zum Gedächtnis von Erich Klibansy* [The Cologne Jawne. On the History of the first Jewish Secondary School and in memory of Erich Klibansky]. Scriba.

Curio, C. (2006). *Flucht, Verfolgung, Rettung. Die Kindertransporte 1938/39 nach Großbritannien [Escape, Pursuit, Salvation: The Child Transports 1938/39 to Great Britain].* Metropol.

Dann, G. (1986–1992). Memoirs of Gertrud Dann (supplement). Available at: https://www.refugeemap.org/map/records/sophie-and-gertrud-dann-1945-1986/gallery/1

Dann, S. (n.d.) Air raid Chart Hampstead Nurseries and Sleeping Chart.

Dann, S. (1960). Beobachtungen an Kleinkindern bei der Anpassung an eine neue Sprache [Observations of toddlers during the adjustment to a new language]. *Schule und Psychologie,* 357–381.

Dann, S. (1978). Zum 3. Reich in Augsburg [On the Third Reich in Augsburg]. *Augsburger Hefter,* 26.

Dann, S. (1979). Juden in Augsburg [Jews in Augsburg]. *Augsburger Blätter,* 11–18.

Dann, S. (1981). Tagebuchnotizen der Fürsorgeschwester der Jüdischen Gemeinde [Journal entries of the nurses in the Jewish community]. *Augsburger Blätter,* 14–18; 81–85.

Dann, S. (1986). Memoirs of Sophie Dann.

Dann, S. (1998a). *Sie lebte nur für andere* [She lived just for others]. Wissner.

Dann, S. (1998b). Unpublished manuscript in English about her life.

Danneberg, E. E. H. (1971). Teamarbeit: Eine Behandlung von Mutter und Sohn [Teamwork: Treatment of a mother and son]. *Psyche, 25*(8), 580–594.

Danziger, L. (1930). Die Beziehung der Pflegemutter zu ihrem Kind [The relationship of mother to her child]. In L. Danziger, H. Hetzer, & H. Löw-Beer (eds), *Pflegemutter und ihr Kind* (pp. 4–100). Hirzel.

Dolce, J. (2020). The Windermere children: Safe at last. Available at: https://quadrant.org.au/magazine/2020/12/the-windermere-children-safe-at-last-joe- dolce/

Eccleshare, J. (2006). Maggie Noach. Hard bargaining agent with a sense of fun. *Guardian.* Available at: www.theguardian.com/news/2006/dec/22/guardianobituaries.booksobituaries https://www.theguardian.com/news/2006/dec/22/guardianobituaries.booksobituaries.

Edgcumbe, R. (2000). *Anna Freud: A View of Development, Disturbance and Therapeutic Techniques.* London: Routledge.

Edgcumbe, R., Kennedy, H., Sandler, J. & Yorke, C (1978). Some reflections on infantile neurosis. In: J. Sandler (ed.) *Bulletin of the Hampstead Clinic,* Volume 1, Part 2, pp. 101–109. The Hampstead Child Therapy Clinic.

Eichelberger, B. (2001). Spurensuche – auf den Lebensspuren von Lili Ester Peller-Roubiczek und der Wiener Montessori-Bewegung. [Tracking – In The Footsteps of Lili Ester Peller-Roubiczek and the Viennese Montessori Movement]. In C. Zwiauer, B. Eichelberger, & H. Picus (eds), *Das Kind ist entdeckt* (pp. 101–118). Picus.

Emde, R. (2011). Regeneration und Neuanfänge: Perspektiven einer entwicklungsbezogenen Ausrichtung der Psychoanalyse [Regeneration and new beginnings: Perspectives of a developmental orientation of psychoanalysis]. *Psyche, 659*, 778–807.

Ermann, M. (2004). Wir Kriegskinder [We war children]. *Forum der Psychoanalyse, 20*(2), 226–239.

Exploring Surrey's Past. (n.d.) Weir Courtney, Lingfield. https://www.exploringsurreyspast. org.uk/themes/subjects/refugees/weircourtney/

Feitscher, P. (1939). Zu den Kleinkindertests von Bühler und Hetzer [On the Bühler and Hetzer tests for small children]. *Archiv für Psychiatrie und Nervenkrankheiten 109*(5), 699–720.

Fonagy, P., Luyten, P., Allison, E. & Campbell, C. (2019). Mentalizing, epistemic trust and the phenomenology of psychotherapy. *Psychopathology, 52*(2), 94–103. https://doi. org/10.1159/000501526

Fonagy, P., Mayes, L. & Target, M. (2018). *Deveopmental Science and Psychotherapy: Integration and Innovation.* London: Routledge.

Fonagy, P., Luyten, P., Allison, E. & Campbell, C. (2019). Mentalizing, epistemic trust and the phenomenology of psychotherapy. *Psychopathology, 52*(2), 94–103. https://doi. org/10.1159/000501526

Fonagy, P., Moran, G. S., Edgcumbe, R., Kennedy, H. & Target, M. (1993). The roles of mental representations and mental processes in therapeutic action. *Psychoanalytic Study of the Child, 48*, 9–48. https://doi.org/10.1080/00797308.1993.11822377

Frankl, L. & Hellman, I. (1962). Symposium on child analysis: II. The ego's participation in the therapeutic alliance. *International Journal of Psychoanalysis, 43*(4–5), 333–337.

Freud, A. (1928a). Four lectures in child analysis. In *The Writings of Anna Freud* (Vol. 1, pp. 3–73). International Universities Press.

Freud, A. (1928b). Zur Theorie der Kinderanalyse [On the theory of child analysis]. *International Zeitschrift für Psychoanalyse, 14*, 153–162.

Freud, A. (1951). Observations on child development. In: *The Writings of Anna Freud* (Vol. 4, pp. 143–162). International Universities Press.

Freud, A. (1952). The mutual influences in the development of the ego and the id: Introduction to the discussion. *Psychoanalytic Study of the Child, 7*, 42–50. https://doi.org/10.10 80/00797308.1952.11823151

Freud, A. (1954). Some remarks on infant observation. *The Psychoanalytic Study of the Child, 8*, 9–19.

Freud, A. (1958). Child observation and prediction of development. In: *The Writings of Anna Freud* (Vol. 5, pp. 102–135). International Universities Press.

Freud, A. (1971). Problems of psychoanalytic training, diagnosis, and the technique of therapy. In: *The Writings of Anna Freud* (Vol. 7). International Universities Press.

Freud, A. (1973a). Monthly Reports of the Hampstead War Nurseries, February 1941–December 1945 In: *The Writings of Anna Freud* (Volume 3). International Universities Press.

Freud, A. (1973b) Tribute to Sara Rosenfeld. Memorial meeting at the Hampstead Child-Therapy Clinic (unpublished).

Freud, A. (1987a). Monthly Report – March 1941. In *The Writings of Anna Freud* (Vol. 2, pp. 375–386). Fischer.

Freud, A. (1987b). Introduction to 'Unpredictability of the mother as a factor in character development, a comparative study of three cases'. *Psychoanalytic Study of the Child, 12*.

Freud, A. & Burlingham, D. T. (1943). *War and Children.* Medical War Books.

Freud, A. & Dann, S. (1951). An experiment in group upbringing. *Psychoanalytic Study of the Child, 6*(1), 127–168. https://doi.org/10.1080/00797308.1952.11822909

Freud, A., Dann, S., & Burlingham, D. (1971). *Heimatlose Kinder. Zur Anwendung psycho-analytischen Wissens auf die Kindererziehung* [Children without homes: On the use of psychoanalytic knowledge in childrearing]. Fischer.

Freud, W. E. (1971). The baby profile. *Psychoanalytic Study of the Child, 26*(1), 172–194. https://doi.org/10.1080/00797308.1971.11822270

Freud-Zentrum Stiftung. (n.d.) Unsere Stiftung. https://www.freud-zentrum.ch/stiftung/ Friedlaender, S., Jarecki, H. & Schonig, B. (1996). *Sophie & Hilde: ein ge-meinsames Leben in Freundschaft und Beruf.* Ed. Hentrich. https://books.google.it/books?id=DKksAQAAIAAJ

Friedlander, H. F. (1947). The recalling of thoughts. *British Journal of Psychology General Section, 37*(2), 87–95. https://doi.org/10.1111/j.2044-8295.1947.tb01124.x

Friedlander, K. (1946). Social factors and mental health; puberty. *Health Education Journal, 4*(4), 172–176. https://doi.org/10.1177/001789694600400408

Friedlander, K. (1947). Neurosis and home background. *The Psychoanalytic Study of the Child, 3*(1), 423–438. https://doi.org/10.1080/00797308.1947.11823096

Friedmann, M. (1986). Alice Goldberger. *Bulletin of the Anna Freud Centre, 9*, 313–314.

Friedmann, M. (1988). The Hampstead Clinic Nursery: The first 20 years (1957–1978). *Bulletin of the Anna Freud Centre, 11*(4), 277–288.

Friedmann, M. (2007). 1933–1939 life in Germany. *'45 Society, 31*, 34–36.

Friedmann, M. (2013). Memories and tributes (Obituary). United States Holocaust Memo-rial Museum. https://collections.ushmm.org/search/catalog/irn512917#?rsc=183630&cv=0&c=0&m= 0&s=0&xywh=-947%2C-1107%2C5651%2C5557

Frohn, A. (2018). Interview zur Geschichte des Anna Freud Centre mit Frau Dr. Inge-Martine Pretorius vom Anna Freud Centre (AFC) und University College London (UCL) [Interview on the history of the Anna Freud Centre with Dr. Inge-Martine Pretorius of the Anna Freud Centre (AFC) and University College London (UCL)] https://www.psychoanalyse-aktuell.de/artikel-/detail?tx_news_pi1%5Baction%5D=detail&tx_news_pi1%5Bcontroller%5D=News&t x_news_pi1%5Bnews%5D=172&cHash=595c979980dfc95f793f3e018db49241

Fuchs, G. (1992). Kriegskinderheime in London 1940–1945. Anna Freud Hampstead Nurseries. [Wartime Children's Homes in London 1940–1945. Anna Freud Hampstead Nurseries]. In U. Benz & W. Benz (Eds), *Sozialisation und Traumatisierung: Kinder in der Zeit des Nationalsozialismus.* Fischer.

Geissman, C. & Geissmann, P. (1998). *A History of Child Psychoanalysis.* Routledge. https://books.google.it/books?id=MxNifrT1auoC

Gilbert, M. (1997). *The Boys: Triumph Over Adversity : The Story of 732 Young Concentra-tion Camp Survivors.* Phoenix. https://books.google.it/books?id=j4LBzgEACAAJ

Göpfert, R. (1999). *Der jüdische Kindertransport von Deutschland nach England 1938/39: Geschichte und Erinnerung.* Campus. https://books.google.it/books?id=wseIN7RILhkC

Grieger, M. (2013). Straus, Moritz. https://www.deutsche-biographie.de/sfz74909.html Gy-omroi, E. L. (1963). The analysis of a young concentration camp victim. *Psychoanalytic Study of the Child, 18*, 484–510. https://doi.org/10.1080/00797308.1963.11822940

Haager, J. (1986). *Kate Friedländer (1902–1949): Leben u. Werk* [Life and Work]. Univer-sität zu Köln. https://books.google.it/books?id=DQRIAQAAIAAJ

Hamilton, M. A. (1944). *Remembering My Good Friends.* Cape.

Hellman, I. (1954). Some observations on mothers of children with intellectual inhibitions. *Psychoanalytic Study of the Child, 9*(1), 259–273. https://doi.org/10.1080/00797308.1954.11822542

Hellman, I. (1962). Hampstead Nursery follow-up Studies. *Psychoanalytic Study of the Child, 17*(1), 159–174. https://doi.org/10.1080/00797308.1962.11822844

Hellman, I. (1964). Assessment of analysability illustrated by the case of an adolescent patient. *Bulletin of the Hampstead Clinic, 1*, 65–73.

Hellman, I. (1983). Work in the Hampstead War Nurseries. *International Journal of Psychoanalysis, 64*(4), 435–439.

Hellman, I. (1990). *From War Babies to Grandmothers: Forty-eight Years in Psychoanalysis*. London: Karnac Books. https://books.google.it/books?id=16J_HqDcBIUC

Hellman, I., Dann, G. & Dann, S. (1942). Annual Report of a Residential War Nursery: A thank-you letter (unpublished manuscript). London: Anna Freud Centre Archives.

Hellman, I., de Monchauy, C. & Ludowyk-Gyomroi, E. (1961). Simultaneous analysis of a mother and her eleven-year-old daughter (unpublished manuscript).

Hellman, I., Friedmann, O. & Shepheard, E. (1960). Simultaneous analysis of mother and child. *The Psychoanalytic Study of the Child, 15*(1), 359–377. https://doi.org/10.1080/00797308.1960.11822582

Hellmann, P. (2009). *Mijn grote verwachtingen: herinneringen*. Augustus. https://books.google.it/books?id=31StPwAACAAJ

Herszberg, J. (1979). *This Is Your Life. Journal of the '45 Aid Society, 6*.

Hirsch, F. (1990). Als nichtjüdischer Lehrer und Erzieher in einem jüdischen Jugendwohnheim für schwererziehbare Jugendliche [In a Jewish Youth Home for difficult youth as a non-Jewish teacher] (*Lehreropposition im NS Staat. Biographische Berichte über den ›aufrechten Gang‹* (pp. 64–82). Fischer.

Hoffmannsthal, H. v. (1967). *Briefe an Paul und Irene Hellmann* [Letters to Paul and Irene Hellmann]. Kröner.

Holocaust Memorial Day Trust (n.d.). Wolf Blomfield. https://www.hmd.org.uk/resource/wolf-blomfield/

Hoyer, T. (2008). *Im Getümmel der Welt: Alexander Mitscherlich, ein Porträt*. Vandenhoeck & Ruprecht. https://books.google.it/books?id=y2fhuNyId9cC

Husserl, Z., Millan, J. & Oppenheimer, R. (2009). 'Lingfielders' Reunion, 2009. *AJR Journal, 9*(5). https://ajr.org.uk/wp-content/uploads/2018/02/2009_september.pdf

Jackson, E. B. (1946). Should mother and baby room together? *American Journal of Nursing, 46*(1), 17–19. https://doi.org/10.2307/3457406

Jackson, E. B. (1948a). General reactions of mothers and nurses to rooming-in. *American Journal of Public Health, 38*(5 Pt 1), 689–695. https://doi.org/10.2105/ajph.38.5_pt_1.689

Jackson, E. B. (1948b). "Rooming-in" gives baby a good start. *The Child*.

Jackson, E. B. & Thoms, H. (1947). The rooming-in plan for mothers and newborn infants. *Connecticut State Medical Journal, 11*(3), 175.

Johler, B., Sommer, M., Steiner-Strauss, A. & Aichhorn, T. (2016). *Anna Freud in Wien: ein Rundgang zu Orten der Psychoanalyse* [Anna Freud in Vienna: A Tour of Places of Psychoanalysis]. Verlag Turia + Kant.https://books.google.it/books?id=Lv1hrgEACAAJ

Kamm, H. (2010). Kriegskinder als Psychoanalytiker. *Forum der Psychoanalyse, 26*(4), 335–349. https://doi.org/10.1007/s00451-010-0044-6

Kennedy, H. (1971). Problems in reconstruction in child analysis. *Psychoanalytic Study of the Child, 26*, 386–402. https://doi.org/10.1080/00797308.1971.11822278

Kennedy, H. (1978a). The analytic treatment of two siblings. A foreword. *Bulletin of the Hampstead Clinic, 1*, 119–120.

Kennedy, H. (1978b). The Hampstead Centre for the Psychoanalytic Study and Treatment of Children. *Bulletin of the Anna Freud Centre 1*, 7–10.

Kennedy, H. (1979). The role of insight in child analysis: A developmental viewpoint. *Journal of the American Psychoanalytic Association, 27* (Suppl.), 9–28.

Kennedy, H. (1980). Hampstead Clinic memorial contributions. *Bulletin of the Hampstead Clinic, 3,* 78–79.

Kennedy, H. (1981a). Die Bedeutung der Einsicht in der Kinderanalyse. In: G. Biermann (ed.), *Handbuch der Kinderpsychotherapie*. Reinhardt Verlag.

Kennedy, H. (1981b). Reports by chairmen on the work of study groups at the Hampstead Clinic: Study Group on developmental disturbances. *Bulletin of the Hampstead Clinic, 4,* 295.

Kennedy, H. (1981c). Vergangenheit und Gegenwart in der Sicht des Kindes: Folgerungen für die Kinderanalyse (Vol. 1). Österreichischen Studiengesellschaft für Kinderpsychoanalyse.

Kennedy, H. (1982a). Die Hampstead Klinic: Ein historischer Überblick. *Studien zur Kinderpsychologie, II,* 129–151.

Kennedy, H. (1982b). El papel del insight. *Psicoanalisis, 1,* 51.

Kennedy, H. (1982c). Questions soulevées par la reconstruction en analyse d'enfant. *La Psychiatrie de l'enfant, 25*(2), 369–386.

Kennedy, H. (1983a). Anna Freud. 1895–1982. *Psychoanalytic Quarterly, 52*(4), 501–506.

Kennedy, H. (1983b). Anna Freud: Funeral tributes. *Bulletin of the Hampstead Clinic, 6,* 11–12.

Kennedy, H. (1984). The "baby at the breast" experience: Memory or fantasy? Some further thoughts on reconstruction. *Bulletin of the Hampstead Clinic, 7,* 15–24.

Kennedy, H. (1985a). For or against child placement: A clinical illustration. *Bulletin of the Hampstead Clinic,* 8), 245–252.

Kennedy, H. (1985b). Growing up with a handicapped sibling. *Psychoanalytic Study of the Child, 40*(1), 255–274. https://doi.org/10.1080/00797308.1985.11823032

Kennedy, H. (1986). Trauma in childhood. Signs and sequelae as seen in the analysis of an adolescent. *Psychoanalytic Study of the Child, 41,* 209–219.

Kennedy, H. (1988). The pre-history of the Nursery School. *Bulletin of the Hampstead Clinic, 11,* 271–275.

Kennedy, H. (1989). Sadomasochistische Perversion in der Adoleszenz. Eine entwicklungsgeschichtliche Betrachtung. *Zeitschrift für psychoanalytische Theorie und Praxis, 46,* 181–198.

Kennedy, H. (1993). Developing resilience in high-risk Nursery School children. In: T. B. Cohen, M. H. Etezady & B. L. Pacella (eds), *The Vulnerable Child* (Vol. 1). International Universities Press.

Kennedy, H. (1994a). Book review: Robert Coles, "Anna Freud: The dream of psychoanalysis". *Psychoanalytic Quarterly, 63,* 587–590.

Kennedy, H. (1994b). Doris Wills, 1908–1993: Memorial tributes. *Bulletin of the Hampstead Clinic 17,* 57–62.

Kennedy, H. (1995). Children in conflict: Anna Freud and the War Nurseries. Paper presented to a conference sponsored by the Anna Freud Centre and the Freud Museum in celebration of the 100th anniversary of the birth of Anna Freud.

Kennedy, H. (1996). Memories of Anna Freud. *American Imago, 53*(3), 205–209. http://www.jstor.org/stable/26304490

Kennedy, H. (2001). The technique of psychoanalysis with the prelatency child. In R. Tyson (ed.), *Analysis of the Under-Five Child* (pp. 262–281). Yale University Press.

Kennedy, H. (2009). Children in conflict: Anna Freud and the War Nurseries. *Psychoanalytic Study of the Child, 64,* 306–319. https://doi.org/10.1080/00797308.2009.11800826

Kennedy, H. (n.d.). *Curriculum vitae* (unpublished).

Kennedy, H. & Moran, G. S. (1984). The developmental roots of self-injury and response to pain in a 4-year-old boy. *Psychoanalytic Study of the Child, 39*, 195–212. https://doi.org/10.1080/00797308.1984.11823426

Kennedy, H. & Yorke, C. (1980). Childhood neurosis vs. developmental deviations. *Dialogue: Journal of Psychoanalytic Perspectives, 4*, 21–33.

Kennedy, H., Moran, G., Wiseberg, S. & Yorke, C. (1985). Both sides of the barrier. *The Psychoanalytic Study of the Child, 40*(1), 275–283. https://doi.org/10.1080/00797308.1985.11823033

Kennedy, H. E. (1950). Cover memories in formation. *Psychoanalytic Study of the Child, 5*(1), 275–284. https://doi.org/10.1080/00797308.1950.11822894

Kennedy, H. E. (1969). Young children in brief separation. *British Journal of Medical Psychology, 42*, 191–193.

Kennedy, S. (2003). Speech on the occasion of the funeral of Hansi Kennedy (unpublished).

Kestenberg, J. S. & Koorland, V. (1993). Als Eure Grosseltern jung waren: mit Kindern über den Holocaust sprechen [Talking to Children about the Holocaust]. Hamburg: Krämer.

Koch, E. (2012). Two supervisors. In N. Malberg (ed.), *The Anna Freud Tradition: Lines of Development – Evolution and Theory and Practice over the Decades* (pp. 376–378). Karnac Books.

Koslowski, J. (2018). *Aus dem Leben der Familie Bonhoeffer. Die Aufzeichnungen von Dietrich Bonhoeffers jüngster Schwester Susanne Dreß* [From the Life of the Bonhoeffer Family. The notes of Dietrich Bonhoeffer's youngest sister, Susanne Dreß]. Gütersloher Verlagshaus.

Krivanek, R. (2014). 'Vertrautheit mit dem Kleinkind ist das Ziel'. Die Arbeit und Forschung in der Jackson-Krippe (Wien 1937/38). ['Familiarity with the infant is the goal'. The work and research in the Jackson nursery (Vienna 1937/38)]. *Luzifer & Amor, 27*(53), 71–107.

Laible, E. (1978). *Anna Freud und die Entwicklung der Psychoanalyse* [Anna Freud and the Development of Psychoanalysis] (Vol. 10). Frommann-Holzboog.

Laible, E. (1982) Anna Freud – von der Arbeit ihres Lebens. 1895–1982 [Anna Freud – From the work of her life. 1895–1982]. *Studien zur Kinderpsychoanalyse, II*: 13–30

Langer, E. (2013). Holocaust survivors reunite with the woman who cared for them after the war. Available at: https://www.washingtonpost.com/lifestyle/style/holocaust-survivors-reunite-with-the-woman-who-cared-for-them-after-the-war/2013/12/25/21112494-61b0-11e3-8beb-3f9a9942850f_story.html (accessed 22 December, 2022).

Lazarus, B., McLoughlin-O'Donnell, M. A. & Holocaust Resource Center (Pomona, NJ) (2008). *Feathers, Smoke, A Shattered Family. A Three Year Old Survivor of Terezin.* Stockton College's Holocaust Resource Centre, Pomona, NJ.

Leibholz-Bonhoeffer, S. (1991). *Weihnachten im Hause Bonhoeffer* [Christmas at the Bonhoeffer house]. Gütersloher Verlagshaus.

Leibholz-Bonhoeffer, S. (2005). *Vergangen, erlebt, überwunden: Schicksale der Familie Bonhoeffer.* Gütersloher Verlag-Haus. https://books.google.it/books?id=cBnxPAAACAAJ

Lichtenstein, J. (2005). Oral history interview with Judith Sherman. United States Holocaust Memorial Museum. https://collections.ushmm.org/search/catalog/irn87431

Lindsay, M. (2013). Joyce Robertson obituary. *Guardian News & Media.* Available at: https://www.theguardian.com/society/2013/may/19/joyce-robertson (accessed 25 June, 2023).

Ludwig–Korner, C. (1998). *Wiederentdeckt. Psychoanalytikerrinnen in Berlin: auf den Spuren ergessener Generationen* [Rediscovered. Women psychoanalysts in Berlin: In the footsteps of forgotten generations]. Gießen: Psychosozial.

Ludwig-Körner, C. (2000). Wegbereiter der Kinderanalyse. Die Arbeit in der »Jackson Kinderkrippe« und den »Kriegskinderheimen« [Pioneers of Child Analysis. The work in the "Jackson Nursery" and the "Wartime Children's Homes"]. *Luzifer-Amor. Zeitschrift zur Geschichte der Psychoanalyse, 25*, 78–104.

Ludwig-Körner, C. (2012). Anna Freud and her collaborators in the early post-war period. In N. T. Malberg & J. Raphael-Leff (eds) *The Anna Freud Tradition: Lines of Development – Evolution of Theory and Practice over the Decades* (pp. 17–29). Karnac Books.

Ludwig-Körner, C. (2013). Wandlerin zwischen Welten. Anneliese Schnurmann [Wanderer between Worlds. Anneliese Schnurmann]. *Forum der Psychoanalyse*(3), 343–355.

Ludwig-Körner, C. (2014). *Wiederentdeckt - Psychoanalytikerinnen in Berlin* [Rediscovered – Female Psychoanalysts in Berlin]. Psychosozial-Verlag. https://books.google.it/books?id= e7RangEACAAJ

Ludwig-Körner, C. (2017). Anna Freud and observation: Memoirs of her colleagues from the Hampstead War Nurseries. *Journal of Infant, Child, and Adolescent Psychotherapy, 16*(2), 131–137. https://doi.org/10.1080/15289168.2017.1307072

Mächtlinger, V. (1984). Anna Freud. Einige persönliche Eindrücke [Anna Freud. Some personal impressions]. *Jahrbuch der Psychoanalyse, 16*, 9–16.

Mahler-Werfel, A. M. (2002). *Tagebuch-Suiten: 1898–1902*. Fischer Taschenbuch Verlag. https://books.google.it/books?id=ZLl3OwAACAAJ

Malberg, N. T. & Raphael-Leff, J. (eds) (2012). *The Anna Freud Tradition: Lines of Development – Evolution and Theory and Practice Over the Decades*. Karnac Books. https://books.google.it/books?id=noVxRR7fEWQC

McGourty, N. (2017). Historic visit honours Dann sisters and the Bulldogs Bank children. *General News*. https://www.annafreud.org/insights/news/2017/06/historic- visit-honours- dann-sisters-and-the-bulldogs-bankchildren

Memory of Nations. (n.d.) Zdenka Husserlová. https://www.memoryofnations.eu/en/ husserlova-zdenka-1939

Meyer, K. (1989). *Keiner will sie haben. Die Exilpolitik in England, Frankreich und den USA zwischen 1933 und 1945 [Nobody wants them. The policy of exile in England, France and the USA between 1933 and 1945]*. Peter Lang.

Midgley, N. (2007). Anna Freud: The Hampstead War Nurseries and the role of the direct observation of children for psychoanalysis. *International Journal of Psychoanalysis, 88*(4), 939–959. https://doi.org/10.1516/v28r-j334-6182-524h

Midgley, N. (2013). *Reading Anna Freud*. Routledge.

Midgley, N. & Pretorius, I.-M. (2014). As creches de guerra Hampstead (1941–1945). Uma perspectiva psicanalitica sobre alcolhimento residencial de criancas e jovens em perigo [The Hampstead War Nurseries (1941–1945): A psychoanalytical perspective on residential care for infants and young children]. In: T. Mendes & P. Santos (eds), *Alcolhimento de criancas e jovens em perigo* (pp. 1–17). Lisbon: Climepsi.

Miller, J. M. & Neely, K. (eds) (2008). *The Psychoanalytic Work of Hansi Kennedy. From War Nurseries to the Anna Freud Centre 1940–1993*. London: Karnac.

Model, E. (1986). Memorial Meeting. *Bulletin of the Anna Freud Centre* (9), 315.

Moskovitz, S. (1983). *Love Despite Hate: Child Survivors of the Holocaust and Their Adult Lives*. Schocken Books. https://books.google.it/books?id=gwlnAAAAMAAJ

Mühlleitner, E. & Reichmayr, J. (1992). *Biographisches Lexikon der Psychoanalyse [Biographic Lexicon of Psychoanalysis]*. Edition Diskord. https://books.google.it/books?id= pkkUAQAAIAAJ

Murray, L. (1988). Effects of post-natal depression on infant development: Direct studies on early mother–infant interactions. In: R. Kumar & I. F. Brockington (eds), *Motherhood and Mental Illness 2: Causes and Consequences* (pp. 159–191). London: Wright.

Murray, L. & Cooper, P. (1997). Effects of postnatal depression on infant development. *Archives of Disease in Childhood*, 77(2), 99–101. https://doi.org/10.1136/adc.77.2.99

National Holocaust Centre and Museum (n.d.) Lingfield House; Report 1951. https://www.holocaust.org.uk/lingfield-house-report

Niederacher, S. (2018). *Dossier zu Gustav Klimt: Der Blinde, ca. 1896. Leopold Museum Privatstiftung.* https://www.leopoldmuseum.org/media/fi le/620_LM_4144_Hellmann.pdf

Nölleke, B. (n.d.). *Women Psychoanalysts in Great Britain.* https://www.psychoanalytik-erinnen.de/greatbritain_biographies.html#Hopkins

Penz, M. (2013). *Der Kindertransport im Spiegel britischer Flüchtlingspolitik* [The Kindertransport as reflected in British refugee policy] Universität Wien. http://othes.univie.ac.at/24768/1/2013-01-03_0408293.pdf

Person, E., Cooper, A., & Gabbard, G. (2005). *Textbook of Psychoanalysis.* American Psychiatric Publishing.

Pollner, M. (2014). Die Familien Redlich und Hellmann in Aussee [The Redlich and Hellmann Families in Aussee]. *Alpenpost*, 22–24.

Pretorius, I.-M. (2012). From the Hampstead War Nurseries to the Anna Freud Centre. In N. Malberg (ed.), *The Anna Freud Tradition: Lines of Development – Evolution of Theory and Practice over the Decades* (pp. 30–37). London: Karnac Books.

Pretorius, I.-M. (2019). Beholding and handling Anna Freud's notes. *Bulletin of the Association of Child Psychotherapists*, 273, 8–10.

Pretorius, I.-M. (2020). Anna Freud's pioneering work in World War 2. In M. Pessler & D. Finzi (eds), *Freud, Bergasse 19, The Origin of Psychoanalysis* (pp. 287–295). Hatje Cantz Verlag GmbH.

Pretorius, I.-M. (2022). Observation: Its role in Anna Freud's developmental approach and parent–toddler groups I. *Journal of Analytical Psychology*, 67(4), 979–998.

Pretorius, I.-M. & Malberg, N. (Guest Eds) (2017). Anna Freud's legacy … The revised provisional diagnostic profile 2016: Historical backdrop and contemporary integration. *Journal of Infant, Child, and Adolescent Psychotherapy*, 16(2) (Special Edition).

Robertson, J. & Robertson, J. (1969). *John, 17 Months: Nine Days in a Residential Nursery.* Film: New York University Film Library.

Robertson, J. & Robertson, J. (1971). Young children in brief separation. A fresh look. *Psychoanalytic Study of the Child*, 26(1), 264–315. https://doi.org/10.1080/00797308.1971.11822274

Robertson, J. & Robertson, J. (1989). *Separation and the Very Young.* Free Association Books.

Römer, G. (1988). *Vier Schwestern* [Four Sisters]. Wißner.

Rosenblum, L. (1967). The Hampstead Psychoanalytic Index: A study of the psychoanalytic case material of a two-year-old child. *Archives of General Psychiatry*, 16(6), 71–772. doi:10.1001/archpsyc.1967.01730240127023

Salo, F. & Friedmann, M. (1988). The Runaway Bunny Mother: The long-term influence of the Nursery School experience. *Bulletin of the Anna Freud Centre*, 1, 57–73.

Sandler, A.-M. (2012). Anna Freud's influence on contemporary thinking about the child. In: N. Malberg (ed.), *The Anna Freud Tradition: Lines of Development – Evolution of Theory and Practice over the Decades* (pp. 47–53). Karnac Books.

Sandler, A.-M., Daunton, E., Schnurmann, A., & Freud, A. (1957). Inconsistency in the mother as a factor in character development: A comparative study of three cases. *Psychoanalytic Study of the Child*, *12*(1), 209–225. https://doi.org/10.1080/00797308. 1957.11822810

Sandler, J. (1965). *The Hampstead Child-Therapy Clinic*

Sandler, J. & Rosenblatt, B. (1962). The concept of the representational world. *Psychoanalytic Study of the Child*, *17*, 128–145. https://doi.org/10.1080/00797308.1962.11822842

Sandler, J., Holder, A. Kawenoka, M., Kennedy, H. A. & Neurath, L. (1969). Notes on some theoretical and clinical aspects of transference. *International Journal of Psychoanalysis*, *50*(4), 633–645.

Sandler, J., Kawenoka, M., Neurath, L., Rosenblatt, B., Schnurmann, A. & Sigal, J. (1962). The classification of superego material in the Hampstead Index. *Psychoanalytic Study of the Child*, *17*(1), 107–127. https://doi.org/10.1080/00797308.1962.11822841

Sandler, J., Kennedy, H. & Tyson, R. L. (1975). Discussions on transference. The treatment situation and technique in child psychoanalysis. *Psychoanalytic Study of the Child*, *30*, 409–441.

Sandler, J., Kennedy, H., Tyson, R. L. & Freud, A. (1980). *The Technique of Child Psychoanalysis: Discussions with Anna Freud*. Hogarth Press and the Institute of Psycho-analysis. https://books.google.it/books?id=gGl-AAAAMAAJ

Schenk-Danziger, L. (1963). Die Grundideen und die theoretischen Fragestellungen in Charlotte Bühlers Lebenswerk. In L. T. Schenk-Danziger, H. (Ed.), *Gegenwartsprobleme der Entwicklungspsychologie. Festschrift für Charlotte Bühler* (Vol. 9–19). Verlag für Psychologie, Dr. C. J. Hogrefe.

Schleffler, J. (1990). Weltstadt und Unterwelt. Urbanisierung, Armenpolitik und Obdachlosigkeit in Berlin 1871–1914 [Cosmopolitan and underworld. Urbanization, poor policy and homelessness in Berlin 1871–1914]. *Internationale wissenschaftliche Korrespondenz zur Geschichte der deutschen Arbeiterbewegung* (Sonderheft Jg. *26*(2), 158–181).

Schlesinger-Kipp, G. (2012). *Kindheit im Krieg und Nationalsozialismus: PsychoanalytikerInnen erinnern sich*. Psychosozial-Verlag. https://books.google.it/books?id= EaI9OqbdebwC

Schnurmann, A. (1947). Observation of a phobia. *Psychoanalytic Study of the Child*, *3*(1), 253–270. https://doi.org/10.1080/00797308.1947.11823087

Schonig, B. (1996). *Sophie und Hilde. Ein Zwillingsbuch. Ein gemeinsames Leben in Freundschaft und Beruf* [Sophie and Hilde. A book about twins. A life together in friendship and profession]. Schriftenreihe AnDenken4. Hg. von der Arbeitsgruppe Pädagogisches Museum e.V. und dem Schulmuseum Berlin. Edition Hentrich.

Sherman, J. (2015). Manna Friedmann. Holocaust survivors. *'45 Aid Society*, *38*. https://45aid.org/wp-content/uploads/2015/05/JOURNAL-2015.pdf

Spillius, E. B., Milton, J., Garvey, P., Couve, C. & Steiner, D. (2011). *The New Dictionary of Kleinian Thought*. Taylor & Francis. https://books.google.it/books?id=XNp2Wb1DPEgC

Stern, D. N. (1998). *The Interpersonal World of the Infant: A View from Psychoanalysis and Developmental Psychology*. Karnac Books. https://books.google.it/books?id= AlhGzAEACAAJ

Target, M. (2010). The psychoanalytic work of Hansi Kennedy: From War Nurseries to the Anna Freud Centre (1940–1993). *Journal of Child Psychotherapy*, *36*(3), 313–316. https://doi.org/10.1080/0075417X.2010.524777

Target, M. & Kennedy, H. (1991). Psychoanalytic work with under-fives: Forty years' experience. *Bulletin of the Anna Freud Centre*, *14*, 5–29.

Taschwer, K. (2020a). Konrad Lorenz' bester Freund. *Der Standard*. www.derstandard.at/story/1381370977060/konrad-lorenz-bester-freund

Taschwer, K. (2020b). *Irene und Paul Hellmann. Fast vergessene Förderer der Salzburger Festspiele.*

Taschwer, K. (2021). Wie wichtige jüdische Förderer der Salzburger Festspiele einfach vergessen wurden. *Der Standard.* https://www.derstandard.de/story/2000127998454/wie- wichtige-juedische-foer-derer-der-salzburger-festspiele-einfach-vergessen-wurden

Thüne, E.-M. (2019). *Gerettet: Berichte von Kindertransport und Auswanderung nach Großbritannien.* Hentrich und Hentrich.

Tucker, N. (2006). Maggie Noach. Literary agent for children's authors. *Independent.* https://www.independent.co.uk/news/obituaries/cormac-mccarthy-books-the-road-blood-meridian-b2360903.html

Vickers, C. (2016). A refugee is seeking a new home: Ilse Hellmann's appeal, 10 June 1939. Freud in Oceania. Histories of psychology and psychoanalysis in the Oceania region https://freudinoceania.com/2016/12/26/a-child-psychologist-refugee-ilse-hellmanns-appeal-for-australia-10-june-1939/

Volke, W. (ed.) (1967) Hugo von Hofmannsthal. Briefe an Irene und Paul Hellmann [Letters to Irene and Paul Helllman]. *Jahrbuch der Deutschen Schillergesellschaft, 11*, 170–224.

Wachtler, B. & Ullrich, P. (2013). »Da wollte man nichts mehr von Hitler wissen«. Nationalsozialismus und Krieg in Berufsbiographien alter deutscher *Psyche, 7.*

Werner, V. (1967). Hugo von Hofmannsthal. Briefe an Irene und Paul Hellmann (*Jahrbuch der Deutschen Schillergesellschaft* (pp. 170–224).

Whitehouse, R. (25 April, 2020). A London cabbie's Holocaust: Taxi driver Jackie Young found out he wasn't who he thought he was. *Tablet Magazine.*

Wiener, J. (2003). Speech, on the occasion of the funeral of Hansi Kennedy (unpublished).

Wies, L. S. (2019). Von ‚Kriegskindern' zu Flüchtlingskindern. Impulse aus Anna Freuds und Dorothy Burlinghams ‚Hampstead War Nurseries' für die psychologische Arbeit mit Flüchtlingskindern heute [From 'war children' to refugee children. Impulses from Anna Freud and Dorothy Burlingham's 'Hampstead War Nurseries' for psychological work with refugee children today]. *Kinderanalyse, 4*, 313–338.

Wildbolz, A. (2012). *Kleine Geschichte des Sigmund-Freud-Zentrums* Bern [A Short History of the Sigmund-Freud Centre Bern]. Available at: https://www.freud-zentrum.ch/wp-content/uploads/2016/06/Kleine-Geschichte-des-FZB.pdf

Wilhelm, H. (2014): Sophie Dann. In: *Augsburgerinnen* (pp. 119–137). Hg. v. Andreas Zellhuber.

Wise, S. A. (2009). Explorations and Responses; Dietrich Bonhoeffer; Jerusalem, Israel. Available at: http://www.thefreelibrary.com/Bigotry+against+Bonhoeffer+in+Jerusalem.-a0205746295

Wolf, K. M. (1945). Evacuation of children in wartime. *Psychoanalytic Study of the Child, 1*(1), 389–404. https://doi.org/10.1080/00797308.1945.11823145

Yad Vashem. (n.d.). The Central Database of Shoah Victims' Names. https://yvng.yadvashem.org/index.html?language=en&s_id=&s_lastName=Goldberger&s_firstName=Max&s_place=Berlin&s_dateOfBirth=&cluster=true

Yorke, C., Kennedy, H. & Stanley, W. (1983). Algunos aspectos clinicos y teoricos de dos lines de desarrolo. *Revista de la Asociación Psicoanalítica de Buenos Aires, 5*(2), 221–248.

Yorke, C., Kennedy, H. & Wiseberg, S. (1991). Clinical and theoretical aspects of two developmental lines In: *The Course of Life, Vol. 3: Middle and Late Childhood.* (pp. 135–160). International Universities Press.

Young-Bruehl, E. (1988). *Anna Freud: A Biography.* Summit Books.

Zwiauer, C. (2001). Emma N. (Spira) Plank (1905–1990). Psychoanalytisch orientierte Montessori-Pädagogik in Wien von 1922–1938 und deren Tradierung in der Emigration. In C. Zwiauer, B. Eichelberger & H. Picus (eds), *Das Kind ist entdeckt. Erziehungsexperimente im Wien der Zwischenkriegszeiten* (pp. 119–181). Picus.

Index of Persons

Aichhorn, August 12, 185, 191
Andrews, Eamonn 34
Andrian-Werburg, Leopold baron of 142
Arlt, Ilse von 144
Astfalck, Eleonore (Nora) 128–130, 139
Auerbach, Alice, married Schnurmann 115

Bahr, Hermann 142
Baker, Judge 144
Baradon, Tessa 200
Bärhold, Katrin, née Richter x
Beer-Hofmann, Richard 142
Benkendorf, Johanna (Hanni), married
    Köhler 13, 132, 169
Bennett, Ivy, married Gwynne-Thomas
    132, 157
Berger, Manfred 139
Bernays, Minna 47
Bernfeld, Siegfried 11, 12
Bernheimer, Simon 115
Bethge, Eberhard 128–130
Bick, Esther, née Wander 145, 146
Blomfield, Wolf 10, 29, 31
Blos, Peter 191
Bonaparte, Maria, Princess George of
    Greece 41
Bonhoeffer, Dietrich 122, 123, 125, 119,
    128, 129, 139
Bonhoeffer, Karl 118
Bonhoeffer, Paula 128
Bonhoeffer, Sabine, married
    Leibholz-Bonhoeffer 123, 139
Bonhoeffer, Susanne, married Dress
    118–126
Bonnard, Augusta 15, 169, 170, 185
Bornstein, Berta 12
Bowlby, John 4, 6, 19, 158
Boyce, E. R. 158
Brecht, Karin 194
Brenner, Nancy 96, 97
Britten, Benjamin 183
Broughton, Carol 200

Bruce, Stanley 149
Bucci, Andra 82, 110, 111
Bucci, Tatiana 110
Budritzki, Eva von 22
Bühler, Charlotte, née Malachowski 5, 6,
    20, 145–7, 149, 150, 159, 160
Bühler, Karl 145, 160
Burlingham, Dorothy i, ix, x, 1–6, 11–13,
    16, 18, 19, 48, 49, 51, 55, 56, 59, 79, 95,
    99, 100, 133, 135, 151–3, 158, 169, 185,
    191, 194, 196, 197
Busch, Adolf 141, 142

Carelbach, Emanuel 112
Clarke, Lady Rebekah 26, 52, 59
Clarke, Sir Ralph Stephenson 52
Cohen, Helen x, 72, 75, 76, 109, 111
Cohen, Theodor (Ted) 179
Colonna, Alice 103, 106, 175
Corbach, Dieter 69, 112
Craddock, Jana x
Crawshaw, Jack 33
Curio, Claudia 9

Daimler, Paul 139
Dann, Albert 37, 41, 45, 57, 60
Dann, Elisabeth (Elishibber) 37–40, 45,
    60, 61
Dann, Fanny, née Kitzinger 37, 45, 60
Dann, Gertrud i, ix, x, 4, 6, 8, 21, 25, 27,
    31, 32, 35–62, 79, 80, 92, 108, 153, 154,
    162, 185
Dann, Lotte, married Treves 37–40, 45, 47,
    60, 61
Dann, Sophie i, ix, x, 4, 11, 26, 27, 37–45,
    47–54, 56–62, 79, 154, 175, 196
Dann, Thea 37–9, 41
Danneberg, Erika 158
Danzinger, Charlotte (Lotte), married
    Schenk-Danziger 145, 146, 159, 160
Deming, Julia 1
Demjanjuk, Ivan (John) 148

Dewey, John 191
Dik, Afine Kornélie (Phiny) 148
Douglas, Diana 154, 155, 158
Drage, Sir Benjamin 11, 27, 34, 36
Dreyfuss, Luis 76
Dührssen, Annemarie 158
Dünkelsbühler, Thekla 46

Eccleshare, Julia 155
Edgcumbe, Rose Marjorie 180, 198
Eichelberger, Brigitte 191
Eichmann, Adolf 8
Emde, Robert 146, 192
Engl, Oskar 163
Eppel, Hedda 158
Erikson, Erik 191

Feitscher, Paul 159
Fichtl, Paula 6, 24, 105
Finton, Lacerta 149
Fischer, Hilde 1
Fonagy, Peter 17, 177, 178, 180, 192
Frankl, Liselotte 15, 20, 32, 133, 134, 145,
    146, 150, 153, 157, 169
Freud, Anna i, ix, x, 1–7, 11–19, 24, 25, 27,
    32–35, 41, 47–53, 58–60, 77, 79, 85,
    88, 89, 91, 93–100, 103–106, 108, 119,
    131–134, 136, 139, 140, 146, 149–143,
    165–171, 173–183, 185, 189–201
Freud, Sigmund 1, 29, 59, 197, 199
Friedlander, Käthe (Kate), née Misch 2,
    11–15, 132–4, 168–70
Friedmann, Ignaz 142
Friedmann, Marta (Manna) née Weindling
    i, ix, x, 3, 11, 14, 22, 24, 25, 27, 29,
    31–35, 55, 56, 58, 63–113, 125, 127,
    136–8, 156, 190, 194
Friedmann, Oskar, alias Oscar Friedman
    11, 25, 26, 29, 82–5, 87, 88, 100–2, 136,
    153, 156
Fuchs-Wertheim, Hertha 1

Gardiner, Muriel 12
Gaulton, Judith 52
Geissmann, Claudine 16
Geissmann, Pierre 16
Gierke, Anna von 126, 128, 129
Gilbert, Martin 27, 53, 84
Glover, Edward 14, 151
Goldberger, Alice i, ix, x, 6, 8, 10, 11, 13,
    21–36, 53, 59, 67, 77, 78, 80, 81, 87, 89,
    95, 106, 132, 175, 194
Gombrich, Ernst 154

Gomperts, Konrad 133
Göpfert, Rebekka 9
Green, Henry 29
Gryn, Hugo 29

Haager, Jutta 2, 12, 14, 15
Hahn-Warburg, Lola 10
Halberstadt, Ernst W., alias W. Ernest Freud
    13, 24, 158, 197
Hamilton, Mary Agnes 142, 149
Hauser, Eva 89
Heimann, Paula 133, 134, 152, 153, 156
Heine, Heinrich 142
Heinig, Christine 149
Hellman, Ilse, married Noach i, ix, x, 5, 11,
    85, 131, 133–5, 141–160, 166, 175, 194
Hellmann, Bernhard (grandfather of Ilse
    Hellman) 159
Hellmann, Bernhard Wolfgang (brother of
    Ilse Hellman) 143, 147, 148, 159, 160
Hellmann, Christiane (Christine) 149
Hellmann, Elisabeth (Jeanette, Lili, Lily),
    married Wärndorfer 142
Hellmann, Ernst Richard 143, 149
Hellmann, Irene, née Redlich 142, 148
Hellmann, Lina 159
Hellmann, Margarete (Gretl) married
    Rémy-Berzencovich de Szilla 159
Hellmann, Paul (father of Ilse Hellman)
    141, 148, 159
Hellmann, Paul (nephew of Ilse Hellman)
    145, 147, 148, 158
Hermann, Anni 91
Herszberg, Jerczy 29, 34
Herzberg, Martha 6, 49
Hetzer, Hildegard 145, 159
Heumann, Karola (Carol) 73
Heymann, Clemy, née Dann 37, 44
Heymann, Sigmund 37
Hirsch, Fritz 84
Hoffer, Hedwig 11–13, 132, 133, 152, 153
Hoffer, Willi 11–13, 152, 156, 185, 195
Hofmannsthal, Hugo von 141, 142
Hohenlohe-Schillingsfürst, Family 141
Horkheimer, Max 130
Husserl (Husserlová), Zdenka 27, 28, 34,
    35, 55, 108

Isaacs, Susan 149, 151, 153, 158
Israels, Martin 156

Jackson, Edith 1, 6, 12
Jacobs, Lydia 15

Jahoda, Maria 160
James, Jessica 200

Kamm, Harald 194
Kearney, Lotte (Lottie) 88, 96
Kennedy, Catherine 184, 185
Kennedy, Gerald Helmut, alias Helmut Kahn 4, 170, 172, 183
Kennedy, Hanna (Hansi) née Engl i, ix, x, 3, 4, 6, 13, 15, 16, 50, 60, 92, 132, 133, 154, 157, 158, 163, 169–184, 192, 199
Kennedy, Steven x, 173, 175, 184, 185
Kennedy, Tony 173
Kent, Princess Alexandra 41, 154
Kestenberg, Judith S. 194
Kisch, Bruno 67, 73, 87, 88, 112
Kisch, Rifka 67
Kitzinger, Berthold 38
Kitzinger, Elisabeth, née Merzbacher 42, 43
Kitzinger, Fritz 38
Kitzinger, Gabriel 42
Kitzinger, Ida, née Dünkelsbühler 38
Kitzinger, Wilhelm 38, 42
Klein, Melanie 134, 152, 197–200
Klibansky, Menachen Erich 67, 69, 112
Klimt, Gustav 159
Köhler, Hanni (Joanna), married Benkendorf 13, 132, 169
Koorland, Vivienne 194
Körner, Jürgen x
Koslowski, Jutta 118–123, 125, 127
Kris, Ernst 20, 196
Kris, Marianne 185
Kröller-Müller, Helene 148
Kut, Sara (Sarah), married Rosenfeld 132, 169, 171, 173, 175

Laible, Eva 12, 189, 197
Lampl de Groot, Jeanne 162, 185
Lantos, Barbara 2, 13, 132, 133
Le Seur, Paul 128
Lenau, Nikolaus 142
Levital, Shula 62
Levy, Katja 85
Liegmann, Heiko x
Lindig, Horst 84
Lion, Hilde Gudilla 130, 131
Livingstone, Maureen 52
Lockot, Regine x
Loeb, Dora 68, 112
Loeber, Tara x
Lorenz, Konrad 159, 160
Ludewyk-Gyömröi, Edith (Edit) 194

Ludwig, Luitpold, Prince Regent of Bavaria 41
Ludwig-Körner, Christiane i, ix, x, 4, 11, 16, 50, 84, 138, 140, 184, 194, 196

Mächtlinger, Veronica 200, 201
Mahler-Werfel, Alma, née Schindler 142, 159
Malberg, Norka 197
Mänchen, Anna, née Aronsohn 199, 201
Mannheim, Julia 13, 132, 133, 140
Mannheim, Karl 130, 134, 139, 140
Mantua, Josef von 37
Mautner, Konrad 142
Mayes, Linda 17
McGourty, Niall 62
McLean, Duncan 200
Meyer, Hilde 8
Meyer, Zoë x
Midgley, Nick 4, 195–7
Milberger, Mizzi 1
Miller, Jill 163, 169, 173, 174, 180–2
Mitscherlich, Alexander 176
Model, Elizabeth 31, 35
Moll, Carl 159
Montefiore, Leonard 10, 84
Montessori, Maria 1, 191
Monteverdi, Claudio 142
Moran, George 177, 180, 182
Moshagen, Elisabeth 21
Moskovitz, Sarah 26–9, 36, 53
Mühlleitner, Elke 1, 185
Müller-Braunschweig, Ada 84, 85
Mussolini, Benito 47

Nacken, Johanna 128–30, 139
Nagera, Humberto 197
Nettl, Claire 11, 19, 20
Neumayer, Max 159
Neurath, Lily (Lili) 13, 132
Niederacher, Sonja 159
Noach, Arnoldus (Arnold) 148, 152, 154, 155, 156
Noach, Maggie, married Williams 142–4, 148, 155–8

Oppenheimer, Rachel 35
Oppenheimer-Todesco, family 142
Orff, Carl 142

Parkinson, John 35
Payne, Sylvia 51, 152, 153
Pears, Peter 183
Penz, Michaela 9

Piaget, Jean 146
Pollner, Martin 141
Pretorius, Inge x, 4, 7, 18, 48, 132, 197, 200
Prewitt, Judith 52
Prussia, Victoria Luise of 41

Raphael-Leff, Joan 153
Redlich, Rosa, née Fanto 141
Reinhardt, Max 141
Richter, Roger x
Riviere, Joan 152
Robertson, James (Jimmy) 3, 4, 6, 7, 19, 158, 168, 175, 193
Robertson, Joyce, née Usher 4, 6, 18, 19, 158, 168, 191, 193
Rogger-Müller, Cornelia 138
Rolnick, Lizzy, née Wallentin 13, 132
Römer, Gernot 37–42, 47, 48, 52, 54, 55, 58–60, 196
Rosenfeld, Eva 13, 191
Roubiczek, Lili Esther, married Roubiczek-Peller 191
Ruben, Margarete 133
Rubens, Joanna, married Millan, alias Bela Rosenthal 27, 28, 35, 62

Salo, Frances 97
Sandler, Anne-Marie ix, x, 91, 178, 180, 185, 193, 194
Sandler, Joseph 17, 133, 134, 179, 182, 197
Schacht, Lore 176
Scheffler, Jürgen 22
Schlesinger-Kipp, Gertraud 194
Schnitzler, Arthur 142
Schnurmann, Anneliese i, ix, x, 7, 13, 15, 23, 48, 95, 96, 102, 108, 114–139
Schnurmann, Claudia x, 102, 103, 107, 137, 139
Schnurmann, Jakob 114, 115
Schnurmann, Samuel 115
Schonig, Bruno 22, 128, 139
Schorr, Friedrich 142
Schultze, Friedrich Siegmund 129
Schwarz, Hedwig (Hedy) 3, 4, 11, 133, 165, 166
Schwehm, Beatrice 28, 53
Shepheard, Elizabeth 85
Sherman, Judith 32, 71, 78, 79, 82, 106, 107, 110, 194
Spitz, René 6, 145, 146, 195, 196
Sterba, Edith 12
Sterba, Richard 18
Stern, Daniel 197
Stern, Elisabeth 41, 60
Stern, Siegfried (Shlomo) 39

Stifter, Adalbert 142
Straus, Leonore, née Schnurmann 116, 120–3
Straus, Moritz 116, 120–3, 132, 139
Strauss, Richard 142
Stross, Josephine (Josefine) 1, 3, 11, 14, 18, 105, 151, 154, 160, 175
Sylvester, Emmy 146

Target, Mary 17, 180–3
Taschwer, Klaus 141, 142, 160
Thomas, Ruth 4, 133
Thüne, Eva-Maria 8
Tillich, Paul 130
Treves, Claudio 40, 60
Treves, Paolo 47, 60
Tyson, Robert 180, 182

Volke, Werner 142

Wachtler, Benjamin 194
Wärndorfer, Fritz 142
Wassermann, Jacob 141, 142
Weindling, Albert 64, 65, 69, 70
Weindling, Auguste (Gusta), née Horowitz 63, 65, 69
Weindling, David 65, 69
Weindling, Devora (Dora) 65, 73, 112
Weindling, Julius (Jodi) 65, 69
Weindling, Nathan 63, 69
Weindling, Paul (Poldi) 65, 69, 72
Weindling, Salo 63, 64, 69, 71–3, 76, 79
Weiss, Julia 3, 137
Wellesz, Egon 142
Wiener, Jan x, 165, 166, 183, 184
Wiesengrund, Theodor (Teddy), alias Theodor Adorno 130
Winnicott, Claire 4
Winnicott, Donald Woods 14, 18, 85, 152
Wismuller-Meyer, Geertruida 8
Wolff, Emmy 23
Wolfison, Maureen 52
Wolkowski, Chava 109, 112
Wolkowski, Eran x, 72, 73, 82, 109, 110, 112
Wolkowski, Norbert-Nathan 112
Wutsch, Sophie (Sofie) 3, 6, 11, 27–9, 31, 35, 49

Yorke, Clifford 153–5, 157, 171, 177, 180, 181
Young, Jackie (Jack), alias Jonah Spiegel 34, 62, 194
Young-Bruehl, Elisabeth 1, 103–6

Zwiauer, Charlotte 1, 191

Index of Terms

action research 195, 196
adoption 35, 80
adoptive: mother 35, 194; parents 26, 28, 34, 35, 53
AFC *see* Anna Freud Centre
air raid 50, 65; and Chart Hampstead Nursery 48, 196; shelter 12
Alsergrund 159
Altaussee 141, 142, 159
Amsterdam 148, 185
Anna Freud Centre x, 3, 13, 16–18, 35, 42, 50, 54, 60, 62, 136, 137, 177, 180–2, 185, 196, 200
Anna Freud National Centre for Children and Families (AFNCCF) 16, 17
applied field research 191
attachment 4, 26, 193, 194; figure 6; research 6, 19; theory 5, 97, 192
Augsburg ix, x, 4, 37–9, 41–6, 50, 61
Auschwitz 21, 27, 36, 78, 148
Australia 34, 149

Babies Rest Centre 2, 4, 5, 19, 151
baby nurse 3, 162
baby profile 158, 197
Bentschen 70, 72
Berlin x, 6, 10, 13, 19, 21–3, 26, 27, 29, 30, 33, 36, 39, 45, 84, 112, 116, 118, 124, 126–9, 131, 133, 139, 160, 163, 185
Birmingham 18, 19, 76, 77
Bismarck Secondary School, Siemensstrasse, Berlin-Grunewald 118
blind children 13, 32, 34, 94, 197
Blitzkrieg 19; blitz 2, 3, 76, 167, 192; *see also* bombing
Bloomsbury House 74, 84
bombing 2, 6, 25, 48, 131, 132, 196
bond 53, 62, 194; bonding 5, 193

Boys Club 19
British Home Office 10
British Psycho-Analytic Society 153, 200
British Psycho-Analytical Institute 133
British Psychotherapy Foundation, BPF 18
Bühler-Hetzer Development Test 11
Bulldogs Bank: as place 8, 11, 26, 28, 52, 53, 57, 196; children 8, 28, 52, 54, 79, 80
Burlingham–Rosenfeld School 191

carer 3, 5, 8, 10, 19, 21, 28, 52, 55, 144, 146, 150, 158
Central British Fund for Jewish Relief and Rehabilitation (CBF) 36
Centre of Excellence 17, 18, 200
chart 48; development 195; observation 196; sleeping 196; *see also* Air Raid Chart Hampstead Nursery
child analysis x, 12, 15, 89, 158, 170, 179, 181, 182, 194, 197–9, 201; candidates 18, 89; technique 11, 180, 197; training 15, 133
child expert 13, 32, 132, 133, 200
child guidance: centre 14, 15; clinic 12, 15, 20, 133, 134, 146, 168, 185; services 14
child transports 7, 9, 10
children's home ix, x, 2, 4–7, 10–12, 19, 22, 44, 45, 48, 50, 65, 66, 69, 83, 150–2, 194; in Hampstead 13, 49; at Weir Courtney 11, 85
Children's House 191
Cologne x, 46, 63, 65–7, 69, 70, 72–5, 100, 103, 112, 137
compensation 22, 58; file 22
concentration camp x, 3, 9–11, 29, 30, 33, 35, 53, 54, 57, 63, 72, 77, 84, 132, 148, 194

consulting 156, 179
Contemporary Freudian Group of the
    British Psychoanalytic Society 156
Crosby-on-Eden 26, 52, 84

daycare 7
death camp 11
deportation 69, 70, 72–4, 112
development-orientated therapeutic
    approach 192
Development Profile Research Group 197
developmental: profile 146; psychology 11,
    18, 150, 160; research 146; test 11
domestic permit 23, 33, 74, 75
donation 2, 13, 17, 27, 29, 66, 139, 190, 200
Dresden-Hellerau 44

early: childhood 83, 155, 158, 195; life 2;
    years 6
East End London Hospital 18, 169
eating disorder 39, 53, 59
emigrate 2, 6, 23, 44, 45, 49, 67, 73, 82,
    85, 130–2, 147, 149, 160, 165, 172,
    175, 185
emigration 22, 68, 69, 130, 131, 165, 173;
    forced 139; see also emigrate
enemy alien 23, 33, 75, 133, 149

foster: care 9; child 8, 160; family 9, 28,
    79, 150; father 78; mother 78, 160;
    parents 78, 185
Foster Parents' Plan for War Children 2,
    19, 151
Foundation for Research in
    Psychoanalysis 13
Frankfurt School 130
Freud Library 59
Freud Museum 18, 41, 42, 154, 174
friendly alien 23, 75
Fürth 37, 38, 42

Göding (today Hodonice), Czech Republic
    141, 142
Grundlsee 142, 159

Hagana 73
Hamburg-Blankenese 44
Hampstead Child Therapy Course and
    Clinic 17, 153, 197
Hampstead Index 197
Hampstead Nursery 19, 49, 89, 181; War
    Nursery 48; see also children's home

Haslemere, Surrey 130, 131, 139
Haus der Kinder see Children's House
Hietzingen 191
Holocaust Memorial Museum, Washington,
    DC 8, 24, 30, 31, 78, 110, 111
Holocaust Museum, Yad Vashem 71
Holocaust survivors 25, 36, 148
home visits 13
housekeeper 4, 24, 48, 67, 105, 106
housekeeping 125–7

Immenhof 139
Index Research Group 179
infant nurse 4, 49, 167; training 42; see also
    baby nurse
infant research 145, 197
internment camp 33
Isle of Man 23–5, 33, 149

Jackson Nursery 1, 4, 12, 48, 53, 191, 192
Jawne reform grammar school, Cologne
    65, 112
Jugendstube see youth centre

Kantor Centre of Excellence see Centre of
    Excellence
kibbutz 73, 82, 83, 106, 112
kindergarten 4, 11–3, 21–3, 36, 44, 45, 50,
    58, 77, 83, 88–94, 96–9, 158, 185, 191,
    195; children 93; psychoanalytic 200;
    teacher 3, 21, 22, 53, 66, 68, 77, 81, 83,
    98, 99, 103, 104, 165, 169, 191; teacher
    training 21, 44, 149, 166; see also
    Montessori; seminar
Kings College 39, 168
Kristallnacht 67; see also Night of Broken
    Glass

Lingfield House: as place 29–31, 55, 57,
    58, 175; children 21, 28, 31, 35, 79, 106
London ix, 2, 4, 6, 7, 9, 11–13, 18–20, 25,
    27–9, 32, 33, 35, 36, 38, 39, 41, 46–9,
    51, 52, 60, 72, 74–7, 82, 84, 85, 87, 89,
    96, 102, 103, 109, 110, 112, 131, 132,
    137–40, 145–50, 154, 156, 158, 160,
    163, 165, 168, 179, 180, 185, 186

maid 6, 38, 41, 47, 49, 66, 67, 75, 76;
    see also housekeeper
Marienthal Study 18, 160
mentalization based treatment 17
Middle Group 18, 85, 153

milk kitchen 4, 12, 48, 166
Montessori 91, 94, 132, 191; kindergarten
    1, 4, 165; method 11; pedagogy 94;
    society 1; teacher 91
Moritz Straus foundation x
mother–child relationship 5, 19, 192
Munich 38, 42, 43, 45, 160

Nazi regime 11, 154, 189
New Barn 2, 6, 7, 25, 35, 49, 51
New Land Foundation 13
newborn 5, 132, 146
Night of Broken Glass 132
NSDAP *see* Nazi Regime
nurse 3, 4, 11, 19, 37, 39, 42, 43, 44, 47–9,
    59, 60, 74, 77, 106, 131, 150, 196; *see
    also* infant nurse
nursery school *see* kindergarten
nursery teacher 96, 97, 128, 196; *see also*
    kindergarten
nursing home 61, 72, 74, 102; at Horncastle
    House 61; at White Horse 158

Obdach *see* shelter
object relations 1
observation 4, 17, 48, 93, 95, 97, 133, 146,
    150, 160, 179, 181, 195–7; baby 18, 146,
    150; child 4, 166, 195, 196; developmental
    192; *see also* chart; infant research
On the Technique of Child Analysis 11
Oranienburg 84; *see also* Sachsenhausen
orphan 21, 152; orphaned 144; war orphan
    5, 7
orphanage 21, 42, 43, 65, 70, 79, 83, 84;
    Mosestift 21; Reichenheim 84
Otwock 71

Palestine 8, 39, 44, 45, 56, 72, 73, 81–3,
    85, 112
playgroup 14, 192
Plzeň (Pilsen) 162
Polish action 69
preschool children 18
prevention 15, 17, 194
Profile Research Group 179
*Psycho-Analysis and Contemporary
    Thought* 158
psychoanalytic training 4, 11, 17, 32, 85,
    88, 95, 151, 179, 185, 200

Questionnaire for the Personnel of all
    Colonies 19, 160

Ravensbrück 78, 106
refugee 3, 8, 9, 18, 23, 29, 34, 53, 56, 149,
    194; camps 8; committee in England 73;
    organization 10; policy 9
Refugee Children's Movement (RCM) 7
research ix, 4, 6, 13, 15, 17–19, 85, 103,
    121, 133, 139, 146, 150, 153, 160,
    178–82, 189, 194–8, 200; assistant 20,
    145, 146, 150, 154; behavioural 160;
    cardiovascular 112; facilities 16, 144;
    historical 102; on the Holocaust 28;
    see also action research; applied field
    research; attachment; Development
    Profile Research Group; developmental;
    Foundation for Research in
    Psychoanalysis; Index Research Group;
    infant; Profile Research Group
retirement 4, 14, 18, 33, 90, 99, 108, 135,
    137, 148, 156, 172, 182, 185
retirement home 35, 107, 111, 138; as
    community 109; *see also* nursing home
Robertson Centre 4
Rockefeller Foundation 160
rooming-in 6
Rotterdam 148, 158

Sachsenhausen 132
Salzburg Festival 141, 142
Schottengymnasium 143, 159
Scout movement 19
second generation 79
seminar 11–15, 132, 133, 140, 146,
    152, 153, 155, 176; clinical 13, 152;
    kindergarten 44, 185; technical 17, 134;
    theoretical 13, 17, 167
separation 4–6, 8, 70, 97, 98, 167,
    168, 192–5; anxiety 168, 192; early
    5; reaction 4, 19, 35; research 19;
    trauma 194
Sharpthorne 61
shelter 2, 3, 6, 21, 22, 148, 167; for air
    raids 12, 19, 48, 135; overnight 22;
    state-run 22
sibling 5, 7, 40, 71, 77–80, 117, 119, 120,
    123, 128, 132, 158
Sigmund Freud Institute 156, 176
Sigmund Freud Museum 18; *see also* Freud
    Museum
Sobibór, Poland 148
social worker 3, 5, 14, 15, 19, 26, 31, 43,
    52, 66, 81, 83–5, 107
Sorbonne 145

Stetten Institute 39
Stoatley Rough 23, 130, 139
substitute: child 108, 125; family 3, 119, 194; home 139; mother 194, 195
superego 1, 183
supervision 17, 133, 134, 153, 156, 177, 179, 180, 183, 197
Surrey 11, 23, 27, 34, 36, 80, 130, 131, 139
synagogue ix, 37, 45, 65; destruction of 45, 67, 69; Goldlers Green 36; West London 11, 27, 29, 34, 36

Tavistock Clinic 4, 6, 19, 185
teacher 3, 13, 33, 39, 44, 65, 66, 70, 77, 78, 84, 93–5, 98, 104, 112, 127, 128, 158, 167, 180, 185, 190, 191, 195; academy 160; certification 68; examination 45; *see also* kindergarten; Montessori; seminar
teaching: analysand 1; analysis 13, 132, 133, 151, 153, 156; analyst 20, 134, 135, 185, 194
Tel Aviv 83, 109, 110, 112
therapeutic: concept 15; technique 175
Theresienstadt, Terezin 26–8, 34, 36, 53; children rescued from 8, 11, 28, 34, 37, 52–4, 59, 62, 108
This is Your Life 33–5
toddler 4, 11, 12, 17, 18, 48, 50–2, 132, 136, 167, 192; *see also* playgroup
trainee 3, 12, 19, 21, 131, 181, 189; traineeship 169; *see also* training candidate
training: candidate 12, 13, 15–18, 33, 89, 92, 94, 95, 153, 176, 191, 195; course 11, 12, 19, 169, 173; *see also* Hampstead Child Therapy Course and Clinic
treatment method 14, 15, 200
twin 65, 123, 135, 157, 175, 196

unemployment 18, 22, 96
University College London (AFC-UCL) 18, 146

USHMM *see* Holocaust Memorial Museum, Washington, DC

Vienna x, 1, 2, 4–6, 11–13, 16, 18–20, 49, 91, 137, 141–8, 151, 159, 160, 162, 163, 165, 178, 185, 191, 199, 201
Vienna Secession 159

Walberswick 56, 100, 101, 170
Wandervogel 41
war children's home ix, 6, 21, 48, 50, 151, 194; *see also* children's home
War Nursery i, ix, 1, 3–7, 11–13, 18, 19, 23, 32, 35, 48, 60, 62, 131–3, 135–7, 157, 166, 168, 169, 171, 173–5, 181, 185, 189, 191, 193–5, 197, 199; in London 25; *see also* Hampstead
Warsaw 70, 71
Wedderburn Road 2, 7, 48, 150, 151, 166
Wednesday evening seminars 13
Weir Courtney 9, 11, 23, 27–31, 34, 36, 52, 53, 71, 77–81, 85, 110, 111; *see also* children's home
Well Baby Clinic 13, 14, 17–19, 97, 175, 191, 192, 197, 200
Westerbrok (Transit Camp) 148
Wiener Werkstätten 142
Windermere 25, 26, 33, 52, 53, 84
Wolberswick 104
Wolzig 84
Women's Voluntary Service 131
Women's Zionist Organization 83
work permit 10, 47, 145
Workers' Education Association 18
world war i; first 19, 22, 37, 63, 76, 142, 144, 185; second 36, 72, 84, 133, 154; outbreak of 33, 150

youth centre 127–30
youth home in Charlottenburg 21
youth welfare office 12

Zionist 73; movement 72